Burkhard Tönshoff and Lars Pape (eds.)
Management of the paediatric kidney transplant recipient

Management of the paediatric kidney transplant recipient

Working Groups Transplantation of the GPN, ESPN and the CERTAIN research network

Edited by Burkhard Tönshoff and Lars Pape

UNIVERSITÄTS-
BIBLIOTHEK
HEIDELBERG

Bibliographic information published by the Deutsche Nationalbibliothek
The Deutsche Nationalbibliothek lists this publication in the Deutsche Nationalbibliografie; detailed bibliographic data are available on the Internet at https://dnb.dnb.de.

UNIVERSITÄTS-
BIBLIOTHEK
HEIDELBERG

Published by heiBOOKS, 2026
Heidelberg University / Heidelberg University Library
heiBOOKS
Grabengasse 1, 69117 Heidelberg, Germany
https://books.ub.uni-heidelberg.de/heibooks
e-mail: ub@ub.uni-heidelberg.de

The electronic open access version of this work is permanently available on the e-book platform of Heidelberg University Library heiBOOKS:
https://books.ub.uni-heidelberg.de/heibooks
URN: urn:nbn:de:bsz:16-heibooks-book-1732
DOI: https://doi.org/10.11588/heibooks.1732

Layout: text plus form, Dresden
Cover illustration: Map of Europe showing the locations of centres of the CERTAIN research network (https://certain-registry.eu). © Kai Krupka and Burkhard Tönshoff.

ISBN 978-3-911056-62-5 (Softcover)
ISBN 978-3-911056-61-8 (PDF)

Introduction

We are pleased to present this book, Management of the Paediatric Kidney Transplant Recipient. The aim of this book is to provide paediatric transplant physicians and associated professional groups with practical recommendations for their daily clinical work in a total of 40 chapters covering 13 thematic areas. Where available, these recommendations are based on international guidelines and clinical practice recommendations or have been compiled by experienced clinicians from our community for our community. A total of 52 authors have contributed to this book, and we would like to take this opportunity to thank them very much for their contributions.

As transplant medicine is subject to rapid change due to advances in knowledge, some of the recommendations will have changed in a few years' time. Please do not hesitate to inform us of any new developments, which we will then incorporate into future editions.

We hope you enjoy reading this book and that it provides you with valuable insights.

Yours sincerely,
Burkhard Tönshoff and Lars Pape

Table of Contents

List of authors

Thurid Ahlenstiel-Grunow, Department of Paediatrics II, University Hospital of Essen, Essen, Germany;

Jan Ulrich Becker, Department of Pathology, University Hospital of Cologne, Cologne, Germany

Kathrin Buder, Department of General Paediatrics and Haematology/Oncology, University Children's Hospital Tübingen

Anja Büscher, Department of Paediatrics II, University Hospital of Essen, Essen, Germany

Daniela Choukair, Heidelberg University, Medical Faculty, Department of Paediatrics I, University Children's Hospital Heidelberg, Germany

Marlies Cornelissen, Department of Paediatric Nephrology, Radboud University Medical Centre, Nijmegen, The Netherlands

Susanne Deininger, Department of Urology, University Hospital Tübingen, Eberhard Karls University, Hoppe-Seyler-Str. 3, 72076, Tübingen, Germany

Jan Dudley, Bristol Royal Hospital for Children, Bristol, United Kingdom

Alexander Fichtner, Heidelberg University, Medical Faculty Heidelberg, Department of Paediatrics I, University Children's Hospital Heidelberg, Germany

Florian Grahammer, III. Department of Medicine, University Hospital Hamburg Eppendorf, Hamburg, Germany

Sandra Habbig, Pediatric Nephrology, Children's and Adolescents' Hospital, University Hospital Cologne, Medical Faculty University of Cologne, Germany

Dieter Haffner, Department of Paediatric Kidney, Liver, Metabolic and Neurological Diseases, Hannover Medical School, Hannover, Germany

Uta Herden, Department of Visceral Transplantation, University Medical Centre Hamburg-Eppendorf, Hamburg, Germany

Britta Höcker, Heidelberg University, Medical Faculty, Department of Paediatrics I, University Children's Hospital Heidelberg, Germany

Ulrike John-Kroegel, Department of Pediatric Nephrology, University Children's Hospital of Jena, Germany

Nele Kanzelmeyer, Department of Paediatric Nephrology, Hepatology, Metabolic and Neurology Diseases, Hannover Medical School, Hannover, Germany

Markus J. Kemper, Asklepios Medical School Hamburg, Department of Paediatrics, AK Hospital Hamburg-North, Germany

Lea Keppner, Heidelberg University Hospital, Institute of Immunology, Heidelberg, Germany

Martina Koch, Department of General, Visceral, and Transplantation Surgery, Johannes Gutenberg University Medical Centre Mainz, Mainz, Germany

Birgitta Kranz, Department of Paediatric Nephrology, University Hospital of Münster, Münster, Germany;

Eberhard Kuwertz-Bröking, Rehabilitation Centre Ederhof, Iselsberg-Stronach, Austria

Sebastian Loos, Department of Paediatric Nephrology and Hepatology, University Hospital Eppendorf, Hamburg, Germany

Britta Maecker-Kolhoff, Hannover Medical School, Pediatric Haematology and Oncology, Hannover, Germany

Anette Melk, Department of Paediatric Nephrology, Hepatology, Metabolic and Neurology Diseases, Hannover Medical School, Hannover, Germany

Christian Morath, Department of Nephrology, University Hospital Heidelberg, Clinic for Internal Medicine, Nephrology, Nuremberg Hospital, Germany

Dominik Müller, Department of Paediatrics, Charité University Hospital, Berlin, Germany

Jun Oh, Department of Paediatric Nephrology and Hepatology, University Hospital Eppendorf, Hamburg, Germany

Lars Pape, Department of Paediatrics II, University Hospital of Essen, Essen, Germany

Christian Patry, Heidelberg University, Medical Faculty, Department of Paediatrics I, University Children's Hospital Heidelberg, Germany

Lien Pham, Heidelberg University Hospital, Institute of Immunology, Heidelberg, Germany

Jenny Prüfe, Department of Paediatrics II, University Hospital of Essen, Essen, Germany

Agnieszka Prytuła, Department of Paediatric Nephrology and Rheumatology, Ghent University Hospital, Ghent, Belgium

Steffen Rausch, Department of Urology and Andrology, Salzburg University Hospital, Paracelsus Medical University, 5020 Salzburg, Austria

Stefan Reuter, University Clinics Münster, Department of Medicine D, Transplant Nephrology

Susanne Rieger, Heidelberg University, Medical Faculty, Department of Paediatrics I, University Children's Hospital Heidelberg, Germany

Raphael Schild, Department of Paediatric Nephrology, Paediatric Hepatology and Paediatric Transplantation, University Medical Centre Hamburg-Eppendorf, Hamburg, Germany

Tomas Seeman, Department of Paediatrics, 2nd Faculty of Medicine, Charles University Prague, Prague 5, Czech Republic; Department of Paediatrics, University Hospital Ostrava and Faculty of Medicine of University of Ostrava, Ostrava, Czech Republic

Claus P. Schmitt, Department of Paediatrics I, University Children's Hospital Heidelberg, Heidelberg, Germany

Rukshana Shroff, Renal Unit, University College London Great Ormond Street Hospital, London, United Kingdom

Maximilian Stich, Heidelberg University, Medical Faculty, Department of Paediatrics I, University Children's Hospital Heidelberg, Germany

Caner Süsal, Heidelberg University, Medical Faculty Heidelberg, Institute of Immunology, Transplantation Immunology, Heidelberg, Germany; Transplant Immunology Research Centre of Excellence, Koç University School of Medicine, Istanbul, Turkey

Barbara Suwelack, University Clinics Münster, Department of Medicine D, Transplant Nephrology

Christina Taylan, Department of Paediatric Nephrology, University Hospital of Cologne, Cologne, Germany

Burkhard Tönshoff, Heidelberg University, Medical Faculty, Department of Paediatrics I, University Children's Hospital Heidelberg, Germany

Thuong Hien Tran, Heidelberg University Hospital, Institute of Immunology, Heidelberg, Germany

Marieke Voet, Amalia Children's Hospital, Department of Anaesthesiology, Radboud University Medical Centre, Nijmegen, The Netherlands

Lutz T. Weber, Pediatric Nephrology, Children's and Adolescents' Hospital, University Hospital Cologne, Medical Faculty University of Cologne, Germany

Marcus Weitz, Department of General Paediatrics and Haematology/Oncology, University Children's Hospital Tübingen

Jens H. Westhoff, Heidelberg University, Medical Faculty, Department of Paediatrics I, University Children's Hospital Heidelberg, Germany

Elke Wühl, Heidelberg University, Medical Faculty Heidelberg, Department of Paediatrics I, University Children's Hospital Heidelberg, Germany

Martin Zeier, Department of Nephrology, University Hospital Heidelberg, Clinic for Internal Medicine, Nephrology, Nuremberg Hospital, Germany

Miriam Zimmering, Rehabilitation Centre Ederhof, Iselsberg-Stronach, Austria

CHAPTER 1
Preparation for kidney transplantation

CHAPTER 1.1 Superiority of kidney transplantation vs. chronic dialysis, indications and contraindications

Burkhard Tönshoff[1] & Lars Pape[2]

[1] Heidelberg University, Medical Faculty Heidelberg, Department of Paediatrics I, University Children's Hospital, Heidelberg, Germany
[2] Department of Paediatrics II, University Hospital of Essen, Essen, Germany

ORCIDs:
Burkhard Tönshoff: https://orcid.org/0000-0002-6598-6910
Lars Pape: https://orcid.org/0000-0002-3635-6418

1 Superiority of kidney transplantation as renal replacement therapy

Chronic dialysis therapy in children and adolescents is associated with a number of complications. In chronic home peritoneal dialysis, the patient is usually confined to the cycler machine for 8–12 hours each night and cannot participate in normal evening leisure activities during adolescence. Chronic in-centre haemodialysis therapy requires the patient to travel to a paediatric dialysis centre, usually far away, for several hours at least 3 times a week, resulting in long periods of absence from school and other activities. Dialysis therapy puts a lot of strain on the circulatory system. Even a good dialysis therapy usually cannot guarantee more than 15% of normal kidney function. As a result, the paediatric dialysis patient has chronic uraemia with a variety of secondary complications, such as

- Growth impairment,
- CKD mineral bone disease,
- Renal anaemia,
- Metabolic acidosis,
- Accelerated atherosclerosis leading to an increased rate of cardiovascular complications from an early age,
- Impaired psychosocial development,

- Inferior quality of life,
- Impaired educational and employment outcomes in children and adolescents.

The survival benefit of kidney transplantation compared to dialysis therapy is demonstrated in a recent analysis of the ERA registry of adult outcomes of childhood kidney replacement therapy in Europe from 2008 to 2019 [1]. Dialysis patients had a higher risk of death than kidney transplant recipients (adjusted hazard ratio 5.44 (95% CI: 3.34–8.86)). Compared with the general population, life expectancy for eighteen-year-old kidney transplant and dialysis patients was 17 and 40 years shorter, respectively.

In addition, the quality of life after successful kidney transplantation is significantly better than during chronic dialysis treatment: patients can lead an almost normal life, with only a few restrictions in daily life apart from the necessary medication intake and outpatient visits. Growth and physical development are also almost normal if the transplant is successful.

2 Indications and contraindications for kidney transplantation

In terms of the size required for a child to be considered for a kidney transplant, most transplant centres require a body weight of at least 8–10 kg, otherwise the graft cannot be safely placed for anatomical reasons. However, in rare cases, recipients weighing 4–6 kg are accepted by specialised centres, for example if chronic dialysis is associated with significant complications or is not technically feasible. In these rare cases, a kidney from a deceased child donor can be transplanted.

In principle, AB0 blood group incompatibility is no longer an immunological contraindication (see Chapter 5.3); the long-term results are similar to those after AB0 blood group compatible transplantation. However, depending on the level of ABOi antibody titres, the organ recipient may require conditioning treatment by antigen-specific immunoadsorption prior to transplantation to remove the blood group antibodies in the recipient. Immunoadsorption is less problematic in older children than in infants due to the device-related extracorporeal volume. In addition, current protocols for AB0 blood group incompatible living kidney donation include more intensive immunosuppressive induction therapy with the B-cell depleting antibody rituximab, which may increase the risk of infection. These factors make ABO blood group transplantation less desirable as first choice.

Absolute contraindications to kidney transplantation:
- ongoing infectious diseases,
- malignant diseases that have not been treated curatively,
- serious comorbidities (e.g., cardiovascular, bronchial, pulmonary and liver disease) that either pose a life-threatening risk during transplantation or jeopardise the long-term success of the transplant.
- In the case of children with a severe physical or mental handicap, an indication for transplantation should be considered after careful assessment of the expected overall life expectancy.

References

1 Montez de Sousa IR, Bonthuis M, Kramer A, et al. Adult outcomes of childhood kidney replacement therapy in Europe from 2008 to 2019: an ERA Registry study. Nephrol Dial Transplant. 2024 Aug 24:gfae189.
2 Tönshoff B, Becker JU, Pape L. Nierentransplantation, pp. 243–74. In: Nierenerkrankungen im Kindes- und Jugendalter, Dötsch J, Weber LT (Hrsg.), Springer Berlin, 2024

CHAPTER 1.2 Kidney transplantation after deceased or living donation

Burkhard Tönshoff[1] & Lars Pape[2]

[1] Heidelberg University, Medical Faculty Heidelberg, Department of Paediatrics I, University Children's Hospital, Heidelberg, Germany
[2] Department of Paediatrics II, University Hospital of Essen, Essen, Germany

ORCIDs:
Burkhard Tönshoff: https://orcid.org/0000-0002-6598-6910
Lars Pape: https://orcid.org/0000-0002-3635-6418

1 Pre-emptive kidney transplantation

In recent years, it has been shown that kidney transplantation performed pre-emptively, i.e. without prior dialysis therapy, can result in

- Better patient survival,
- Superior short- and long-term graft survival compared to the results after prior prolonged dialysis therapy.
- Complete avoidance of dialysis-associated medical and psychosocial complications

However, in most developed countries, pre-emptive transplantation remains the minority. In Germany, for example, only 15–20% of transplantations in children and adolescents are currently performed before the need for dialysis is reached with a residual kidney function (estimated glomerular filtration rate, eGFR) of approximately 5–10 mL/min/1.73 m^2. Depending on the waiting time in the different allocation systems, most pre-emptive transplantations are carried out from living donors. The exact criteria for the timing of a pre-emptive transplantation have not yet been clearly defined; the date should be determined on a case-by-case basis, taking into account medical and psychosocial aspects.

2 Listing for deceased donation and organ allocation

If the patient is in a transplantable condition, he or she is registered on a waiting list through the responsible transplant centre. A national list is maintained with country-specific algorithms for allocation of available organs.

In the Eurotransplant sytem, transplant kidneys are allocated

1. on the basis of histocompatibility criteria, and
2. according to the patient's immunisation status and waiting time.

This allocation procedure is widely accepted in Europe, as there is a large body of data demonstrating the superior role of histocompatibility in early and late graft survival. In Germany, children under the age of 18 years are given priority in organ allocation due to the risk of physical and psychological developmental disorders during dialysis therapy. Today, the goal of early transplantation of a deceased kidney cannot be achieved in many cases due to the high number of dialysis patients, the decreasing willingness of the population to donate organs and the resulting increase in the waiting time until transplantation.

HLA matching

It is important to ensure a good HLA match,

- relevant for the longest possible kidney graft survival,
- relevant to avoid HLA sensitisation for a second or third transplant that may be required in the future,
- a good HLA match also allows for less intensive drug immunosuppression, thus avoiding infectious and oncological complications such as post-transplant lymphoproliferative disorder (PTLD),
- kidney transplants with 2 mismatches at the HLA-DR locus should only be accepted in exceptional cases.

Donor age

Deceased donation: Long-term data show that transplantation of donor kidneys from older deceased donors > 50 years is associated with poorer graft survival, so that, if possible, only a donor kidney from a deceased donor < 50 years should be accepted for a paediatric recipient. However, this principle is not always adhered to, as the average age of organ donors in Germany is steadily increasing and the number of organ donors is decreasing.

Living donation: The age limit of 50 years does not apply to living donors, and after careful selection of kidney-healthy living donors, possibly also grandparents, quite good long-term results can be achieved.

Young paediatric donors: The extent to which donor organs from young children < 5 years of age should be accepted for paediatric recipients is controversial, as transplantation of these very small organs into young recipients is associated with an increased rate of arterial and venous thrombosis due to difficult vascular anastomoses in anatomically small vessels, which may lead to early organ loss. Ultimately, the success of such high-risk transplants depends on the vascular surgical expertise of the transplant surgeon.

According to Eurotransplant guidelines, kidneys from paediatric donors aged < 2 years must be removed *en bloc,* and *en bloc* removal is recommended for donors aged between 2 and < 5 years. Some transplant surgeons recommend a recipient with a body weight of 20–50 kg for *en bloc* kidney transplantation, as smaller or larger recipients may have less favourable outcomes. In experienced centres, *en bloc* kidneys are often split into two kidneys that can be used for two smaller recipients.

3 Listing for living donation

Currently, about 30% of kidney transplants in children and adolescents up to the age of 18 years in Germany are performed with kidneys from living donors, usually the parents. Donations from other related and unrelated people who have a close emotional relationship with the recipient are also possible. This law is currently under review in Germany with the intention of changing to less stringent rules. Recently, the trend towards living donation has increased.

Transplantation of a kidney from a living donor has the following advantages over transplantation from a deceased donor:

- the donor is usually young and healthy,
- the procedure can be well timed,
- the immunological tolerance is usually better than with a deceased kidney because of the haploidenticity of parent and child, so the intensity of the immunosuppressive drug regimen and consequently their side effects are lower,

- there is no need for prolonged preservation of the organ; so the structure and function of the graft are better preserved.

These factors contribute to the fact that 5-year graft survival after living kidney donation is about 10% better than after deceased kidney donation. The average kidney graft survival (half-life) after deceased donation is currently about 19 years, which is about 5 years shorter than the graft survival after living donation (currently about 24 years). In addition, living donor transplantation can be more easily performed pre-emptively (before the need for dialysis therapy), thus avoiding potential dialysis-related complications.

The advantages of living kidney donation are offset by the surgical risk for the donor, although this is very low (see chapter 1.4). The perioperative mortality risk associated with living kidney donation is very low, at 0.03%. After kidney donation, the donor's kidney function is about 80% of baseline. Therefore, annual follow-up of living donors is mandatory in order to detect renal dysfunction or arterial hypertension in time. Annual follow-up includes a 24-hour ambulatory blood pressure monitoring, kidney function testing, protein excretion, sonography of the remaining autologous kidney, quality of life questionnaires or counselling, and psychological support if needed.

References

1 Boyer O, Pape L Is ABO Incompatible Living Donor Kidney Transplantation in Children a Better Option than the Use of Optimal Grafts From Deceased Donors? A Plea for Better Prioritization of Deceased Kidney Grafts for Children. Transpl Int. 2023;36:11911.

2 Heidotting NA, Ahlenstiel T, Kreuzer M, Franke D, Pape L. The influence of low donor age, living related donation and pre-emptive transplantation on end-organ damage based on arterial hypertension after paediatric kidney transplantation. Nephrol Dial Transplant. 2012;27(4):1672–6

3 Tönshoff B, Becker JU, Pape L. Nierentransplantation, pp. 243–74. In: Nierenerkrankungen im Kindes- und Jugendalter, Dötsch J, Weber LT (Hrsg.), Springer Berlin, 2024

4 Tönshoff B. Nierenlebendspende bei Kindern, Kapitel 5, pp. 49–81. In: Organtransplantation mit Lebendspende, Settmacher U, Rauchfuß F (Hrsg.), Springer Verlag, 2023

CHAPTER 1.3 Criteria for selecting a deceased donor

Raphael Schild[1] & Florian Grahammer[2]

[1] Department of Paediatric Nephrology, Paediatric Hepatology and Paediatric Transplantation, University Medical Centre Hamburg-Eppendorf, Hamburg, Germany
[2] III. Department of Medicine, University Hospital Hamburg Eppendorf, Hamburg, Germany

ORCIDs:
Raphael Schild: https://orcid.org/0000-0002-0416-6142
Florian Grahammer: https://orcid.org/0000-0002-7851-754X

There are no guidelines for the selection of a deceased donor kidney. However, the transplant team must make a quick decision to accept or reject the offered organ. The aim is to ensure the best chance of a successful transplant and long graft survival, while minimising the waiting time spent on dialysis. Long-term graft survival is particularly important for paediatric recipients due to their higher life expectancy. Therefore, organ quality criteria are generally more stringent than for older recipients. On the other hand, the burden and health consequences of dialysis are particularly high in this age group, and complications or co-morbidities increase with time on dialysis.

Quality of the donor and the organ

Donor organs can be classified according to the risk of subsequent graft failure. The ideal donor after brain death (DBD) is a donor with isolated brain trauma and no pre-existing conditions such as diabetes or hypertension.

- "Ideal" standard criteria donor (SCD): < 35 years; terminal S-creatinine < 1.5 mg/dl, no hypertension or diabetes, no cerebrovascular cause of death
- Expanded criteria donors (ECD): > 60 years or > 50 years *with at least 2 of the following:* hypertension, diabetes, cerebrovascular cause of death or terminal S-creatinine > 1.5 mg/dl. Paediatric recipients of these organs have an increased risk of graft loss (adjusted hazard ratio (aHR) 1.6 compared with matched non-ECD recipients) and also show no survival benefit over remaining on the waiting list [1]. However, in special cases (high sensitisation, long waiting time, dialysis problems) they may offer an advantage even in children.

- Donor age: Paediatric donors show better long-term graft function and superior growth and are therefore preferably allocated to children. However, in donors under 5 years of age, the risk of early graft loss increases to up to 10% while long-term graft survival remains comparable. In specialised paediatric surgical centres, these kidneys can give excellent results. En bloc transplantation may be appropriate for larger recipients and has been shown to provide a survival benefit over survival benefit over remaining on the waiting list and waiting for an organ from an adult donor [2–4].
- Cause of death, time without circulation ("down time") and need for cardiopulmonary resuscitation are other important factors in donor selection. In addition, diseases that affect renal prognosis such as hypertension (left ventricular hypertrophy as an indicator), stroke, diabetes and diseases that pose a risk to the recipient (malignancy, infection) should be identified and assessed. For the latter, European recommendations exist to guide management (Council of Europe, Guide to the quality and safety of organs for transplantation 8th edition; https://www.edqm.eu/en/guide-quality-and-safety-of-organs-for-transplantation).
- **Kidney function and acute kidney injury in the donor:** Although donor terminal serum creatinine > 1.5 mg/dL is considered a risk factor for delayed graft function (DGF) and graft loss, the results are inconsistent. Recent studies in both adult and paediatric recipients have failed to confirm terminal serum creatinine > 2 mg/dL as an independent risk factor for DGF. Therefore, the acceptance of particularly young donors with non-high-grade acute kidney injury (AKI) (< stage 3) may be considered also for children in individual cases [5, 6]. It is important to look for signs of pre-existing chronic kidney disease (proteinuria, high baseline serum creatinine and creatinine trajectory) and to differentiate from reversible causes of AKI (resuscitation, rhabdomyolysis).
- **Pre-transplant risk prediction tools:** Several risk prediction tools have been developed, but their limitations to adult recipients or substantial differences between countries reduce their usefulness for European recipients.
  - **Kidney Donor Profile Index (KDPI):** Provided by the Organ Procurement and Transplantation Network (OPTN) and is based on U.S. data. It has replaced the SCD/ECD classification for organ allocation. While it has been primarily validated in adult recipients, paediatric studies have shown that paediatric recipients of high (> 85) KDPI kidneys have a survival advantage over remaining on the waiting list (aHR 0.41

for death) [1]. The usefulness for non-US recipients is reduced due to country differences in the donor population.

- **A Dutch pre-transplant risk prediction tool** has shown good performance in predicting monthly graft survival from pre-transplant donor and recipient variables, including data on HLA matching and living vs. deceased donation [7]. While it only performs well in the Dutch population, country-specific variants for France and Germany have recently been developed, which also show good performance (AUC 0.73–0.77) [8]. These tools could in the future support clinical decision making as well as shared decision making with patients and families.

Human Leukocyte Antigen (HLA) Matching

- In current studies, poorer HLA matching is still associated with a higher risk of graft loss (aHR 1.43 in 3–6 mismatches vs. 0–2 mismatches). It also increases the risk of de novo HLA-DSA formation and leads a longer waiting time for retransplantation. Good HLA matching is therefore particularly important for paediatric recipients [6].
- Each transplant centre can determine the criteria for HLA matching. A common minimum requirement is to require at least 2 matches in the systems relevant to allocation (A-B-DR), with at least 1 match in the DR system (= maximum of 4 mismatches, including a maximum of 1 DR mismatch). HLA typing in C and DQ is performed but not used for allocation, and DP typing of the donor is not routinely performed in the ET region.
- In addition, pre-formed HLA antibodies in the recipient may need to be registered as non-acceptable HLA antigens (NAHA) in the potential donor, as they pose an increased risk for long-term graft survival, even with a negative crossmatch [9]. The resulting virtual panel reactivity (vPRA) reduces the number of potential donors and increases the waiting time, so that a critical selection and regular re-evaluation of these unacceptables are required in collaboration with the local HLA laboratory is necessary, taking into account the urgency of the transplantation [10].

Other recipient factors: Criteria for the urgency of the transplantation, which may lead to a potential benefit even if a non-ideal organ is accepted, are particularly relevant here: Previous waiting time, expected waiting time (sensitisation, planned living donation) and clinical condition on dialysis (vascular situation, peritonitis episodes).

Cold ischaemia time (CIT): The cold ischaemia time is the time between kidney retrieval and initiation of cooling until transplantation. The shorter the CIT, the rarer the occurrence of DGF and the better the graft survival. Current data show that the risk of graft failure and patient death increases proportionally by 8% for each additional 6 hours of CIT beyond 6 hours [11]. Recipients of organs with CIT > 18 hours vs. < 18 hours have a 21% higher risk of graft failure.

References

1 Kizilbash SJ, Evans MD, Chinnakotla S, Chavers BM. Use of expanded-criteria donors and > 85 KDPI kidneys for pediatric kidney transplantation in the United States. Am J Transplant. Mar 2021;21(3):1160–1170. doi: 10.1111/ajt.16162

2 Schild R, Carvajal Abreu K, Buscher A, et al. Favorable Outcome After Single-kidney Transplantation From Small Donors in Children: A Match-controlled CERTAIN Registry Study. Transplantation. Aug 1 2024;108(8):1793–1801. doi: 10.1097/TP.0000000000004993

3 Kizilbash SJ, Evans MD, Chinnakotla S, Chavers BM. Survival Benefit of En Bloc Transplantation of Small Pediatric Kidneys in Children. Transplantation. Nov 2020;104(11):2435–2443. doi: 10.1097/TP.0000000000003158

4 Chesnaye NC, van Stralen KJ, Bonthuis M, et al. The association of donor and recipient age with graft survival in paediatric renal transplant recipients in a European Society for Paediatric Nephrology/European Renal Association-European Dialysis and Transplantation Association Registry study. Nephrol Dial Transplant. Nov 1 2017;32(11):1949–1956. doi: 10.1093/ndt/gfx261

5 Chopra B, Sureshkumar KK. Limitation of Terminal Serum Creatinine as a Kidney Donor Profile Index Variable in Predicting Long-Term Kidney Transplant Outcomes. Transplant Proc. Jun 2018;50(5):1272–1275. doi: 10.1016/j.transproceed.2018.03.019

6 Solomon S, Hayde N. Utilization of Donor Kidneys With Acute Kidney Injury in Pediatric Kidney Transplant Recipients. Transplantation. Mar 2020;104(3):597–602. doi: 10.1097/TP.0000000000002827

7 Oomen L, de Jong H, Bouts AHM, et al. A pre-transplantation risk assessment tool for graft survival in Dutch pediatric kidney recipients. Clin Kidney J. Jul 2023;16(7):1122–1131. doi: 10.1093/ckj/sfad057
8 Oomen L, de Wall LL, Tönshoff B, et al. International validation of a pre-transplant risk assessment tool for graft survival in pediatric kidney transplant recipients. Clinical Kidney Journal. 2025; doi: 10.1093/ckj/sfaf031
9 Ziemann M, Altermann W, Angert K, et al. Preformed Donor-Specific HLA Antibodies in Living and Deceased Donor Transplantation: A Multicenter Study. Clin J Am Soc Nephrol. Jul 5 2019;14(7):1056–1066. doi: 10.2215/CJN.13401118
10 de Ferrante H, Smeulders B, Tieken I, et al. Immunized Patients Face Reduced Access to Transplantation in the Eurotransplant Kidney Allocation System. Transplantation. Oct 1 2023;107(10):2247–2254. doi: 10.1097/TP.0000000000004687
11 Debout A, Foucher Y, Trebern-Launay K, et al. Each additional hour of cold ischemia time significantly increases the risk of graft failure and mortality following renal transplantation. Kidney Int. Feb 2015;87(2):343–9. doi: 10.1038/ki.2014.304

CHAPTER 1.4 Selection and examination of the living kidney donor

Stefan Reuter & Barbara Suwelack

University Clinics Münster, Department of Medicine D, Transplant Nephrology

ORCIDs:
Stefan Reuter: https://orcid.org/0000-0003-3180-6245
Barbara Suwelack: https://orcid.org/0000-0002-4082-3074

1 Introduction

Living kidney donation is a complex medical and ethical procedure that requires thorough evaluation, strict adherence to legal standards, and well-structured post-donation care. The following recommendations for the evaluation and management of living kidney donation are primarily based on the 2023 Manual developed by the "Arbeitsgemeinschaft der Nierentransplantationszentren Nordrhein-Westfalens", a not-for-profit collaboration of transplant centres in North Rhine-Westphalia and collaborating centres in Germany. This manual (written in German) is freely available on the websites of both the German Transplant Society and the German Society of Nephrology: https://d-t-g-online.de/inhalte/gesetze-leit-richtlinien/manual-ag-nierentransplantation-nrw.

This chapter provides essential guidelines for transplant teams to evaluate, counsel, and support both kidney donors and recipients before, during, and after transplantation or donation. It provides a standardised approach to ensure rigorous medical assessment, ethical protocols, and comprehensive postoperative care. Each section is designed for flexibility, allowing institutions to adapt protocols as needed to meet specific local or regional regulations.

The following recommendations are based on current German legal regulations as of October 2024. Changes, such as allowing crossover living kidney donation or anonymous altruistic kidney donation or chain donation, are currently being planned but have not yet been finalised and are therefore not considered in this chapter.

2 Donor evaluation for living kidney donation

Ensure that the donor meets medical, psychological, and regulatory criteria to minimise health risks after donation. Key eligibility requirements include legal adulthood, voluntary consent, and a personal relationship with the recipient, as defined in the Transplantation Act.

2.1 Eligibility Criteria

Medical examination:

- *Comprehensive health evaluation:* A complete medical examination assesses cardiovascular health, surgical fitness, cancer risk, and any chronic infections. This evaluation ensures that the donor's body can handle the procedure and that there are no underlying conditions that could be aggravated by the donation.
- *Psychological assessment:* A psychological evaluation is mandatory to verify the donor's willingness, mental stability and health, and the absence of coercion.

Laboratory tests:

- *Immunological testing:* This includes blood group determination, HLA typing, and Cross-Match tests to assess compatibility and reduce the risk of rejection.
- *Infectious disease testing:* Mandatory tests screen for hepatitis B and C, HIV, and other transmissible infections. Additional serological tests may be performed based on the individual's medical and travel history.
- *Renal function tests:* estimated glomerular filtration rate (eGFR), preferably calculated using the CKD-EPI formula, serum creatinine and cystatin c, and kidney function tests (ideally more than one; could be imaging-based [DTPA or MAG3 clearance], CT/MRT kidney volumetry, or creatinine clearance) determine whether the donor has optimal renal health.

Imaging and diagnostic tests:

- *Ultrasound (sonography) of the abdomen:* Assesses kidney anatomy and any structural abnormalities.

- *Advanced imaging:* CT or MRI scans of the abdomen, possibly with contrast media, provide detailed images of renal blood vessels and surrounding organs, which are essential for planning surgery.

2.2 Contraindications to living kidney donation

The basis for certain donor contraindications according to the German Transplantation Act and to expert opinion, is the medical assessment of whether the donor is likely to be endangered beyond the risk of the operation or severely impaired beyond the immediate consequences of the organ removal. Contraindications are divided into absolute and relative categories, with absolute contraindications excluding donation and relative contraindications requiring careful consideration or further testing.

Absolute contraindications

- *Age* < 18 years
- *Pregnancy:* It is recommended that women donate a kidney only after family planning has been completed.
- *Renal function:* estimated glomerular filtration rate (eGFR) or measured GFR < 60 mL/min x 1.73 m^2, function of one kidney less than 30%.
- *Haematuria:* persistent glomerular haematuria
- *Proteinuria:* persistent proteinuria > 300 mg/g creatinine
- *Nephrocalcinosis, bilateral kidney stones*
- *Pathological kidney anatomy:* Horseshoe kidney, significant arteriosclerosis, fibromuscular dysplasia; evaluation for presence of cysts ≥ Bosniak 2F is required.
- *Arterial hypertension:* Blood pressure levels > 140/90 mmHg (on ≥ 2 antihypertensive medications), hypertension-related clinically relevant end-organ damage
- *Diabetes mellitus*
- *Active infections:* Conditions such as HIV, active tuberculosis, or viral hepatitis prevent donation.
- *Cancer risk:* Any current cancer (despite local tumours with no risk of metastasis) is a contraindication due to the potential risk of transmission to the recipient. If there is a history of cancer, an oncologist or tumour board should be consulted to assess suitability.

- *Hereditary kidney disease:*
  Polycystic kidney disease (PKD): Proven cases of ADPKD or ARPKD are an absolute contraindication to donation. This also applies to related donors under 30 years of age with a PKD mutation, even if no cysts are visible on imaging.
  Alport syndrome: In X-linked Alport syndrome, female donors (e.g. mothers of affected males) should generally avoid donation because of the risk of renal dysfunction in the donor. Heterozygous relatives of autosomal recessive Alport have a lower risk and can donate if renal function and proteinuria are normal. Severe renal disease should be excluded by biopsy and the use of RAAS blockade after transplantation is recommended. Genetic testing is recommended.
  Complement-mediated thrombotic microangiopathy/atypical haemolytic uremic syndrome: Absolute contraindication for related living donors with a proven complement mutation.
- *Psychosocial barriers:* Active psychiatric conditions, substance abuse, or any hint of coercion disqualify candidates to ensure that the donor's decision is fully informed, voluntary, and does not further harm mental health.

Relative contraindications
- *High body mass index (BMI):* A BMI over 35 is discouraged but not always prohibitive; weight loss may help some individuals meet eligibility requirements.
- *Cardiovascular risks:* Higher cardiovascular risk, such as hypertension or heart disease, requires further evaluation to prevent undue health risks to the donor.
- *Renal function:* Relative contraindication: eGFR 60–79 mL/min x 1.73 m^2, decide on a case-by-case basis
- *Proteinuria:* Persistent albuminuria > 30 mg/g creatinine
- *Pre-diabetes:* impaired fasting glucose and pathological glucose tolerance (OGTT-blood sugar BZ 140–199 mg/dL after 2 hours)
- *Smoking:* Strongly recommended to stopped before living kidney donation.

2.3 Surgical considerations

- *Kidney structure:* Detailed imaging ensures that each kidney has sufficient function and size. Donors with certain structural abnormalities may not be suitable candidates.

3 Donor postoperative care

3.1 Follow-up protocols

- *Immediately after donation:* Donors receive regular follow-up to monitor kidney function, assess surgical recovery, and manage any complications.
- *Long-term monitoring:* Annual medical check-ups monitor kidney function, blood pressure, and overall physical and mental health. Routine tests such as serum creatinine and eGFR help monitor renal health, while cardiovascular evaluations help manage long-term risks.
- *Psychosocial support:* Donors have access to psychosocial services, which can be vital for some people after donation. Counselling or support groups can help donors adjust, especially those with pre-existing psychological problems.

3.2 Medical examinations

- *Monitoring kidney function:* Regular blood tests will assess serum creatinine levels and eGFR as indicators of kidney function.
- *Urinalysis:* Routine urine tests can help detect early signs of kidney disease.
- *Blood pressure monitoring:* Hypertension management and cardiovascular evaluation are essential, as kidney donors may be at higher long-term risk.
- *Health counselling:* Donors receive lifestyle counselling to support their long-term health, with advice on diet, exercise, self-monitoring of blood pressure, and avoidance of nephrotoxic medications.

4 ABO incompatible living kidney donation

4.1 Overview

ABO incompatible (ABOi) living kidney donation allows transplantation across the blood type barrier by using pre-transplant plasma exchange or immunoadsorption to reduce blood type-specific antibodies, particularly isoagglutinins (IgG, IgM), thereby minimizing the risk of rejection. Because of the higher immunological risk and the need for a more intensive immunosuppressive regimen, donors and recipients must provide specific consent for this option.

4.2 Selection and counselling

- *Donor-recipient counselling:* Both parties are fully informed of the risks, benefits, and procedures involved in ABOi transplantation. If other ABO-compatible donors are available, they are generally preferred.
- *Immunological evaluation:* The recipient's isoagglutinin titres are measured to assess the likelihood of success. High titres may indicate the need for more intensive treatment.

4.3 Immunological preparation

- *Rituximab and immunoadsorption:* To reduce the immune response, recipients may receive rituximab and undergo immunoadsorption or plasmapheresis, depending on individual needs and titres.
- *Regulatory approval:* The donor must meet with the regional transplant commission, which verifies eligibility and ensures informed, voluntary consent.

5 Consent and mutual disclosure

5.1 Consent forms and documentation

Both donor and recipient must sign consent forms acknowledging the risks and agreeing to the mutual disclosure of relevant medical information. This transparency is essential for informed decision making and trust. If there is a language barrier, a qualified interpreter must be present during the counselling sessions. According to the German Transplantation Act, a neutral doctor must also observe the counselling session.

5.2 Counselling topics

Donors and recipients are informed about potential complications, long-term health impacts, and the importance of compliance with post-operative care.

5.3 Documentation

Signed and witnessed consent forms are required to ensure compliance with medical and legal standards. These forms outline potential risks, post-transplant expectations, and voluntary participation.

References

2023 Manual developed by the "Arbeitsgemeinschaft der Nierentransplantationszentren Nordrhein-Westfalens": https://d-t-g-online.de/inhalte/gesetze-leit-richtlinien/manual-ag-nierentransplantation-nrw

CHAPTER 1.5 Preparation of the recipient for kidney transplantation

Thurid Ahlenstiel-Grunow[1], Birgitta Kranz[2] & Christina Taylan[3]

[1] Department of Paediatrics II, University Hospital of Essen, Essen, Germany
[2] Department of Paediatric Nephrology, University Hospital of Münster, Münster, Germany
[3] Department of Paediatric Nephrology, University Hospital of Cologne, Cologne, Germany

ORCIDs:
Thurid Ahlenstiel-Grunow: https://orcid.org/0009-0007-6193-7015
Christina Taylan: https://orcid.org/0000-0001-9585-054X

1 Special aspects and general assessments

Special aspects of paediatric kidney transplantation

- In Germany, paediatric patients with an eGFR < 20 mL/min/1.73 m^2 can already be registered with Eurotransplant for pre-emptive kidney transplantation [1].
- Kidney transplantation from a living related donor (e.g. one of the parents) should be discussed and assessed in advance (note: better graft survival and lower complication rate with pre-emptive living donor transplantation).
- A detailed donor profile often needs to be defined in terms of body height, underlying disease, special anatomical characteristics, etc.
- Where appropriate, the risk of disease recurrence in the transplanted kidney (e.g. FSGS, IgA nephritis, aHUS) should be considered when choosing between living and deceased donation.
- In paediatric transplant recipients, histocompatibility and avoidance of sensitisation are of particular interest in view of the expected need for repeated kidney transplantations during their lifetime.
- Modalities of fluid, nutrition and medication intake are of particular interest in children, considering, for example, the inability to swallow tablets or the need for tube feeding.
- The cognitive maturity of the paediatric patient and the willingness and ability of the parents/caregivers to support their child have a significant impact on adherence to treatment (note: assessment of need for support by care services and/or youth services).

- An individual treatment concept for each recipient should be defined by an interdisciplinary agreement with paediatric nephrology, transplant surgery, urology, immunology, etc.
- Prior to transplantation, a personalised immunosuppressive regimen should be planned for each paediatric recipient, taking into account age, comorbidities and individual risk of infection, rejection, disease recurrence, etc.
- Detailed education of paediatric patients and their parents/caregivers (including psychosocial counselling) is essential to improve adherence and avoid complications after transplantation.

Timing for initiation of preparation for pediatric kidney transplantation

- If possible before starting chronic dialysis therapy (e.g. with an eGFR of around 20–25 mL/min/1.73 m^2), in order to allow pre-emptive registration on the Eurotransplant waiting list (with an eGFR < 20 mL/min/1.73 m^2) and/or to realize a pre-emptive living donor kidney transplantation.

General assessments

- If not already done clarification of underlying renal disease (e.g. genetics)
- Assessment of co-morbidities (e.g. portal hypertension due to chronic liver disease, diabetes mellitus, heart disease, lung disease, neurological impairment, additional malformations, etc.)
- Documentation of co-medication (with regard to possible interactions with the immunosuppressive drugs)
- Documentation of pre-existing allergies
- Documentation of previous blood transfusions
- Documentation of immunisation status
- Assessment of vaccination status (recommendation: complete pre-transplant vaccination status, especially live vaccinations!)
- Documentation of residual diuresis volume
- Clarification of (medical) custody

Aspects for planning of the individual surgical procedure

- Urological aspects: urogenital malformations, bladder dysfunction, ureterocutaneostomy, etc.
- Evaluation of the indication for nephrectomy of the native kidneys (e.g. increased risk of Wilms tumour).
- Assessment of the need for explantation of previous kidney transplants, if applicable.

- Vascular malformations/thrombosis/stenosis:
  - Abdominal vascular malformations/thrombosis/stenosis related to the vascular anastomosis of the transplant.
  - Cervical vascular malformations/thrombosis/stenosis related to a central line for laboratory controls, fluid management, etc.
- Dialysis access management: e.g. peritoneal catheter extirpation during or after transplantation.
- Where appropriate assessment of the possibility/need for combined liver and kidney transplantation (e.g. autosomal recessive polycystic kidney disease [ARPKD]).

2 Diagnostics

Physical examination

- Height, weight, head circumference (if appropriate)
- Full physical examination including pubertal status (skeletal deformities? reduced mobility?)

Laboratory diagnostics

- Complete blood count (including leukocyte differential count and reticulocytes)
- Blood gas analysis
- Electrolytes (sodium, potassium, chloride, calcium, magnesium, phosphate), creatinine, urea, uric acid, cystatin C, creatine kinase (CK), GOT (ASAT), GPT (ALAT), GLDH, alkaline phosphatase (AP), gamma GT, total bilirubin, direct bilirubin, LDH, amylase, lipase, glucose, total protein, albumin, C-reactive protein (CRP), iron, ferritin, transferrin, transferrin saturation, triglycerides, total cholesterol, LDL cholesterol, HDL cholesterol, lipoprotein (a), homocysteine
- Immunoglobulins (IgA, IgG, IgM, IgE)
- Endocrinology: TSH, fT4, fT3, IGF-I, IGFBP-3, parathyroid hormone (PTH), 25-OH vitamin D, HbA1c, LH, FSH, testosterone ♂ or estradiol ♀
- Coagulation: prothrombin time (Quick), aPTT, thrombin time, fibrinogen, antithrombin III (ATIII), factor II, factor V, factor VIII
- Thrombophilia diagnostics: protein C, protein S, MTHFR mutation, factor II mutation, factor V mutation, activated protein C resistance (APC

resistance), lupus anticoagulants, anti-phospholipid antibodies (e.g. anti-cardiolipin, anti-beta-2-glycoprotein I, anti-phosphatidylserine)

- Blood group
- HLA typing (note: Confirmation by HLA re-typing in another blood sample required!)
- HLA antibody screening (note: Repeat every 3 months!)
- Virology: HIV-1/2 screening, anti-HAV, HBs-Ag, anti-HBs, anti-HBc, anti-HCV, anti-CMV, CMV-DNA, anti-EBV, EBV-DNA, anti-HSV, anti-VZV, anti-measles, anti-mumps, anti-rubella
- QuantiFERON test (interferon-gamma release assay; if ≥ 5 years) or tuberculin skin test (if < 5 years)
- As appropriate extended (auto-)immune diagnostics and complement diagnostics (e.g. in autoimmune diseases, haemolytic uraemic syndrome)
- Urinalysis: urine status, urine culture, urine creatinine, urine protein, urine albumin, urine alpha-1 microglobuline, urine calcium, urine glucose

Instrumental diagnostics

- Abdominal ultrasound (including Doppler ultrasound of the aorta, vena cava inferior and iliac vessels); (if necessary) abdominal MRI (especially in case of very young children with small abdominal vessels)
- Doppler ultrasound of the neck vessels (note: repeat after each central venous catheter!)
- Ultrasound of the urinary tract (measurement of residual urine)
- As required extended urological diagnostics: uroflowmetry, micturition cystourethrogram (MCU), cystoscopy, cystomanometry
- Chest x-ray
- X-ray of the left hand (bone mineralisation, bone ageing)
- Echocardiography (ECHO), electrocardiogram (ECG)
- 24-hour ambulatory blood pressure monitoring (ABPM)
- Audiometry
- Electroencephalogram (EEG)
- Pulmonary function tests (PFTs) (if the child is cooperative)

Further diagnostics

- Ophthalmologic examination including fundoscopy (hypertensive retinopathy? cataracts?)
- ENT (ear, nose and throat) examination (looking for focus of infection)
- Dental examination (looking for focus of infection)

- Gynaecological examination (if applicable)
- Psychosocial assessment
- Neuropsychological assessment (developmental diagnostics)
- Neurological evaluation (if appropriate)
- Hepatic and/or gastrointestinal evaluation including endoscopic examination (if appropriate)

All dynamic examination results (laboratory parameters, imaging after specific events) should be repeated regularly.

References

1 Richtlinien der Bundesärztekammer für die Wartelistenführung und Organvermittlung zur Nierentransplantation (gemäß § 16 Abs. 1 S. 1 Nrn. 2 und 5 TPG): https://www.bundesaerztekammer.de/baek/ueber-uns/richtlinien-leitlinien-empfehlungen-und-stellungnahmen/transplantationsmedizin/wartelistenfuehrung-und-organvermittlung (Stand 27.06.2023)

CHAPTER 1.6 Transplantation immunology work-up

Thuong Hien Tran, Lea Keppner & Lien Pham

Heidelberg University Hospital, Institute of Immunology, Heidelberg, Germany

ORCID:
Thuong Hien Tran: https://orcid.org/0000-0001-8587-5989

1 Introduction

The registration of a patient on the waiting list for a deceased donor kidney transplantation requires certain immunological diagnostic tests. The immunological work-up requirements for transplant recipients of kidneys allocated by Eurotransplant (ET) are described in the ET Manual. The recommendations released by ET must be implemented after being approved and published in guidelines by the respective national authorities (e.g. the German Medical Association "BÄK" in Germany). As all European tissue typing laboratories providing histocompatibility data in this framework must be accredited by the European Federation for Immunogenetics (EFI), EFI Standards also apply. This chapter summarises the pre-transplant immunological work-up of a recipient for deceased donor kidney transplantation, mainly based on the latest valid versions of the ET Manual, Chapter Histocompatibilty [1], the BÄK Guideline for Organ Recipient Safety [2] and the EFI Standards, Section Renal and/or Pancreas Transplantation [3]. Other relevant literature is also considered (see references).

Four key pre-transplant immunological tests are required for a recipient to be placed on the waiting list:

- ABO blood group (section 2)
- Human leukocyte antigen (HLA) typing (section 3)
- HLA antibody screening (section 4)
- Autologous crossmatch (section 5)

Other serological tests (e.g., detection of non-HLA antibodies such as anti-endothelial cell antibodies [4], MICA antibodies [5] or the measurement of soluble CD30 levels [6]) are not widely used in routine practice.

Based on the results of HLA antibody screening, unacceptable antigens are defined and reported to ET (section 6). If a donor is available, potential recipients are selected by virtual crossmatching (section 7). For recipients who receive a kidney offer, an additional physical crossmatch is performed (section 8).

2 ABO Blood Group Determination

Kidney transplants from deceased donors with ABO-incompatibility are not permitted. The recipient's blood group must be determined and verified in two independent blood samples before being placed on the waiting list. Recipient and donor blood groups must be confirmed immediately before transplantation.

3 Human Leukocyte Antigen (HLA) Typing

For the registration with ET, each recipient must be typed for at least HLA-A, -B, -C, -DRB1 and -DQB1 (in Germany, also HLA-DPB1) using DNA-based typing techniques. Preferably, HLA-DRB3/4/5, -DQA1 and -DPA1 should also be typed (a total of 11 HLA loci), as the potential donor is usually typed at 11 HLA loci for allocation, and the commercially available antibody kits are able to detect antibodies against all these loci. Typing resolution is usually one-field, but for certain HLA subgroups or patients with allele-specific antibodies, two-field unambiguous typing for the respective HLA locus should be obtained. HLA-Bw4/Bw6 are reported on the basis of the HLA-B antigens. HLA typing of the recipient should be performed on two different blood samples. The HLA typing data are translated into matching determinants by ET algorithms for allocation.

4 HLA Antibody Screening

4.1 Screening schedule

For wait-listing, the patient must be tested for HLA-specific antibodies. While on the waiting list, the patient must be screened for HLA antibodies every three months. The frequency of the repeated HLA antibody screening is necessary to avoid the use of an outdated serum for crossmatching at the time of organ offer. According to the ET Manual [1], a serum is outdated if it is older than 180 days from the date of blood drawing. In Germany, however, the national guidelines [2] consider a serum to be outdated if it is more than 150 days old.

The responsible physicians (dialysis centres, transplant centres) must inform their HLA laboratories about previous immunising events (transfusions, pregnancies, previous transplants) or graft removal. This information is important not only for the plausibility check of the test results, but also for the immunological risk stratification based on which detected HLA antibodies are evaluated for reporting as unacceptable antigens (see section 6). HLA antibody screening should be performed after each immunising event or graft explantation (in addition to regular screening). In these cases, ET recommends a repeat antibody screening two and four weeks after the event.

4.2 Antibody testing methods

Regarding the method used for HLA antibody screening, ET requires different applications depending on the time point and the sensitisation status of the patient. The degree of sensitisation is determined using virtual panel-reactive antibodies (vPRA) (see section 6).

- The complement-dependent cytotoxicity (CDC) test, also known as the lymphocytotoxicity test (LCT), is used to detect complement-fixing antibodies, which are known to correlate with hyperacute/acute rejection. A CDC-PRA of > 5% is considered positive. HLA specificities to which the patient has preformed CDC-positive IgG alloantibodies must therefore be reported as unacceptable antigens. The addition of dithiothreitol (DTT), which disrupts the disulfide bonds of IgM, may help to recognise an IgM-related positive test result. IgM antibodies may be transplant-irrelevant antibodies (e.g. IgM autoantibodies) or IgM HLA alloantibodies. The impact of pre-transplant IgM HLA alloantibodies on graft rejection and failure is controversial [7, 8]. CDC antibody screening must be performed for each new patient on the waiting list. If the patient is classified as immunised (vPRA > 0%), CDC antibody screening must be repeated at least annually. For non-immunised patients (vPRA = 0%), annual CDC screening is not required by ET. In Germany, CDC antibody screening is usually performed at least once a year for all patients on the waiting list for a kidney and pancreas transplantation.

- Solid phase assays (e.g. bead microarray assays on a Luminex platform) show higher sensitivity and specificity than CDC tests [9]. The commercial test formats offer methods for detection (screening for the presence or absence) and identification (differentiation of the specificities) of HLA antibodies. Currently, the Luminex Single Antigen Bead assays are the most sensitive methods for the detection of HLA class I and class II antibodies. All sera used for solid phase assays must be pre-treated by EDTA, heat inactivation, DTT, or dilution to avoid complement interference/prozone effect. HLA antibody screening with solid phase assays is required every three months. In Germany, it is recommended that at least all patients with positive screening results at the time of registration and at annual follow-up be tested with the Single Antigen Beads assay. In case of changes in antibody profile/signal strength or implausibility of the results, additional tests should be performed. New antibody testing is required in all patients after a sensitising event (see section 4.1).

5 Autologous Crossmatch

Autoantibodies may cause false positive results in CDC antibody screening and/or crossmatching. Therefore, the detection/exclusion of autoantibodies must be performed for each patient by autologous CDC crossmatch (incubation of the patient's lymphocytes with his/her own serum) with and without DTT, usually prior to wait-listing. Autologous cross-matching is also useful during the waiting period for patients who show reactivity in CDC antibody screening tests (often without accompanying specific HLA antibodies detected in the solid phase assays). In patients known to have IgM autoantibodies, the allogeneic CDC crossmatch (incubation of donor lymphocytes with patient serum) with and without DTT must be performed at the time of a kidney offer.

6 Unacceptable HLA Antigens

If HLA antibodies are detected, they will be evaluated whether they should be reported to ET as "unacceptable HLA antigens". Unacceptable HLA antigens are prohibited donor HLA mismatches (see section 7). The assignment of an HLA antibody specificity as an unacceptable HLA antigen is centre- and patient-dependent. Therefore, the criteria for defining unacceptable antigens must be discussed between the transplant centre and the affiliated HLA laboratory.

After entering the unacceptable antigens in the ET software ENISNext, the virtual PRA (vPRA) value is automatically calculated, indicating the frequency of the unacceptable HLA antigens in the ET donor pool. A vPRA of > 0% indicates that a patient is sensitised. In addition, based on the unacceptable antigens and ABO blood group of a patient, the donor frequency calculator in ENISNext can also calculate the likelihood of receiving an offer for an ABO identical or compatible kidney transplant.

There are some general considerations published by ET [1] and the German Society for Immunogenetics [10] regarding the determination of unacceptable HLA antigens. All HLA antigens to which antibodies are found in the CDC screen must be reported as unacceptable antigens. Often antibodies are found in the solid phase assays, but not in the CDC test. Therefore, a careful plausibility check of these antibody reactions in the solid phase assays (including non-specific response patterns due to antibodies against denatured antigens or "natural antibodies") and individually adapted stratification of immunological risks (taking into account the patient's history of alloimmunisation) must be integrated into the evaluation. The disadvantage of reporting antigens as "unacceptable" and thus prolonging the waiting time for an organ offer must be weighed against the risk of not reporting them and thus resulting in an HLA incompatible transplant with subsequent short- and long-term post-transplant complications.

Highly sensitised patients (vPRA ≥ 85% in two different sera) often have a low chance of receiving a crossmatch negative kidney offer. Such patients may be eligible for inclusion in the Acceptable Mismatch (AM) programme of ET.

7 Virtual Crossmatch

If a kidney donor is available and expresses HLA antigens that are indicated as unacceptable antigens in a patient, ET will not make a kidney offer to that patient. This exclusion during the allocation process is called a positive virtual crossmatch.

Recipients with a negative virtual crossmatch may be offered the kidney and, if accepted, a physical crossmatch must be performed by the HLA laboratory affiliated with the transplant centre. The virtual crossmatch is performed for all kidney, pancreas and combined kidney-pancreas transplantations.

8 Physical Crossmatch

A physical crossmatch is performed as a decisive crossmatch (also called transplantation crossmatch) after the virtual crossmatch (see section 7) is negative. It is usually performed with the CDC technique, using recipient serum and donor lymphocytes (isolated from either the donor's peripheral blood, lymph nodes or spleen). To increase the sensitivity of the CDC crossmatch, B lymphocytes can be used in addition to T lymphocytes or unseparated lymphocytes. It is important that the serum is representative of the current immunisation status of the recipient: either the most recent serum in the quarterly screening scheme (while avoiding outdated sera – see above) from a non-immunised patient, or a fresh serum if the patient is immunised or has had a recent immunising event. In immunised patients, transplantation can only be performed if the prospective decisive crossmatch is negative. In Germany, for first-transplant, non-immunised recipients (with confirmed negative HLA antibody tests and with no immunising event since the last antibody screening), a decisive crossmatch may be performed either prospectively or in parallel with the transplantation.

A decisive crossmatch must be performed for all kidney, pancreas and combined kidney-pancreas transplantations. Due to the limited tolerance to ischaemia, crossmatching for a pancreas recipient is usually performed at the donor centre and for a kidney recipient at the recipient centre by the affiliated HLA laboratory.

References

1 Eurotransplant Manual – version 5.5; July 9, 2024; Chapter 10 Histocompatibility Testing.
2 German Medical Association Guideline for Organ Recipient Safety (RL BÄK Empfängerschutz), version September 10, 2021, fully effective starting January 24, 2023.
3 European Federation for Immunogenetics – Standards for Histocompatibility & Immunogenetics Testing; version 8.1, effective from January 1st 2024.
4 Fichtner A, Süsal C, Höcker B, Rieger S, Waldherr R, Westhoff JH, Sander A, Dragun D, Tönshoff B. Association of non-HLA antibodies against endothelial targets and donor-specific HLA antibodies with antibody-mediated rejection and graft function in pediatric kidney transplant

recipients. Pediatr Nephrol. 2021 Aug;36(8):2473–2484. doi: 10.1007/s00467-021-04969-1. Epub 2021 Mar 24.

5 Carapito R, Aouadi I, Verniquet M, Untrau M, Pichot A, Beaudrey T, Bassand X, Meyer S, Faucher L, Posson J, Morlon A, Kotova I, Delbos F, Walencik A, Aarnink A, Kennel A, Suberbielle C, Taupin JL, Matern BM, Spierings E, Congy-Jolivet N, Essaydi A, Perrin P, Blancher A, Charron D, Cereb N, Maumy-Bertrand M, Bertrand F, Garrigue V, Pernin V, Weekers L, Naesens M, Kamar N, Legendre C, Glotz D, Caillard S, Ladrière M, Giral M, Anglicheau D, Süsal C, Bahram S. The MHC class I MICA gene is a histocompatibility antigen in kidney transplantation. Nat Med. 2022 May;28(5):989–998. doi: 10.1038/s41591-022-01725-2. Epub 2022 Mar 14.

6 Süsal C, Döhler B, Ruhenstroth A, Morath C, Slavcev A, Fehr T, Wagner E, Krüger B, Rees M, Balen S, Živčić-Ćosić S, Norman DJ, Kuypers D, Emonds MP, Pisarski P, Bösmüller C, Weimer R, Mytilineos J, Scherer S, Tran TH, Gombos P, Schemmer P, Zeier M, Opelz G. Donor-specific antibodies require preactivated immune system to harm renal transplant. A Collaborative Transplant Study. EBioMedicine. 2016 Jul; 9: 366–371. doi: 10.1016/j.ebiom.2016.06.006. Epub 2016 Jun 5.

7 Babu A, Andreou A, Briggs D, Krishnan N, Higgins R, Mitchell D, Barber T, Daga S. Clinical Relevance of Donor-Specific IgM Antibodies in HLA Incompatible Renal Transplantation: A Retrospective Single-Centre Study. Clin Transpl. 2016; 32: 173–179.

8 Everly MJ, Rebellato LM, Haisch CE, Briley KP, Bolin P, Kendrick WT, Kendrick SA, Morgan C, Maldonado AQ, Harland RC, Terasaki PI. Impact of IgM and IgG3 anti-HLA alloantibodies in primary renal allograft recipients. Transplantation. 2014; 97(5): 494–501.

9 Tait BD, Süsal C, Gebel HM, Nickerson PW, Zachary AA, Claas FH, Reed EF, Bray RA, Campbell P, Chapman JR, Coates PT, Colvin RB, Cozzi E, Doxiadis II, Fuggle SV, Gill J, Glotz D, Lachmann N, Mohanakumar T, Suciu-Foca N, Sumitran-Holgersson S, Tanabe K, Taylor CJ, Tyan DB, Webster A, Zeevi A, Opelz G. Consensus guidelines on the testing and clinical management issues associated with HLA and non-HLA antibodies in transplantation. Transplantation. 2013 Jan 15;95(1):19–47.

10 Ziemann M, Suwelack B, Banas B, Budde K, Einecke G, Hauser I, Heinemann FM, Kauke T, Kelsch R, Koch M, Lachmann N, Reuter S, Seidl C, Sester U, Zecher D. Determination of unacceptable HLA antigen mismatches in kidney transplant recipients. HLA. 2022 Jul; 100(1):3–17.

CHAPTER 2
Carrying out the transplant

CHAPTER 2.1 Anaesthesiological and perioperative management

Marieke Voet[1] & Marlies Cornelissen[2]

[1] Amalia Children's Hospital, Radboud University Medical Centre, Department of Anaesthesiology, Nijmegen, The Netherlands
[2] Amalia Children's Hospital, Radboud University Medical Centre, Department of Paediatric Nephrology, Nijmegen, The Netherlands

ORCIDs:
Marieke Voet: https://orcid.org/0000-0003-3017-5410
Elisabeth Cornelissen: https://orcid.org/0000-0002-1156-5264

Introduction

Anaesthesia care not only ensures insensitivity and unawareness during surgery, but, even importantly, also involves the monitoring and support of vital organ functions. Reduced physiological reserve has significant implications for anaesthetic management. As the systemic effects of end-stage renal disease impair the function of multiple organs, a comprehensive preoperative assessment – focusing on evaluation of metabolic changes and assessment of end-organ damage – is crucial for determining perioperative risks.[1] A thorough preoperative work-up, including the optimisation of fluid status, electrolyte balance, lung function and cardiovascular status, can help reduce perioperative complications. Table 1 outlines the pathophysiological changes in each organ system and the recommended preoperative tests and preparations.

Table 1 Preoperative assessment in pediatric kidney transplantation: tests and considerations

Organ system	Encountered problems	Preoperative Tests	Preoperative preparation
Pulmonary function	Pulmonary edema Lung fibrosis Obstructive and/or restrictive lung function	Lung function tests	Perioperative bronchodilator therapy when indicated
Cardiac function	Hypertension Left ventricular hypertrophy, diastolic dysfunction, structural lesions	Blood pressure Cardiac ultrasound	Anti-hypertensive medication usually stopped on day before surgery, to prevent intra-operative hypotension
Neurologic Development	Cognitive impairment Uremic neurotoxicity		
Electrolytes	Hyperphosphatemia Hypocalcemia Hypomagnesemia Hyperkalemia Acidemia	Serum electrolyte analysis Blood gas analysis	Diet, Cation exchangers, Phosphate binders, Calcium, Magnesium supplements; all stopped on day of surgery Sodium bicarbonate; continued until surgery

Table 1. *(continued)*

Organ system	Encountered problems	Preoperative Tests	Preoperative preparation
Fluids and feeding	Residual diuresis or anuria Fluid restriction Malnutrition, feeding difficulties	Glucose (in)tolerance	Gastric tube for feeding and medication Fluid restriction Glucose containing fluids when at risk for hypoglycemia
General evaluation	Urologic impairment, risk of postrenal failure Vascular patency Immunologic status	Full urology assessment Imaging of abdominal organs and vasculature Serology for past infections	Voiding training Immunization
Hormones	Reduced erythropoietin Hyperparathyroidism Renal osteodystrophy; brittle teeth and bones Growth hormone deficiency	Anemia, full blood count Serum calcium and phosphate	Erythropoietin therapy Growth hormone therapy in growth retardation Dental care
Nephrological disease	Nephrotic Syndrome Glomerulonephritis Renal agenesis or dysplasia	Fluid and protein status Hypotension Hypertension	Nephrectomy prior to transplantation in active nephrotic syndrome Adequate fluid status and electrolyte control
Urologic disease	Obstructive uropathies	Anuria in utero: lung hypoplasia Congenital cardiac disease	Urologic work up Cardiologic work up

Anaesthesia during Kidney Transplantation

Kidney transplantation requires general anaesthesia with endotracheal intubation and controlled mechanical ventilation. It is important to recognise that children with chronic kidney disease (CKD) often have impaired growth and may have brittle bones and teeth. Tube and catheter sizes should be adjusted accordingly. In patients with pre-existing pulmonary restrictions, mechanical ventilation should be tailored according to lung-protective strategies.[2]

Monitoring and supporting circulation is essential to ensure optimal (re)perfusion of the donor kidney and to minimise ischaemia-reperfusion injury. Significant haemodynamic changes are expected, especially in young children receiving a relatively large (adult) donor kidney.[3] In cases of post-mortem donation and prolonged cold ischaemia times, haemodynamic instability may be pronounced due to the vasodilatory effects of cytokines released into the circulation after reperfusion.[4]

A relatively high blood pressure is recommended after reperfusion, as the ischaemic period may lead to cellular oedema and a compromised vasculature in the donor kidney.[5] Due to the vasodilatory effects of anaesthetics and cytokines, temporary use of vasopressors, such as norepinephrine, may be necessary. However, it is important to ensure optimal fluid status when administering vasopressors. To avoid both fluid overload and hypovolemia, fluid administration should be guided by a monitor capable of detecting changes in flow or stroke volume following fluid loading. Isotonic, balanced crystalloid fluids are recommended as the fluid of first choice.[4, 6]

In patients with systolic dysfunction, inotropes may be required to support cardiac output. However, diastolic dysfunction is more common and requires careful monitoring to prevent fluid overload.[7] Therefore, advanced haemodynamic monitoring is recommended in children who are expected to experience haemodynamic instability during transplantation. This monitoring should be able to track changes in blood flow, as well as the effects of fluid administration, vasopressors, and inotropes on flow or stroke volume.[1] Appendix 1 provides an algorithm that summarises the above recommendations.

Table 2 summarises the potential organ impairments that may arise during anaesthesia and provides recommendations for monitoring these complications.

Table 2 Anaesthesia care during paediatric kidney transplantation: checklist of considerations and advise (continues on the next page)

	Considerations & Advice	Monitoring
Airway	Adjust tube and catheter sizes to patient's size, not to age	
Breathing	Lung protective ventilation (TV 6–8 ml/kg, PEEP 5–10 cm H_2O); A reduced oxygen reserve might be present	Airway pressures Pulse oximetry Capnometry
Circulation	Reduced vascular compliance Left ventricle hypertrophy Diastolic dysfunction Anesthesia induced hypotension Set target arterial blood pressure, add vasopressors if fluid loading is insufficient	ECG (Intra-arterial) blood pressure Cardiac output and/or fluid responsiveness
Anesthesia & Analgesia	No clear advantages of one anesthetic over another; choose best cardiovascular profile No succinylcholine in hyperkalemia Preference for hepatic clearance or inactive metabolites if delayed graft function is anticipated	Neuromuscular monitoring

Table 2. *(continued)*

	Considerations & Advice	**Monitoring**
Electrolytes	Consider sodium bicarbonate solution as part of fluid therapy Treat hyperkalemia with calcium gluconate and/or glucose/insulin Prevent hyponatremia and brisk osmolality shifts	Regular serum electrolyte and blood gas analysis
Fluids	Reduce basic fluids in patient with anuria Beware of hypoglycemia when patient is on continuous feeding Fluid loading before graft reperfusion with isotonic solutions and mannitol Withhold fluid loading when signs of fluid overload appear: increased central venous pressure or pulmonary edema Compensate fluid losses; beware of poly-uric phase in first hours after transplantation	Regular glucose control Fluid responsiveness Central venous pressure Urine output after reperfusion
Blood	Anemia; lower threshold to transfusion	Full blood count
Medication	Antibiotic prophylaxis; dose adjusted to body surface area Immune suppressive medication Thrombosis prophylaxis when indicated No rationale for diuretics or dopamine Mannitol; dose adjusted to body surface area	

Postoperative care

Close monitoring of respiratory function, blood pressure, diuresis, electrolytes, fluid balance, and pain management is essential in the postoperative period. The postoperative care unit should be equipped with the appropriate facilities and expertise for this level of care, often being an intensive care unit (ICU).

The decision to keep the child intubated and on mechanical ventilation depends on the child's age and the haemodynamic and metabolic changes that occur during anaesthesia and surgery. Young children receiving a relatively large donor kidney often remain sedated and on ventilatory support in the ICU until their haemodynamic and metabolic status has stabilised. If possible, the aim is to withdraw sedation and ventilatory support within 24 hours. This approach minimises the risk of circulatory compromise due to positive pressure ventilation and the vasodilatory effects of sedatives.

Continuous monitoring:

- Administration of fluids and vasopressors guided by an advanced haemodynamic monitor, together with continuous assessment of diuresis.
- Frequent checks of blood gas analysis, glucose and electrolytes.

Additional monitoring may be required if diuresis decreases despite optimal haemodynamic support. For example, Doppler ultrasound may be used to assess vascular patency or to rule out post-renal obstruction.

Postoperative pain management:

Pain can be managed with paracetamol and opioids. Non-steroidal drugs are not recommended as they compromise renal capillary blood flow. Opioids are usually given intravenously, either continuously or on demand, depending on the child's age and cooperation. In cases of delayed graft function, reduced opioid clearance may increase the risk of apnoea. Therefore, careful monitoring of consciousness and respiration is recommended in all children receiving intravenous opioids. Epidural anaesthesia is less commonly used for postoperative pain management because of its potential effects on blood pressure and the increased risk of bleeding in patients with kidney failure.

References

1 Voet M, Cornelissen EAM, van der Jagt MFP, Lemson J, Malagon I. Perioperative anesthesia care for the pediatric patient undergoing a kidney transplantation: An educational review. Paediatric anaesthesia. 2021;31(11):1150–60.
2 Kneyber MC. Intraoperative mechanical ventilation for the pediatric patient. Best Pract Res Clin Anaesthesiol. 2015;29(3):371–9.
3 Voet M, Nusmeier A, Lerou J, Luijten J, Cornelissen M, Lemson J. Cardiac output-guided hemodynamic therapy for adult living donor kidney transplantation in children under 20 kg: A pilot study. Paediatric anaesthesia. 2019;29(9):950–8.
4 Weiss SL, Peters MJ, Alhazzani W, Agus MSD, Flori HR, Inwald DP, et al. Surviving sepsis campaign international guidelines for the management of septic shock and sepsis-associated organ dysfunction in children. Intensive Care Med. 2020;46(Suppl 1):10–67.
5 Gingell-Littlejohn M, Koh H, Aitken E, Shiels PG, Geddes C, Kingsmore D, Clancy MJ. Below-target postoperative arterial blood pressure but not central venous pressure is associated with delayed graft function. Transplant Proc. 2013;45(1):46–50.
6 Collins MG, Fahim MA, Pascoe EM, Hawley CM, Johnson DW, Varghese J, et al. Balanced crystalloid solution versus saline in deceased donor kidney transplantation (BEST-Fluids): a pragmatic, double-blind, randomised, controlled trial. Lancet. 2023;402(10396):105–17.
7 Lindblad YT, Axelsson J, Balzano R, Vavilis G, Chromek M, Celsi G, Barany P. Left ventricular diastolic dysfunction by tissue Doppler echocardiography in pediatric chronic kidney disease. Pediatr Nephrol. 2013;28(10):2003–13.

Appendix 1: Hemodynamic monitoring and support algorithm

Basic hemodynamic management

- administer crystalloid solution* according to body weight to cover basic fluid requirements
- give $NaHCO_3$ 1.4% solution: 5 mL kg^{-1} in case of metabolic acidosis, especially in patients on $NaHCO_3$ supplements before transplantation
- administer mannitol 10%: 500 mL 1.73 m^{-2}, 20 minutes before reperfusion of donor kidney
- transfuse erythrocytes to maintain hemoglobin > 8 g dL^{-1}

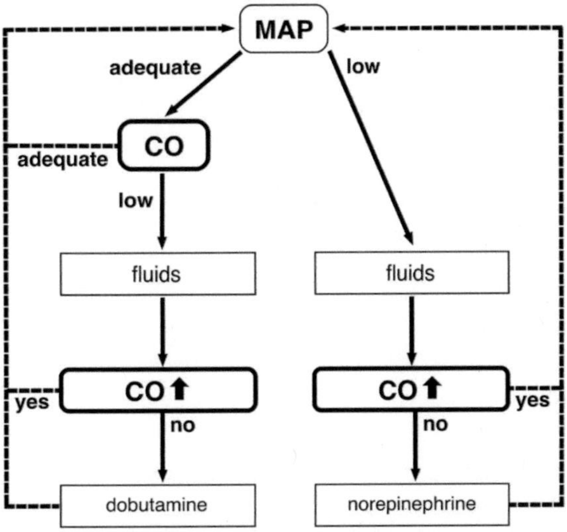

Cardiac output strategy

- target values
  - before reperfusion: CI > 3.0 L min^{-1} m^{-2}
  - after reperfusion : CI > 3.5 L min^{-1} m^{-2}
- administer boluses of 10 mL kg^{-1} crystalloid solution* when CI is too low; stop when patient is no fluid responder
- start dobutamine at 2 mcg kg^{-1} min^{-1} if target CI is not met after fluid loading
- adjust dobutamine dosing if target CI is not achieved but reduce dose when patient becomes tachycardic

Blood pressure strategy

- target values
  - before reperfusion: MAP > 70% of base line value
  - after reperfusion : MAP = 65 - 100 mmHg depending on donor blood pressure and visual judgment of renal perfusion during surgery
- administer boluses of 10 mL kg^{-1} crystalloid solution* when MAP is too low; stop if patient is no fluid responder
- start norepinephrine infusion at 0.05 mcg kg^{-1} min^{-1} when MAP is too low and fluid loading is ineffective
- adjust norepinephrine dosing to reach target MAP

CHAPTER 2.2 Surgical-operative procedure in paediatric kidney transplantation

Uta Herden[1] & Martina Koch[2]

[1] Department of Visceral Transplantation, University Medical Centre Hamburg-Eppendorf, Hamburg, Germany
[2] Department of General, Visceral, and Transplantation Surgery, Johannes Gutenberg University Medical Centre Mainz, Mainz, Germany

ORCIDs:
Uta Herden: https://orcid.org/0000-0003-2921-7943
Martina Koch: https://orcid.org/0000-0001-8151-422X

Selection of graft type

The standard organ in paediatric kidney transplantation is a single kidney graft from a living or deceased adult donor. Not only is there a shortage of age- and size-matched paediatric donors in paediatric kidney transplantation. Data show an increased risk of technical complications and early graft loss in children using organs from small (≤ 20 kg body weight) and especially very small (≤ 10 kg body weight) paediatric donors. However, after surviving the critical initial period, paediatric kidney grafts transplanted into children show a very good growth and superior long-term function compared to adult grafts. It is possible to transplant both kidneys en-bloc from paediatric donors (especially in small donors < 12–15 kg body weight). However, in contrast to adult recipients, there is no clear advantage over single kidney transplantation because of the negative impact on the risk of surgical complications and the small increase in nephron mass in paediatric recipients.

Graft placement

Routinely, the kidney graft is placed heterotopically into the iliac fossa. This allows good placement of the transplant, access to the large vessels and proximity to the urinary bladder. The right side is preferred, especially in smaller children, because of its proximity to the vena cava. In very small children and the resulting size mismatch, intraabdominal placement of the kidney protects the graft from increased pressure and reduced graft perfusion. Although there is no general age or weight limit for paediatric kidney transplantation, most centres prefer a minimum weight of 8–10 kg for the recipient child.

Native nephrectomy

Native kidneys can usually be left in place. Indications for native nephrectomy in children are based on the underlying diagnosis, namely recurrent urinary tract infection, malignant predisposition, resistant hypertension, persistent nephrotic syndrome or polyuria. The decision regarding the timing of surgery (pre-transplant vs. peri-transplant vs. post-transplant), the number of kidneys removed (one vs. both) and the order of removal (same procedure vs. staged procedure) should be discussed individually. The decision should take into account preservation of residual kidney function and residual pretransplant diuresis, avoiding opening of the peritoneal cavity and preserving peritoneal dialysis capability, avoiding unnecessary multiple operations and anaesthesia, creating space for the kidney transplant and removing the focus of infection.

Surgical technique

Access is made in the right (left) lower to mid-abdomen through a J-shaped incision ("hockey stick"). The peritoneum is shifted medially and upwards, and the transplant cavity is prepared extraperitoneally. The distal aorta and vena cava or the iliac vascular axis are dissected, protecting the surrounding lymphatic vascular plexus. First, the venous anastomosis is made between the renal vein and the vena cava as an end-to-side anastomosis. The arterial anastomosis is then made between the renal artery and the aorta in small children or with the common iliac vessels in older recipients. In the case of multiple kidney arteries, each artery must be anastomosed to avoid poor perfusion and function. In particular, the polar arteries of the lower pole are important because they provide blood flow to the ureter. These arteries can be reconstructed and reperfused sequentially after reperfusion to avoid long warm ischaemic times. All vascular anastomoses are made with fine (6-0 or 7-0), monofilament, absorbable sutures to allow for growth. At least the transplant ureter is directly connected to the bladder by a ureterocystostomy. Technique and pitfalls are described more in detail in chapter 2.3 [1–7].

Management of complications

The likelihood of complications after paediatric kidney transplantation depends on patient and donor factors such as age and size, immunosuppression, and surgical technique. In paediatric transplantation, the size and weight of the recipient and donor have an important impact on surgical complications. Complications rates are particularly high in small recipients [8]. Perioperative complications requiring revision are reported to occur in 15% of patients at a large German transplant centre [9]. Typical complications include:

Injury to other organs and structures

As with all surgery, nerves, blood vessels, or organs in the surgical area may be injured. Because kidney transplantation is usually performed retroperitoneally, injuries to the bowel or other viscera are rare. In small children, the kidney may be placed intra-abdominally. This increases the risk of injury to abdominal organs, adhesions or other intestinal problems. In rare cases, boys may have damage to the spermatic cord. Typically, injury to the lymphatic vessels can occur during dissection of the pelvic arteries. This can lead to lymphocele, some of which may need to be drained. The rate of lymphocele requiring drainage has been reported to be 4–10% in larger studies [10]. In small children, the vascular anastomoses are usually sutured to the vena cava and aorta, so injury to the great vessels is a major concern.

Vascular disorders

Vascular anastomoses can be challenging, especially in small children. As adult kidneys are usually transplanted into children, the donor renal artery may be larger in diameter than the child's aorta. In addition, children often have low blood pressure, which can present an anaesthetic and surgical challenge in perfusing the graft. Graft thrombosis is, therefore, the most feared complication. Vascular complications are higher than in adult kidney transplantation and have been reported in up to 10% of paediatric recipients [8, 10]. Vascular complications need to be rapidly identified by duplex sonography and clinic examination if the graft is to be salvaged [11].

Bleeding

Large blood vessels are connected during kidney transplantation. In addition, the kidney is an organ with a strong blood supply, which means that bleeding may occur during and after surgery, requiring replacement of blood loss with blood transfusions/blood products.

The need for plasmapheresis or immunoadsorption, for example in the case of ABO incompatible transplantation or high immunological risk, can also increase the risk of bleeding [12]. Fortunately, these conditions are very rare in children. Intra- and postoperative bleeding complications are reported in less than 5% of paediatric patients [10].

Complications of the ureter-bladder anastomosis

Several children require transplantation because of congenital anomalies of the kidney and urinary tract (CAKUT). In these patients, the ureter-bladder anastomosis can be challenging [13] (see chapter 2.3). Although urethral leaks are rare, they usually require surgical intervention. This is also true for early ureteral/anastomotic stenosis, such as those caused by torsion of the ureter.

The incidence of ureteral complications has been reported to be 5–9% in adults in a review and was lower with the most common Lich-Gregoir extravesical technique than with an intravesical technique, and lower with a double J (DJ) stent than without [14, 15]. Data in children show comparable results [10], but ureteral complications are significantly higher in recipients with pre-existing bladder pathology [13]. If a DJ stent has been used, it should not be left behind but removed by cystoscopy. Mono-J ureteral stents are more commonly used in small children as they can be removed without this procedure.

Wound healing problems

In contrast to adult recipients, wound healing problems in children are very rare (<2%) [10]. In small children, abdominal wall closure sometimes requires the interposition of a resorbable (Vicryl-)mesh. However, hernias in children are fortunately rare.

Risk of infection from blood products and the donor organ

As with blood transfusions, the risk of disease transmission from the donor organ cannot be completely excluded. In individual cases, fatal diseases (e.g., rabies, melanoma) have been transmitted through organ donation.

Summary

Vascular complications are more common in paediatric kidney transplantation than in adults. Duplex sonography and careful clinical assessment (e.g., urine output, pain, haematuria) are important to detect vascular problems as early as possible. Children with CAKUT are at higher risk of urological complications and require multidisciplinary management.

References

1 Crawford B, Kizilbash S, Bhatia VP, Kulsum-Mecci N, Cannon S, Bartosh SM. Native nephrectomy in advanced pediatric kidney disease: indications, timing, and surgical approaches. Pediatr Nephrol. 2024;39(4): 1041–1052.
2 Etesami K, Hogen R, Lestz R. Pediatric kidney transplantation, a technical update. Curr Opin Organ Transplant. 2021;26(4): 356–359.
3 Mo H, Ko H, Chung CTY, Kim HK, Han A, Min S, Ha J. Single versus en bloc kidney transplant from donors less than or equal to 15 kg to pediatric recipients. Pediatr Transplant. 2021;25(2): e13719.
4 Pape L, Hoppe J, Becker T, Ehrich JH, Neipp M, Ahlenstiel T, Offner G. Superior long-term graft function and better growth of grafts in children receiving kidneys from paediatric compared with adult donors. Nephrol Dial Transplant. 2006;21(9): 2596–2600.
5 Sampaio MS, Lum EL, Homkrailas P, Gritsch HA, Bunnapradist S. Outcomes of small pediatric donor kidney transplants according to donor weight. Transpl Int. 2021;34(11): 2403–2412.
6 Schild R, Carvajal Abreu K, Buscher A, Kanzelmeyer N, Lezius S, Krupka K, Weitz M, Prytula A, Printza N, Berta L, Saygili SK, Sellier-Leclerc AL, Sparta G, Marks SD, Kemper MJ, Konig S, Topaloglu R, Muller D, Klaus G, Weber S, Oh J, Herden U, Carraro A, Dello Strologo L, Ariceta G, Hoyer P, Tonshoff B, Pape L. Favorable Outcome After Single-kidney Transplantation From Small Donors in Children: A Match-controlled CERTAIN Registry Study. Transplantation. 2024;108(8): 1793–1801.
7 Yaffe HC, Friedmann P, Kayler LK. Very small pediatric donor kidney transplantation in pediatric recipients. Pediatr Transplant. 2017;21(5).

8 Prudhomme T, Mesnard B, Abbo O, Banuelos B, Territo A, Transplantation EAUYAUgoK, the EAUYAUgoPU. Postoperative surgical complications after pediatric kidney transplantation in low weight recipients (< 15 kg): a systematic review. Curr Opin Organ Transplant. 2023;28(4): 297–308.
9 Beetz O, Weigle CA, Nogly R, Klempnauer J, Pape L, Richter N, Vondran FWR. Surgical complications in pediatric kidney transplantation-Incidence, risk factors, and effects on graft survival: A retrospective single-center study. Pediatr Transplant. 2021;25(2): e13871.
10 Kim JK, Lorenzo AJ, Farhat WA, Chua ME, Ming JM, Koyle MA. Assessment of perioperative surgical complications in pediatric kidney transplantation: A comparison of pre-emptive and post-dialysis recipients. Clin Transplant. 2018;32(12): e13421.
11 Gander R, Asensio M, Royo GF, Molino JA, Garcia L, Madrid A, Ariceta G, Lopez M. Vascular thrombosis in pediatric kidney transplantation: Graft survival is possible with adequate management. J Pediatr Urol. 2018;14(3): 222–230.
12 Koch M, Kantas A, Ramcke K, Drabik AI, Nashan B. Surgical complications after kidney transplantation: different impacts of immunosuppression, graft function, patient variables, and surgical performance. Clin Transplant. 2015;29(3): 252–260.
13 Morrison CD, Shannon R, Rosoklija I, Nettey OS, Superina R, Cheng EY, Gong EM. Ureteral Complications of Pediatric Renal Transplantation. J Urol. 2019;201(4): 810–814.
14 Mangus RS, Haag BW. Stented versus nonstented extravesical ureteroneocystostomy in renal transplantation: a metaanalysis. Am J Transplant. 2004;4(11): 1889–1896.
15 Slagt IK, Klop KW, Ijzermans JN, Terkivatan T. Intravesical versus extravesical ureteroneocystostomy in kidney transplantation: a systematic review and meta-analysis. Transplantation. 2012;94(12): 1179–1184.

CHAPTER 2.3 Urological surgical procedure and management of complications

Susanne Deininger[1, 2] & Steffen Rausch[1]

[1] Department of Urology and Andrology, Salzburg University Hospital, Paracelsus Medical University, Salzburg, Austria
[2] Department of Urology, University Hospital Tübingen, Eberhard Karls University, Tübingen, Germany.

ORCIDs:
Susanne Deininger: https://orcid.org/0000-0003-3541-6973
Steffen Rausch: https://orcid.org/0000-0002-6398-8701

1 Urological evaluation of kidney transplant recipients and management of underlying urinary tract anomalies

Congenital kidney anomalies account for 42% of end-stage kidney disease in paediatric patients, making them the leading cause [1]. Therefore, a careful preoperative workup of the anatomical and physiological conditions of the urinary tract is essential. A detailed patient history, including a voiding diary if diuresis is still present, physical examination, and ultrasound are basic investigations. If necessary, these may be followed by urodynamics, voiding cystourethrogram, or cystoscopy [2]. Successful kidney transplantation (KTx) has been reported in cases of bladder dysfunction [3]. Secondary small-capacity bladders may regain volume after transplantation and with increased urine output [4].

KTx in cases of neurogenic bladder can be successful with the use of anticholinergics, and intermittent sterile catheterisation [2]. In cases of very small bladder volume, bladder augmentation can be performed using native dilated ureters or bowel segments. In addition, KTx may be considered in the presence of an ileal conduit or Mitrofanoff stoma. Timing is critical: bladder augmentation should be performed at least 3 months before transplantation or after transplantation (while the patient is on ongoing immunosuppression) [4].

2 Urological surgical technique

In some cases, it may be necessary to remove the native kidneys of paediatric patients prior to KTx (massive proteinuria, polyuria, refractory hypertension, recurrent urinary tract infection (UTI), malignancy or space-limiting cystic kidney disease [2]). Nephrectomy can be performed either simultaneously with the kidney transplantation or in a staged approach, with the subsequent lack of bladder filling potentially reducing bladder volume. For KTx itself, the organ is usually placed intraperitoneally in children under 10 kg. Depending on the source, kidney transplantation can be performed extraperitoneally in patients weighing between 8 and 15 kg [2].

After graft placement, the ureteroneocystostomy (UCN) is performed. Several points are important here: while the perfusion of the distal ureter should not be compromised, unobstructed urine flow from the ureter to the bladder is also crucial, as is the formation of an anti-reflux mechanism. The use of anti-reflux techniques in ureteroneocystostomy (UNC) was first described by V. Politano in the 1950s. Since then, this technique has been modified several times, and other techniques have been developed. The Politano-Leadbetter (PL) technique involves the following steps: an anterior cystostomy is performed to create an intravesical submucosal tunnel (2–3 cm). The new ureter is then introduced through this tunnel and sutured in place [5, 6]. In contrast, the Lich-Gregoir (LG) technique uses an extravesical approach. A 4 cm incision is made in the bladder wall, the ureter is sutured to the bladder mucosa, and the muscularis layer is then closed over the ureter [6]. In contrast, the Woodruff technique also involves an extravesical bladder incision, but unlike the Lich-Gregoir technique, the muscularis is not closed after the spatulated ureter is implanted into the bladder mucosa [7]. Several studies and meta-analyses have shown that the LG technique results in significantly lower rates of urological complications such as urinary leakage, uretero-vesical junction obstruction, and haematuria compared to the PL technique in adult patients [6, 8].

For paediatric patients, the optimal technique remains unclear. Anti-reflux techniques may increase the risk of UVJO, and Ranchin et al. demonstrated a VUR incidence of up to 58% in paediatric patients despite the use of anti-reflux techniques [9]. Furthermore, VUR remains asymptomatic in most organ recipients. The perioperative placement of a double-J ureteral stent is controversial in paediatric KTx: while the risk of urological complications is reduced [10], the risk of BK polyoma viremia and UTIs seems to be increased [11].

3 Management of urological complications in kidney transplant recipients

Ureteral stricture

Ureteral strictures occur in about 8% of children after KT. It usually manifests within the first 100 days after KTx and may be caused by ureteral ischaemia due to loss of distal perfusion from graft explantation, pre-existing anatomical anomalies (i.e. posterior urethral valves [12]), haematoma, lymphocele, stones, tumours, or scarring [13]. Initial treatment typically involves placement of a ureteral stent or nephrostomy, followed by further definitive operative treatment (endoscopic or open/laparoscopic ureteral reimplantation, or Psoas- or Boari hitch technique). Endoscopic options include laser or cold incision and/or balloon dilation followed by double-J stent placement.

Christman et al. (2012) treated 17 paediatric patients with primary obstructive megaureter using retrograde balloon dilatation (for strictures < 2 cm) or laser incision combined with balloon dilatation (for strictures > 2 cm), achieving resolution of obstruction in all cases. These techniques can also be effective in more proximal strictures [14–17]. If the retrograde approach is difficult, percutaneous access with dilatation can also be successful in such cases: Bachtel et al. reported a 75% success rate using antegrade balloon or Amplatz sequential dilatation for early postoperative strictures (< 6 months post-transplant) in paediatric patients. However, this technique was never successful in strictures older than one year [12].

Vesicoureteral reflux

The incidence of vesicoureteral reflux (VUR) after kidney transplantation varies from 10.5% to 86% depending on the implantation technique, with deceased donor organs having a higher risk than living donor organs [18, 19]. However, some studies suggest that VUR does not appear to adversely affect bacteriuria, renal function, or graft survival [20]. Nevertheless, VUR can cause complications that may initially go unnoticed: dimercaptosuccinic acid (DMSA) scans of paediatric KTx with VUR and recurrent UTI revealed that 69% had renal scarring [21]. Active treatment may be required in such cases. Similar to VUR in the native kidney, antibiotic prophylaxis may reduce the frequency of infections in cases of recurrent UTIs [22]. Injecting a bulking agent such as dextranomer/hyaluronic acid copolymer (Dx/HA) beneath the ureteral orifice or in the ureteral tunnel can effectively treat urinary reflux in certain cases. In paediatric patients, the injection has been well studied: a single injection is usually sufficient, with only 3% experiencing febrile urinary tract infections over time [23]. The use of Dx/HA has also been studied in KTx patients with VUR. While Pichler et al. [24] observed a significant reduction in UTI frequency in adult kidney transplant recipients with VUR following Dx/HA injection, Wu et al. reported a success rate of only 22% for Dx/HA in paediatric patients with VUR post-transplant [22]. In cases of renal dysfunction, recurrent infection and failed endoscopic therapy, anti-reflux techniques such as ureteral reimplantation may be required.

Urolithiasis

Following KTx, paediatric patients may develop urinary stones: according to Khositseth et al., 5% of paediatric KTx patients developed urinary stones within the first 19 ± 22 months post-transplant [25]. The most common stone compositions were calcium phosphate and calcium oxalate, mixed calcium phosphate and oxalate, and struvite. Risk factors for stone formation in KTx patients include certain suture techniques, recurrent UTIs, urinary obstruction [25], and comorbidities associated with chronic kidney disease, such as hyperparathyroidism, hypercalciuria, hypocitraturia, or hypophosphatemia [26, 27]. Due to renal denervation during explantation, stone passage may sometimes be asymptomatic. For definitive stone management, endoscopic therapy with antegrade or retrograde flexible ureteroscopy appears to be a safe and successful approach [28, 29]. Percutaneous nephrolithotomy (PCNL) or mini-PCNL can be easily carried out for larger calculi due to the location of the kidney in the iliac fossa In the paediatric cohort studied by Khositseth et al. [25], spontaneous stone passage occurred in only 20% of the patients. The remaining patients required surgical intervention, with 55% undergoing retrograde endoscopic procedures, and the remainder treated by open or laparoscopic surgery. Boissier et al. (2023) reported in a meta-analysis that in adult KTx patients, the stone-free rates (SFR) at 3 months were 96% with open surgery, 95% with antegrade ureteroscopy, 86% with percutaneous nephrolithotomy (PNL), 81% with retrograde ureteroscopy, 75% with shock wave lithotripsy (SWL), and 62% with medical treatment.

Urinoma

Urinomas occur in less than 10% of kidney transplant patients, usually within the first 3 months after transplantation [30, 31]. All parts of the urinary tract can be affected, and management with nephrostomy or antegrade stenting is the treatment of choice for symptomatic urinomas, as the retrograde approach can be challenging. Larger fluid collections may also require percutaneous drainage under CT or ultrasound guidance may also be necessary [32]. A transurethral catheter may be placed to minimise reflux across the double-J stent [33, 34]. Surgical revision, such as ureteral reimplantation or lesion repair, is rarely required [35].

Lymphocele

Lymphocele formation after kidney transplantation is a common complication, occurring in up to 22% of cases [11], due to dissection of donor or recipient lymphatic vessels during surgery. It typically occurs within the first week after KT. Risk factors include immunosuppression with sirolimus, older age, higher BMI, number of transplantations and surgical technique [11, 36]. Most cases are asymptomatic, but some patients require intervention due to pain or graft dysfunction. Patients requiring treatment for lymphoceles are at higher risk of graft rejection or delayed function [37]. Gander et al. showed that percutaneous drainage, with or without sclerotherapy (especially with povidone-iodine), is a safe approach for symptomatic lymphoceles in paediatric patients [38]. If minimally invasive therapy fails, open or laparoscopic lymphocele fenestration is used [39].

Recurrent urinary tract infections

Urinary tract infections (UTIs) are the most common type of infection after transplantation, occurring in up to 47% of cases. The risk of UTI is particularly high in the first month post-transplant [40]. Risk factors for UTI post-KTx include female sex, race, immunosuppression (i.e. azathioprine or cyclosporin A) [41], history of acute rejection, cytomegalovirus infection, UVJO [42], re-transplantation [43], polycystic kidney disease [44], diabetes mellitus [45], VUR in the native kidneys, male sex (2–5 years of age) and female sex ($\leq$ 1 year of age) [41]. Prophylactic antibiotics are recommended for acute cases and primary recurrences, but it is also important to evaluate for potential allograft pathology. The risk of graft loss is significantly increased in all children after early UTI (< 6 months post-transplant; $P < 0.001$), but not after late UTI ($\geq$ 6 months post-transplant; $P = 0.27$) [41].

The most common pathogens in paediatric organ recipients are E. coli, Pseudomonas aeruginosa, Klebsiella, and Enterococci [46]. Candida infections are also possible, and some centres recommend prophylactic antifungal treatment during antibiotic therapy. Paediatric patients typically receive prophylactic antibiotics for the first 3–6 months after KT, including prophylaxis for Pneumocystis jirovecii, although this practice is controversial, and some studies have found that it only exacerbates resistance patterns in UTIs [46, 47].

Any underlying anatomical or functional problems should be addressed. Residual urine should be managed with intermittent sterile self-catheterisation. Behavioural measures include high oral fluid intake, hygienic practices – especially for sexually active women – and management of constipation [46].

Additional measures, such as herbal therapies (e.g., Canephron® or Angocin®, Utribro®), cranberry products, D-mannose, urinary acidification, and vaccination (e.g., Uro-Vaxom®, StroVac®), have not been specifically studied in paediatric kidney transplant patients, but can be discussed.

References

1 McEnery, P.T., et al., Renal transplantation in children. A report of the North American Pediatric Renal Transplant Cooperative Study. N Engl J Med, 1992. 326(26): p. 1727–32.
2 Gunawardena, T., et al., Surgical considerations in paediatric kidney transplantation: an update. Renal Replacement therapy 2021. 54.
3 Serrano, D.P., et al., Transplantation into the long-term defunctionalized bladder. J Urol, 1996. 156(3): p. 885–8.
4 Salvatierra, O., Jr., M. Millan, and W. Concepcion, Pediatric renal transplantation with considerations for successful outcomes. Semin Pediatr Surg, 2006. 15(3): p. 208–17.
5 Politano, V.A. and W.F. Leadbetter, An operative technique for the correction of vesicoureteral reflux. J Urol, 1958. 79(6): p. 932–41.
6 Thrasher, J.B., D.R. Temple, and E.K. Spees, Extravesical versus Leadbetter-Politano ureteroneocystostomy: a comparison of urological complications in 320 renal transplants. J Urol, 1990. 144(5): p. 1105–9.
7 Starzl, T.E., et al., A new technique of extravesical ureteroneocystostomy for renal transplantation. Transplant Proc, 1989. 21(5): p. 3856–8.
8 Alberts, V.P., et al., Ureterovesical anastomotic techniques for kidney transplantation: a systematic review and meta-analysis. Transpl Int, 2014. 27(6): p. 593–605.
9 Ranchin, B., et al., Vesicoureteral reflux after kidney transplantation in children. Nephrol Dial Transplant, 2000. 15(11): p. 1852–8.

10 Kumar, A., et al., Evaluation of the urological complications of living related renal transplantation at a single center during the last 10 years: impact of the Double-J* stent. J Urol, 2000. 164(3 Pt 1): p. 657–60.
11 Oomen, L., et al., Pearls and Pitfalls in Pediatric Kidney Transplantation After 5 Decades. Front Pediatr, 2022. 10: p. 856630.
12 Smith, K.M., et al., Risk factors and treatment success for ureteral obstruction after pediatric renal transplantation. J Urol, 2010. 183(1): p. 317–22.
13 Sandhu, C., Renal transplantation dysfunction: the role of Interventional Radiology Clinical Radiology, 2002. 57: p. 772–783.
14 Gdor, Y., et al., Success of laser endoureterotomy of ureteral strictures associated with ureteral stones is related to stone impaction. J Endourol, 2008. 22(11): p. 2507–11.
15 Lane, B.R., et al., Long-term efficacy of holmium laser endoureterotomy for benign ureteral strictures. Urology, 2006. 67(5): p. 894–7.
16 Tran, H., et al., Evaluation of risk factors and treatment options in patients with ureteral stricture disease at a single institution. Can Urol Assoc J, 2015. 9(11–12): p. E921–4.
17 Rabenalt, R., et al., Retrograde balloon dilation >10 weeks after renal transplantation for transplant ureter stenosis – our experience and review of the literature. Arab J Urol, 2011. 9(2): p. 93–9.
18 Molenaar, N.M., et al., Vesicoureteral Reflux in Kidney Transplantation. Prog Transplant, 2017. 27(2): p. 196–199.
19 Jung, G.O., et al., Clinical significance of posttransplantation vesicoureteral reflux during short-term period after kidney transplantation. Transplant Proc, 2008. 40(7): p. 2339–41.
20 Favi, E., et al., Long-term clinical impact of vesicoureteral reflux in kidney transplantation. Transplant Proc, 2009. 41(4): p. 1218–20.
21 Coulthard, M.G. and M.J. Keir, Reflux nephropathy in kidney transplants, demonstrated by dimercaptosuccinic acid scanning. Transplantation, 2006. 82(2): p. 205–10.
22 Wu, H.Y., W. Concepcion, and P.C. Grimm, When does vesicoureteral reflux in pediatric kidney transplant patients need treatment? Pediatr Transplant, 2018. 22(8): p. e13299.
23 Stenberg, A. and G. Lackgren, Treatment of vesicoureteral reflux in children using stabilized non-animal hyaluronic acid/dextranomer gel (NASHA/DX): a long-term observational study. J Pediatr Urol, 2007. 3(2): p. 80–5.

24 Pichler, R., et al., Endoscopic application of dextranomer/hyaluronic acid copolymer in the treatment of vesico-ureteric reflux after renal transplantation. BJU Int, 2011. 107(12): p. 1967–72.

25 Khositseth, S., et al., Urolithiasis after kidney transplantation in pediatric recipients: a single center report. Transplantation, 2004. 78(9): p. 1319–23.

26 Mamarelis, G., et al., Lithiasis of the renal allograft, a rare urological complication following renal transplantation: a single-center experience of 2,045 renal transplantations. Transplant Proc, 2014. 46(9): p. 3203–5.

27 Harper, J.M., et al., Risk factors for calculus formation in patients with renal transplants. Br J Urol, 1994. 74(2): p. 147–50.

28 Hyams, E., et al., Ureteroscopy for transplant lithiasis. J Endourol, 2012. 26(7): p. 819–22.

29 Swearingen, R., W.W. Roberts, and J.S. Wolf, Jr., Ureteroscopy for nephrolithiasis in transplanted kidneys. Can J Urol, 2015. 22(2): p. 7727–31.

30 Isa, W.A., et al., [Urologic complications in 237 recipients of cadaveric kidney transplantation]. Actas Urol Esp, 1991. 15(4): p. 351–6.

31 Buresley, S., et al., Postrenal transplantation urologic complications. Transplant Proc, 2008. 40(7): p. 2345–6.

32 Titton, R.L., et al., Urine leaks and urinomas: diagnosis and imaging-guided intervention. Radiographics, 2003. 23(5): p. 1133–47.

33 Streeter, E.H., et al., The urological complications of renal transplantation: a series of 1535 patients. BJU Int, 2002. 90(7): p. 627–34.

34 Shoskes, D.A., et al., Urological complications in 1,000 consecutive renal transplant recipients. J Urol, 1995. 153(1): p. 18–21.

35 Shokeir, A.A., et al., Salvage of difficult transplant urinary fistulae by ileal substitution of the ureter. Scand J Urol Nephrol, 1993. 27(4): p. 537–40.

36 Ranghino, A., et al., Lymphatic disorders after renal transplantation: new insights for an old complication. Clin Kidney J, 2015. 8(5): p. 615–22.

37 Bzoma, B., et al., Treatment of the Lymphocele After Kidney Transplantation: A Single-center Experience. Transplant Proc, 2016. 48(5): p. 1637–40.

38 Gander, R., et al., Treatment of Post-transplant Lymphocele in Children. Urology, 2017. 103: p. 218–223.

39 Iwan-Zietek, I., et al., Minimally invasive methods for the treatment of lymphocele after kidney transplantation. Transplant Proc, 2009. 41(8): p. 3073–6.

40 Ranganathan, M., et al., Infective complications associated with ureteral stents in renal transplant recipients. Transplant Proc, 2009. 41(1): p. 162–4.
41 Dharnidharka, V.R., L.Y. Agodoa, and K.C. Abbott, Effects of urinary tract infection on outcomes after renal transplantation in children. Clin J Am Soc Nephrol, 2007. 2(1): p. 100–6.
42 Alangaden, G.J., et al., Infectious complications after kidney transplantation: current epidemiology and associated risk factors. Clin Transplant, 2006. 20(4): p. 401–9.
43 Golebiewska, J., et al., Urinary tract infections in renal transplant recipients. Transplant Proc, 2011. 43(8): p. 2985–90.
44 Illesy, L., et al., Autosomal Dominant Polycystic Kidney Disease Transplant Recipients After Kidney Transplantation: A Single-center Experience. Transplant Proc, 2017. 49(7): p. 1522–1525.
45 Almond, P.S., et al., Risk factors for chronic rejection in renal allograft recipients. Transplantation, 1993. 55(4): p. 752–6; discussion 756–7.
46 John, U. and M.J. Kemper, Urinary tract infections in children after renal transplantation. Pediatr Nephrol, 2009. 24(6): p. 1129–36.
47 Green, H., et al., Antibiotic prophylaxis for urinary tract infections in renal transplant recipients: a systematic review and meta-analysis. Transpl Infect Dis, 2011. 13(5): p. 441–7.

CHAPTER 3 Immediate postoperative monitoring

CHAPTER 3.1 Perioperative volume and blood pressure management and concomitant medications

Burkhard Tönshoff & Jens H. Westhoff

Heidelberg University, Medical Faculty Heidelberg, Department of Paediatrics I, University Children's Hospital, Heidelberg, Germany

ORCIDs:
Burkhard Tönshoff: https://orcid.org/0000-0002-6598-6910
Jens H. Westhoff: https://orcid.org/0000-0002-9837-9383

1 Perioperative volume and blood pressure management

The difference in size between an adult kidney and a child's body must be taken into account after surgery. This is particularly true in young children. After transplantation of an adult donor kidney, the intravascular volume of a paediatric recipient can increase by up to 20%, meaning that the circulating blood volume must be replenished by administering infusion solutions. A paediatric haemodialysis catheter, or a central venous line in older children, is usually placed preoperatively into the internal jugular vein and, less commonly, into the subclavian vein. The purpose of this is to: monitor central venous pressure; ensure rapid and safe fluid administration; enable the administration of catecholaminergic drugs; and allow for renal replacement therapy in case of delayed graft function. Young transplant recipients usually require an arterial line for invasive arterial blood pressure measurement.

During surgical preparation, balanced isotonic crystalloid solutions and 5% human albumin are used for fluid replacement. The initial target value for central venous pressure is 5–10 mmHg. During preparation of the renal vascular anastomoses, however, higher values of 10–14 mmHg are targeted by administering balanced crystalloid solutions, 5% human albumin and red blood cell concentrate, if necessary (haematocrit target: 25–30%). Please note that patients with pre-existing cardiomyopathy may require different values. To achieve a mean arterial blood pressure of 70–80 mmHg during the preparation of vascular anastomoses, catecholaminergic drugs may be required. During reperfusion of the transplanted kidney, particularly in young children, it is essential to closely monitor and maintain stable arterial blood pressure and central venous pressure. Furosemide is administered continuously in this phase of surgery. Following reperfusion, the mean arterial pressure should be maintained above 80 mmHg. The fluid requirement following reperfusion is 4–6 ml per kg of body weight per hour, and this should be adapted according to diuresis. Depending on thrombophilic risk, unfractionated heparin can be administered either before abdominal wall closure or six hours after reperfusion (see Chpater 3.2).

For recipients weighing less than 20 kg, a higher volume supply is mandatory, and the risk of cardiovascular instability following reperfusion of an adult donor kidney must be considered.

General recommendations for perioperative fluid management:

- Fluid intake = excretion plus perspiratio insensibilis (400 mL/m^2 body surface area per day).
- In case of polyuria (> 2000 mL/m^2 per day): Replacement with two/thirds balanced isotonic crystalloid solution (e.g., STEROFUNDIN ISO), one third glucose 5%, or in case of hyperglycaemia, a pure balanced isotonic solution; switch to a semi-isotonic solution after a few days.
- In case of oliguria (< 1 ml/kg per hour): Replace with a solution of 2/3 sodium chloride 0.9% and 1/3 glucose 5%.
- Replace drainage fluid with a balanced isotonic solution and 5% albumin at a ratio of 1:1.
- Body weight should be 5–10% above the "dry weight" achieved during dialysis. Note: many patients are overhydrated before transplantation.
- Target central venous pressure: 5–7 mmHg. Target systolic blood pressure: 100–140 mmHg.
- Initially, check urine output hourly and replace accordingly.
- Check body weight twice daily.
- Check serum chemistry twice daily.
- In case of primary graft dysfunction: Perform a Doppler ultrasound of the renal allograft vessels within the first hour post-transplant to rule out vascular thrombosis.
- If primary graft dysfunction persists, repeat the Doppler ultrasound of the renal allograft vessels daily.
- Maintain haemoglobin concentration above 8 g/dL. If necessary, transfuse CMV-negative blood using a leukocyte filter.

- Maintain plasma total protein concentration above 50 g/L and albumin concentration above 30 g/L.

Specific recommendations for young children under 6 years of age who have received a kidney from an adult donor (aged over 15 years):

- Children weighing less than 20 kg require a particularly high volume of fluids. During preparation, administer 10–20 ml/kg of balanced crystalloids and 5% albumin (10–20 mL/kg) per hour. Aim for a central venous pressure of 7–10 mmHg at this stage.
- During placement of the vascular anastomoses (approx. 30 min) and before opening the aortic clamp, administer crystalloid volume (see above) and, if necessary, administration of erythrocyte concentrates to achieve a target central venous pressure of > 10–14 mmHg and a target haematocrit of 25–30% (caveat: patients with pre-existing cardiomyopathy).
- In consultation with the transplant surgeon, administer heparin 10 IU/kg before clamping the aorta and anastomosing the renal artery.
- Target mean arterial blood pressure of > 80 mmHg in this phase; catecholamines are usually required to achieve this goal (give Akrinor®; in case of prolonged hypotension, give noradrenaline/suprarenin at a starting dose 0.1 µg/kg body weight per minute). Perfusors must be pre-run at the time of declamping.
- Close communication with the surgeon is required for gradual opening of the aortic clamp.
- After opening the anastomosis, there is a risk of a sharp drop in blood pressure and central venous pressure, particularly in young children, due to the redistribution of the blood volume into the transplanted adult kidney. Maintaining haemodynamics at the above levels is particularly critical in this phase (note: avoid warm ischaemia; do not tolerate drops in blood pressure). A drop in central venous pressure of up to 50% can be expected for up to 2 hours after declamping.
- Initial fluid requirements: 4–6 ml/kg per hour Sterofundin ISO, then adjusted according to diuresis. In the case of primary graft function, there will be a high fluid requirement of up to 70% of body weight.
- In the first 24 hours post-transplant, aim for a central venous pressure of 7–10 mmHg and a mean arterial blood pressure of > 80 mmHg.
- Continuation of catecholamine therapy and recording of circulatory parameters is also mandatory during transport from the operating theatre to the intensive care unit.

- After 48 hours, polyuria decreases as the adult kidney adapts to the child's circulation.

Following surgery, the patient is monitored in the Paediatric Intensive Care Unit (PICU) for at least 24 hours. Initially, there are hourly checks of central venous and blood pressure, as well as precise fluid balance facilitated by urine drainage through a suprapubic bladder catheter. Postoperative ventilation may sometimes be necessary for a few hours due to the high fluid load during surgery, particularly in young children. If the operation goes smoothly, the patient is extubated immediately afterwards.

If a child's own kidneys still have good residual diuresis, total diuresis is not a reliable indicator of successful kidney transplantation. Therefore, to better assess and continuously monitor the diuresis of the kidney transplant, it is recommended that the transplanted kidney be selectively splinted with a single-J catheter for about 1 week.

Following a kidney transplant from a deceased donor, cold ischaemic time (during which the organ is transported without blood supply and kept on ice) often leads to acute tubular damage. This can initially cause anuria, followed by "forced polyuria" and considerable water and electrolyte losses. If the transplanted kidney fails to function properly for an extended period, dialysis therapy may be required. This can be performed as peritoneal dialysis using an intraperitoneal indwelling catheter (Tenckhoff catheter), or as haemodialysis using a Shaldon catheter. This complication occurs in around 10% of patients, particularly if the ischaemia time is prolonged and the quality of the organ is poor.

2 Concomitant medications

In most centres, furosemide is administered postoperatively as a continuous intravenous infusion, depending on diuresis. Low-dose furosemide (1–3 mg/kg/day) also has a tubuloprotective effect. The dose is tapered depending on the clinical course after 1–3 days and switched to oral administration. Furosemide is discontinued in the event of anuria for more than 24 hours or polyuria. Some centres recommend the calcium channel blocker diltiazem (dose: 1 mg/kg/day intravenously or orally for the first 10 days post-transplant) for tubuloprotection.

After the anastomosis is opened, acidic valences are often released from the transplanted kidney. The resulting metabolic acidosis inhibits the kidney's immediate functional uptake. Buffering with 8.4% sodium bicarbonate is then required. Perioperative antibiotic prophylaxis with a broad-spectrum antibiotic, such as ceftriaxone, is also administered. Antifungal prophylaxis with oral nystatin is recommended for the duration of the antibiotic prophylaxis. Specific prophylaxis against cytomegalovirus (CMV) and Pneumocystis jirovecii is described in chapters 7.1 and 7.4. The recommended anticoagulation is described in chapter 3.2.

Ulcer prophylaxis is also recommended, for example in younger children with esomeprazole, at the following dosages: patients aged 1–11 years with a body weight of 10–20 kg: 10 mg/day; with a body weight of > 20 kg: 20 mg/day; patients aged 12–18 years: 20–40 mg/day or in older children with pantoprazol (20–40 mg/day). If there are no gastrointestinal symptoms, esomeprazole should be stopped two weeks post-transplant.

References

Tönshoff B, Becker JU, Pape L. Nierentransplantation, pp. 243–74. In: Nierenerkrankungen im Kindes- und Jugendalter, Dötsch J, Weber LT (Hrsg.), Springer Berlin, 2024

CHAPTER 3.2 Prophylactic antithrombotic management in kidney transplantation

Marcus Weitz & Kathrin Buder

Department of General Paediatrics and Haematology/Oncology, University Children's Hospital Tübingen

ORCIDs:
Marcus Weitz: https://orcid.org/0000-0002-1696-5646
Kathrin Buder: https://orcid.org/0000-0002-5425-0772

Background

With a reported incidence of 0–13%, arterial or venous thrombosis of kidney allografts is a major cause of allograft loss, mostly within the first week after paediatric kidney transplantation (KTx) [1–3].

Body of evidence

Antithrombotic prophylaxis with heparin (anticoagulation) or acetylsalicylic acid (ASA) (platelet aggregation inhibition) appears to be beneficial in preventing arterial and venous kidney graft thrombosis (Figure 1) [4].

The following evidence-based and pathophysiological considerations may be helpful in the decision-making process:

- The risk of thrombosis is higher in paediatric than in adult KTx [5].
- Antithrombotic prophylaxis should be considered in patients with a positive history of thromboembolic events [6, 7].
- Congenital and acquired prothrombotic risk factors due to chronic kidney disease should be considered [3, 6, 7].
- The risk of kidney transplant thrombosis is highest in the first week after KTx [8]. Therefore, it seems reasonable to initiate antithrombotic prophylaxis pre- or intraoperatively and to discontinue it within a few weeks (< 4–6 weeks) after KTx [9, 10].
- Platelet aggregation plays a crucial role in the early phase of coagulation activation [11, 12]. The administration of ASA immediately before or during

Figure 1 Results of a systematic review and meta-analysis of antithrombotic strategies to prevent allograft thrombosis in paediatric and adult kidney transplantation: heparin monoprophylaxis unless otherwise stated (*acetylsalicylic acid [ASA] monoprophylaxis, #ASA/heparin dual prophylaxis). However, the poor quality of the available data and inconsistent management protocols do not allow an unrestricted recommendation of antithrombotic prophylaxis for paediatric KTx. In addition, the uncertain evidence does not allow reliable conclusions to be drawn on several clinical issues: Choice of drug class or agent, mono- or combination therapy, dosage, timing and duration of prophylaxis, route of administration, dosing according to thrombosis risk, drug monitoring and adverse effects.

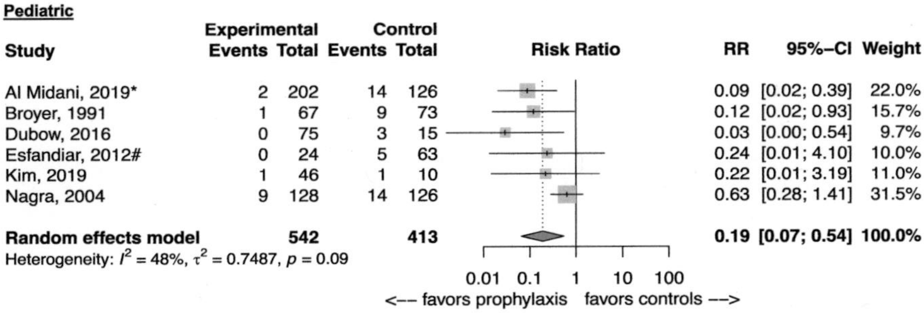

KTx is avoided due to the lack of antidotes and the limited therapeutic drug monitoring compared to heparin. Nevertheless, the perioperative bleeding risk of ASA can be classified as low to moderate [12–15].

- The most commonly used drugs are (in decreasing order):
  - Unfractionated heparin (UFH) intravenously + low molecular weight heparin (LMWH) subcutaneously
  - LMWH subcutaneously + ASA per os
  - UFH intravenously
  - LMWH subcutaneously
  - ASA per os
  - UFH intravenously + ASA per os

  (if 2 drugs are specified: sequential use) [16].
- In the presence of impaired graft function, altered pharmacokinetics with an increased risk of accumulation (LMWH) and risk of bleeding should be considered [17, 18].

The data on antithrombotic agents and doses in paediatric kidney transplantation from a systematic review and an international survey are summarised in the following table [4, 16]:

Results of the systematic review

Active ingredient (group) + mode of application	Dose	Timing	Duration	Study
ASA p.o.	1 mg/kg, max. 75 mg OD	d 0	≥ 4 weeks	[19]
LMWH s.c.	Start: 0.5 mg/kg initial dose Continuation: 0.4 mg/kg BD	d −1 d +1	21 d	[20]
UFH i.v. continuously **UFH i.v. bolus** (in case of concerns for increased risk of thrombosis)	10 IU/kg/h 10 IU/kg	d 0 d 0 (intraoperatively)	5–7 d	[21]
UFH s.c.	<15 kg: 1000 IU TD 15–20 kg: 1500 IU TD 20–40 kg: 2500 IU TD	d 0	Until mobilisation	[22]
<u>**Low thrombosis risk:**</u> **UFH i.v. continuously** **ASA p.o.**	 10 IU/kg/h 3–5 mg/kg/d 3 x/week	 Postoperatively Subsequently	 7 d 1 year	[23]*
<u>**High thrombosis risk:**</u> **UFH i.v. continuously** **LMWH (Enoxaparin) s.c.** **ASA p.o.**	 10 IU/kg/h 1 mg/kg OD 3–5 mg/kg OD 3 x/week	 Postoperatively Subsequently Subsequently	 7 d 8 weeks 1 year	

* Study publication after completion of the systematic review, therefore not included in the latter and presented separately. Abbreviations: ASA, acetylsalicylic acid; BD, twice a day; d, day; h, hour; IU, international units; i.v., intravenously; kg, kilograms (body weight); LMWH, low molecular weight heparin; mg, milligrams; OD, once a day; p.o., per os; s.c., subcutaneously; TD, thrice a day; UFH, unfractionated heparin; 0 = day of transplantation

International survey results compared with general dosing recommendations [16, 24]

Active ingredient (group) + mode of application	Dosage	
	Survey results	**Dosing recommendations from a paediatric formulary**
ASA p.o.	1–5 mg/kg OD	1 month–18 years: 3–5 mg/kg OD, max. 80 mg/d [11, 25]
UFH i.v. bolus intraoperatively	5000 IU once 20–40 IU/kg once	–
UFH i.v. continuously	100–400 IU/kg/d	(perioperative thrombosis prophylaxis) 1 month–18 years: 10 IU/kg/h [24]
LMWH s.c. (Enoxaparin)	0.5–1 mg/kg OD or divided in BD	(Indication: prophylaxis) 2 months–18 years: 0.5 mg/kg BD (= 100 IU/kg/d) [26]

Abbreviations: ASA, acetylsalicylic acid; BD, twice a day; d, day; h, hour; IU, international units; i.v., intravenously; kg, kilograms (body weight); LMWH, low molecular weight heparin; mg, milligrams; OD, once a day; p.o., per os; s.c., subcutaneously; UFH, unfractionated heparin; 0 = day of transplantation

References

1 Chua A, Cramer C, Moudgil A, Martz K, Smith J, Blydt-Hansen T, et al. Kidney transplant practice patterns and outcome benchmarks over 30 years: The 2018 report of the NAPRTCS. Pediatr Transplant. 2019;23(8):e13597.

2 Gander R, Asensio M, Royo GF, Molino JA, Garcia L, Madrid A, et al. Vascular thrombosis in pediatric kidney transplantation: Graft survival is possible with adequate management. J Pediatr Urol. 2018;14(3):222–30.

3 Ponticelli C, Moia M, Montagnino G. Renal allograft thrombosis. Nephrol Dial Transpl. 2009;24(5):1388–93.

4 Bapistella S, Zirngibl M, Buder K, Toulany N, Laube GF, Weitz M. Prophylactic antithrombotic management in adult and pediatric kidney transplantation: A systematic review and meta-analysis. Pediatr Transplant. 2021;25(4):e14021.
5 Rodricks N, Chanchlani R, Banh T, Borges K, Vasilevska-Ristovska J, Hebert D, et al. Incidence and risk factors of early surgical complications in young renal transplant recipients: A persistent challenge. Pediatr Transplant. 2017;21(7).
6 Bock ME, Bobrowski AE, Bhat R. Utility of thrombophilia screening in pediatric renal transplant recipients. Pediatr Transplant. 2019;23(1):e13314.
7 Parajuli S, Lockridge JB, Langewisch ED, Norman DJ, Kujovich JL. Hypercoagulability in Kidney Transplant Recipients. Transplantation. 2016;100(4):719–26.
8 Smith JM, Stablein D, Singh A, Harmon W, McDonald RA. Decreased risk of renal allograft thrombosis associated with interleukin-2 receptor antagonists: a report of the NAPRTCS. Am J Transplant. 2006;6(3):585–8.
9 Penny MJ, Nankivell BJ, Disney AP, Byth K, Chapman JR. Renal graft thrombosis. A survey of 134 consecutive cases. Transplantation. 1994;58(5):565–9.
10 Singh A, Stablein D, Tejani A. Risk factors for vascular thrombosis in pediatric renal transplantation: a special report of the North American Pediatric Renal Transplant Cooperative Study. Transplantation. 1997;63(9):1263–7.
11 Monagle P, Chan AKC, Goldenberg NA, Ichord RN, Journeycake JM, Nowak-Gottl U, et al. Antithrombotic therapy in neonates and children: Antithrombotic Therapy and Prevention of Thrombosis, 9th ed: American College of Chest Physicians Evidence-Based Clinical Practice Guidelines. Chest. 2012;141(2 Suppl):e737S–e801S.
12 Murphy GJ, Taha R, Windmill DC, Metcalfe M, Nicholson ML. Influence of aspirin on early allograft thrombosis and chronic allograft nephropathy following renal transplantation. Br J Surg. 2001;88(2):261–6.
13 Aboul-Hassan SS, Stankowski T, Marczak J, Peksa M, Nawotka M, Stanislawski R, et al. The use of preoperative aspirin in cardiac surgery: A systematic review and meta-analysis. J Card Surg. 2017;32(12):758–74.
14 Burger W, Chemnitius JM, Kneissl GD, Rucker G. Low-dose aspirin for secondary cardiovascular prevention – cardiovascular risks after its perioperative withdrawal versus bleeding risks with its continuation – review and meta-analysis. J Intern Med. 2005;257(5):399–414.

15 Halvorsen S, Mehilli J, Cassese S, Hall TS, Abdelhamid M, Barbato E, et al. 2022 ESC Guidelines on cardiovascular assessment and management of patients undergoing non-cardiac surgery. Eur Heart J. 2022;43(39):3826–924.
16 Buder K, Zirngibl M, Bapistella S, Nadalin S, Tönshoff B, Weitz M, et al. Current practice of antithrombotic prophylaxis in pediatric kidney transplantation – Results of an international survey on behalf of the European Society for Paediatric Nephrology. Pediatr Transplant. 2020;24(7):e13799.
17 Parker K, Hartemink J, Saha A, Mitra R, Lewis P, Power A, et al. A systematic review of the efficacy and safety of anticoagulants in advanced chronic kidney disease. J Nephrol. 2022;35(8):2015–33.
18 Kohli R, Platton S, Forbes S, Thuraisingham R, Tan J, Green L, et al. Renal transplant and hemostasis: early postoperative changes in recipients and donors. Res Pract Thromb Haemost. 2023;7(4):100168.
19 Al Midani A, Rudarakanchana N, Nagra A, Fidan K, Tugtepe H, Matthias M, et al. Low-Dose Aspirin Reduces the Rate of Renal Allograft Thrombosis in Pediatric Renal Transplant Recipients. Exp Clin Transplant. 2020;18(2):157–63.
20 Broyer M, Gagnadoux MF, Sierro A, Fischer AM, Revillon Y, Jan D, et al. Prevention of vascular thromboses after renal transplantation using low molecular weight heparin. Ann Pediatr (Paris). 1991;38(6):397–9.
21 Kim JK, Chua ME, Teoh CW, Lee MJ, Kesavan A, Hebert D, et al. Assessment of prophylactic heparin infusion as a safe preventative measure for thrombotic complications in pediatric kidney transplant recipients weighing < 20 kg. Pediatr Transplant. 2019;23(6):e13512.
22 Nagra A, Trompeter RS, Fernando ON, Koffman G, Taylor JD, Lord R, et al. The effect of heparin on graft thrombosis in pediatric renal allografts. Pediatr Nephrol. 2004;19(5):531–5.
23 Beatrice JM, Takahashi MS, Celeste DM, Watanabe A, Koch VHK, Carneiro JDA. Thromboprophylaxis after kidney transplantation in children: Ten-year experience of a single Brazilian center. Pediatr Transplant. 2021;25(8):e14101.
24 https://www.kinderformularium.de/ [Internet].
25 Giglia TM, Massicotte MP, Tweddell JS, Barst RJ, Bauman M, Erickson CC, et al. Prevention and treatment of thrombosis in pediatric and congenital heart disease: a scientific statement from the American Heart Association. Circulation. 2013;128(24):2622–703.

26 Klaassen ILM, Sol JJ, Suijker MH, Fijnvandraat K, van de Wetering MD, Heleen van Ommen C. Are low-molecular-weight heparins safe and effective in children? A systematic review. Blood Rev. 2019;33:33–42.

CHAPTER 4
Immunosuppressive therapy and monitoring

CHAPTER 4.1 Immunosuppressive induction therapy

Burkhard Tönshoff[1], Lars Pape[2] & Jan Dudley[3]

[1] Heidelberg University, Medical Faculty Heidelberg, Department of Paediatrics I, University Children's Hospital, Heidelberg, Germany
[2] Department of Paediatrics II, University Hospital of Essen, Essen, Germany
[3] Bristol Royal Hospital for Children, Bristol, United Kingdom

ORCIDs:
Burkhard Tönshoff: https://orcid.org/0000-0002-6598-6910
Lars Pape: https://orcid.org/0000-0002-3635-6418
Jan Dudley: https://orcid.org/0000-0002-8066-6739

1 Basiliximab

The humanised anti-interleukin-2 receptor antibody basiliximab (Simulect®) is available for the prophylaxis of acute rejection episodes as part of induction therapy and is routinely administered in some countries (e.g., the United Kingdom [UK]) for prevention of acute rejection. Binding of IL-2 to the IL-2 receptor initiates a cascade of intracellular signals leading to functional differentiation of T cells and cell proliferation. The association of the constitutively expressed alpha-chain of the receptor and beta-chain is required for the formation of the IL-2 binding site, but this is only expressed on activated T cells and a subpopulation of B cells and antigen-presenting cells. Therapy with anti-IL-2 receptor antibodies therefore only blocks the antigen-activated T cells.

Studies of cyclosporine- and steroid-based maintenance immunosuppressive regimens without MMF or everolimus have shown that basiliximab reduces acute rejection compared with no induction (Cransberg et al. 2008; the Network meta-analysis of RCTs in adults). However, no prospective studies have shown that basiliximab has the same effect on reducing the incidence of acute rejection, when the maintenance regimen is based on tacrolimus and/or MMF.

In fact, two prospective randomised trials in paediatric kidney transplant recipients at low or moderate immunological risk failed to demonstrate an additional benefit of basiliximab in preventing acute rejection compared with a regimen of tacrolimus, azathioprine and steroids or a regimen of cyclosporine A, mycophenolate mofetil (MMF) and steroids (Grenda et al 2006, Offner et al 2008). In Europe, basiliximab is particularly indicated when other immunosuppressive drugs, e.g., glucocorticoids, are to be stopped early, i.e., from day 5 post-transplant (see Chapter 5.1). Some centres give basiliximab induction therapy with early use of low-dose CNI in combination with everolimus.

Recommended dose: in children > 35 kg is 20 mg, in children ≤ 35 kg 10 mg basiliximab as a short infusion over 30 min given intravenously 1 hour preoperatively; the second dose is given on day 4 after transplantation.

Half-life of basiliximab in children and adolescents receiving MMF is approximately 10 weeks, without MMF approximately 5 weeks (Höcker et al 2008).

Side effects: Rare. Severe acute (within less than 24 hours) hypersensitivity reactions were observed both on initial application of basiliximab and on re-application during a further treatment cycle. These included anaphylactoid reactions such as rash, urticaria, pruritus, sneezing, wheezing, hypotension, tachycardia, dyspnoea, bronchospasm, pulmonary oedema, heart failure, respiratory insufficiency and capillary leak syndrome. If a severe hypersensitivity reaction occurs, treatment with basiliximab must be discontinued permanently and no further application must be carried out. There is a small risk of hypersensitivity reactions in a subgroup of patients who receive further doses of basiliximab for subsequent transplants.

2 Lymphocyte-depleting antibodies

The two polyclonal anti-thymocyte globulin (ATG) preparations Thymoglobulin® and Grafalon® (formerly ATG-Fresenius®) and the monoclonal anti-B-cell antibody rituximab are currently available as lymphocyte-depleting antibodies in transplantation medicine in Europe. Thymoglobulin® is produced from rabbits immunised with human thymocytes; the antithymoglobulin recognises and destroys human T-lymphocytes and thus acts by removing T-lymphocytes from the bloodstream, modulating T-cell activation and so-called T-cell homing. The production of Grafalon® is based on the immunisation of rabbits with the Jurkat T-lymphoblast cell line.

A network meta-analysis of RCTs in adults showed that ATG (Thymoglobulin®) reduces acute rejection compared with treatment without induction, but treatment is longer and more complex than with basiliximab, and that adults having Thymoglobulin® have more adverse events (including post-transplant lymphoproliferative disorder) than those having basiliximab (NICE 2017). For this reason, indications for ATG as induction agents are limited to those at high immunological risk of an early acute rejection reaction.

ATG contains a variety of antibodies with broad specificity and therefore does not have a single mechanism of action. In addition to T cell-specific antibodies (CD2, CD3, CD4, CD5, CD8, CD25, CTLA-4), which suppress the T cell-mediated immune response, ATG contains specific antibodies against activated B cells (CD19, CD20, CD21), but also against adhesion molecules (CD11a, CD18) and cell line-unspecific markers such as ß2-microglobulin and HLA-DR. In addition, ATG contains antibodies against monocytes, natural killer cells and transduction molecules (CD45). Many of the antibodies in ATG, despite purification, also recognise antigens expressed on non-lymphoid cells such as erythrocytes, neutrophils, platelets and endothelial cells. Thus, despite the name implying lymphocyte specificity, ATG is not specific for any cell type.

Indications:

- high immunological risk of an early acute rejection, such as highly immunised patients with a panel-reactive HLA antibody titre > 80% (see Chapter 5.2).
- steroid-resistant rejection that do not respond to intravenous bolus administration of glucocorticoids (see Chapter 6.1).

The dosage of Thymoglobulin® is patient-adjusted with cell monitoring to successfully treat rejection while avoiding excessive immunosuppression. The initial dose is 1.5 mg/kg per day, with subsequent doses administered on alternate days over 3–5 days based on total lymphocyte count or total T-lymphocyte count (CD3+).

Recommended dosage:

1st loading dose: 1.5 mg/kg Thymoglobulin®,
2nd maintenance dose (administer over 3–5 days on alternate days):

Maintain dose if:	Total lymphocytes > 100/µl <300/µl or CD3+ or CD2+ > 10/µl < 50/µl.
Reduce the dose if:	Leucocyte count between 2,000 and 3,000 Platelet count between 50,000 and 75,000
Stop the dose if:	Total lymphocytes < 100/µl or CD3+ or CD2+ < 10/µl Leukocyte count below 2,000 Platelet count below 50,000
Increase the dose (e.g., 2 mg/kg) if:	Total lymphocytes > 300/µl or CD3+ or CD2+ > 50/µl.

The maximum cumulative dose of 8 mg/kg thymoglobulin should not be exceeded. If limit values such as total lymphocytes 120/µl or CD3+ 20/µl are measured, the dose may be reduced to 0.75 mg/kg.

Important:

- An ongoing infection should be ruled out before administration: medical history, physical examination, differential blood count, C-reactive protein, urinalysis, chest x-ray if necessary.
- Treatment with this drug requires close clinical monitoring of the patient: The first dose of Thymoglobulin® should be administered in the intermediate or intensive care unit. Some centers recommend that the patient should be fasting in the morning. The infusion is placed and started by the physician. During the infusion period, the patient is monitored as follows and vital signs are recorded on a monitoring sheet:
  - Monitor until the following morning,
  - Blood pressure taken initially every 15 minutes, then every 30 minutes until 2 hours after completion of the infusion,
  - Temperature taken at least twice.

According to the calculated dose, administer per manufacturer instructions via a central vein catheter for 4 hours (or longer if there is a hypersensitivity reaction (see below)).

Co-medication:

- All patients should receive an antihistamine (clemastin 0.04 mg/kg body weight i.v.) one hour prior to thymoglobulin administration.
- (Methyl)prednisolone 2–7 mg/kg i.v. should be given at least 30 minutes before the first dose of thymoglobulin.
- If the first dose is well tolerated, methylprednisolone can be omitted for the subsequent doses on days 3 and 5.
- At least 30 minutes before thymoglobulin administration, esomeprazole (Nexium®, dosage: patients aged 1–11 years: 10–20 kg bw – 10 mg/d; > 20 kg bw – 10–20 mg/d, patients aged 12–18 years: 20–40 mg/d) is given as short infusion.
- Paracetamol should be administered at least 30 minutes prior to the administration of thymoglobulin:
    - In children > 3 months and < 10 kg bw: 7.5 mg Paracetamol/kg as a short infusion
    - for body weight of 10–50 kg: 15 mg Paracetamol/kg as short infusion
    - for body weight of > 50 kg: 1 g Paracetamol as a short infusion

Adverse effects:

Immediately at the start, during or shortly after the infusion of thymoglobulin, anaphylactoid reactions may occur, such as a drop in blood pressure, a feeling of tightness in the chest, fever and urticaria. These symptoms are usually more severe with the first infusion of thymoglobulin and disappear with subsequent infusions. However, if the reactions are clinically significant, thymoglobulin treatment must be discontinued and anaphylaxis or shock therapy initiated. Similar to the use of other heterologous antisera, serum sickness may occur after 8 to 14 days of thymoglobulin treatment. If the symptoms are mild and reversible, there is no need to discontinue thymoglobulin therapy.

Infection prophylaxis:

- Except for CMV-negative donors and CMV-negative recipients, prophylaxis with valganciclovir in a prophylactic dosage for 6 months is required for all other constellations (see Chapter 7.1).
- Pneumocystis jirovecii prophylaxis with cotrimoxazole for 6 months (see Chapter 7.4).

References

1 Cransberg K, Bouts AH, Cornelissen EA, Lilien MR, Van Hoeck KJ, Hop WC, Nauta J. Recovery of graft function in pediatric kidney transplantation is not affected by delayed introduction of cyclosporine. Transplantation. 2008 Nov 15;86(9):1199–205
2 Grenda R, Watson A, Vondrak K, et al. A prospective, randomized, multicenter trial of tacrolimus-based therapy with or without basiliximab in pediatric renal transplantation. Am J Transplant. 2006;6(7):1666–72
3 Höcker B, Kovarik JM, Daniel V, et al. Pharmacokinetics and immunodynamics of basiliximab in pediatric renal transplant recipients on mycophenolate mofetil comedication. Transplantation. 2008;86(9):1234–40.
4 Offner G, Tönshoff B, Höcker B, et al. Efficacy and safety of basiliximab in pediatric renal transplant patients receiving cyclosporine, mycophenolate mofetil, and steroids. Transplantation. 2008;86(9):1241–8.
5 National Institute for Health Care Excellence. Immunosuppressive therapy for kidney transplantation in children and adolescents (technology appraisal guidance 484); 2017
6 Pape L. State-of-the-art immunosuppression protocols for pediatric renal transplant recipients. Pediatr Nephrol. 2019;34(2):187–194.
7 Tönshoff B, Becker JU, Pape L. Nierentransplantation, pp. 243–74. In: Nierenerkrankungen im Kindes- und Jugendalter, Dötsch J, Weber LT (Hrsg.), Springer Berlin, 2024
8 Tönshoff B. Immunosuppressive therapy post-transplantation in children: what the clinician needs to know. Expert Rev of Clin Immunol 2020;16:139–154.
9 Tönshoff B. Immunosuppressants in Organ Transplantation. In: Handbook of Experimental Pharmacology, S. 441–469, Kiess W, Schwab M, van den Anker J (Eds.), Springer Berlin, 2020

CHAPTER 4.2 Immunosuppressive maintenance therapy

Burkhard Tönshoff[1], Lars Pape[2] & Jan Dudley[3]

[1] Heidelberg University, Medical Faculty Heidelberg, Department of Paediatrics I, University Children's Hospital, Heidelberg, Germany
[2] Department of Paediatrics II, University Hospital of Essen, Essen, Germany
[3] Bristol Royal Hospital for Children, United Kingdom

ORCIDs:
Burkhard Tönshoff: https://orcid.org/0000-0002-6598-6910
Lars Pape: https://orcid.org/0000-0002-3635-6418
Jan Dudley: https://orcid.org/0000-0002-8066-6739

1 Introduction

Immunosuppressive therapy after kidney transplantation is carried out with a combination of drugs that affect the immune system at different points in the cascade of lymphocyte activation and proliferation. It is therefore useful to combine these drugs. In this way, the dose of the individual drug can be reduced and side effects avoided or at least reduced. Drugs used for maintenance immunosuppression include calcineurin inhibitors (tacrolimus, cyclosporin A), mycophenolate mofetil (MMF) or enteric-coated mycophenolate sodium as a more effective replacement for azathioprine, glucocorticoids and, for specific indications, mammalian target of rapamycin (mTOR) inhibitors such as everolimus and sirolimus. To avoid both under- and over-immunosuppression, the dosage of immunosuppressive drugs must be adjusted individually. This is usually done by measuring blood levels (therapeutic drug monitoring, see also Chapter 4.3) and adjusting the dosage of the drugs used accordingly. The *de novo* appearance of donor-specific HLA antibodies can be interpreted as a biomarker for under-immunosuppression. Various biomarkers are currently being investigated in transplantation medicine to enable even better individualisation of immunosuppressive therapy in the future.

2 Tacrolimus

Tacrolimus is a more potent immunosuppressant than cyclosporin A. A randomised prospective study of the efficacy and safety of tacrolimus compared with cyclosporin A in paediatric kidney transplant recipients showed a lower rate of rejection, better GFR and also better graft survival at 4 years in the tacrolimus group (Filler et al 2005), so most paediatric kidney transplant centres internationally now use tacrolimus as the primary immunosuppressant.

Immediate-release tacrolimus (Prograf®, 0.5, 1 and 5 mg capsules; Modigraf®, 0.2 mg granules for oral suspension)

Dosage:

- Children < 40 kg: 0.3 mg/kg body weight (bw) per day p.o. in 2 divided doses,
- Children > 40 kg: 0.2 mg/kg bw per day p.o. in 2 divided doses.
- Start within 6 hours of transplantation. Tacrolimus dose adjustment according to whole blood trough level 12 hours after intake immediately before morning administration.
- In the UK, tacrolimus is prescribed (initial dosing) at 0.15 mg/kg twice daily with a maximum initial dose of 5 mg twice daily for all children and adolescents, regardless of weight (Dudley et al 2021)

Target trough levels (measured in whole blood by mass spectrometry), if given in combination with MMF or azathioprine:

- Day 0–21: 8–12 ng/mL
- Day 22–month 6: 7–10 ng/mL
- Month 6–12: 5–8 ng/mL (depending on overall immunosuppression and individual immunological risk)
- After month 12: 5–8 ng/mL

UK target tacrolimus levels:

- Day 0–56: 8–12 ng/mL
- Day 57–365: 5–8 ng/mL
- Beyond the first year, tacrolimus levels may be individualized (e.g., 3–5 ng/mL)

Dose adjustments: Usually in 25% increments, with a maximum of 2 dose adjustments per week (long half-life of approximately 16 hours). However, in the early post-transplant period and in individual cases, however, daily dose adjustments may be required.

Living kidney donation: Tacrolimus dosing may be started 5 days before transplant; target trough level before transplant: 8–12 ng/mL.

Tacrolimus Monitoring by Mini-AUC (Limited Sampling Strategy (LSS))
Indication: Patients, in whom trough levels in the target range cannot be achieved with a relatively high body weight-based dose (in children < 40 kg, > 0.3 mg tacrolimus/kg per day; in children > 40 kg > 0.2 mg tacrolimus/kg per day); i.e., tacrolimus rapid metabolisers, infants and young children. In this situation, a more accurate determination of tacrolimus exposure using a mini-AUC should be performed to avoid toxicity or underexposure.

Practical implementation: A light, low-fat breakfast is permitted on the day of the mini-AUC; no large meal should be eaten in the first hour after taking tacrolimus. A blood sample is taken (via an indwelling intravenous catheter) before tacrolimus administration (C_0) and 1 (C_1), 2 (C_2) and 4 hours (C_4) after oral administration.

Algorithm for calculating the mini-AUC:
Tacrolimus-AUC = 4.15390 + 3.17385 x C0 + 1.28131 x C1 + 0.75475 x C2 + 5.35301 x C4 [Filler G et al 2002]

Target tacrolimus exposure (target AUC)
The target tacrolimus exposure depends on the time period post-transplant and the immunological or infectious risk:
Week 1–4 (early post-transplant period): 150–200 µg · h/L (in conjunction with an MPA-AUC > 40 mg · h/L) [Scholten EM et al., 2005, Lee and Butani 2007]
Month 1–3: 120–150 µg · h/L
> Month 3 (stable period): 75–150 µg · h/L

Modigraf® 0.2 mg and 1 mg for suspension preparation
For young children who cannot swallow Prograf® capsules, use Modigraf® granules for oral suspension. Modigraf® should be dissolved in a minimum of 2 mL

and a maximum of 50 mL of liquid. This suspension can also be used for administration by nasogastric tube.

Intravenous administration of tacrolimus

Only in exceptional cases, when oral or enteral therapy by gastric tube is not possible, intravenous continuous infusion of 0.06 mg/kg per day over 24 hours. During this time, the tacrolimus blood levels should be between 10–25 ng/mL.

Premedication for intravenous administration due to possible anaphylactic reaction:
Clemastine (Tavegil®) 0.04 mg/kg; Esomeprazole (Nexium®), dosage: patients aged 1–11 years or 10–20 kg b.w.: 10 mg esomeprazole per day; patients > 20 kg b.w.: 10–20 mg esomeprazole per day, patients aged 12–18 years: 20–40 mg esomeprazole per day as a short infusion over 30 minutes.

- Avoid intravenous administration of tacrolimus for more than 3 days due to increased risk of PTLD.
- After intravenous administration, give the first oral dose 12 hours after stopping the infusion.
- If repeat intravenous therapy is required, 20% of the previous p.o. dose should be given.

Common side effects of tacrolimus

Metabolic acidosis, hyperkalaemia, hypomagnesaemia, hyperuricaemia, bone pain, impaired renal function, hypertension, neurological complications (headaches, tremor), gastrointestinal complaints, blood count changes, diabetes mellitus (dose-dependent, generally reversible), etc. (see Drug product information package insert).

- Caution in EBV-seronegative children < 5 years of age receiving a kidney transplant from an EBV-positive donor, as there is an increased risk of PTLD in the event of seroconversion.
- Caution: Paradoxical increase in tacrolimus exposure (trough levels) with severe diarrhoea (gastroenteritis); therefore, close monitoring of tacrolimus trough levels is recommended.

Relative contraindications (cautions) for tacrolimus: Diabetes mellitus (DM) type I (possibly also type II) or disturbed glucose tolerance (consider also DM in first-degree relatives), cardiomyopathy or prolonged QT interval.

Pharmacokinetics

- Rapid absorption after oral administration, t_{max} 1.5–3 hours.
- Take at least 1 hour before or 2 hours after a meal (not with grapefruit juice!).
- Note large inter-individual variability in bioavailability, therefore individualised dosing based on measured blood levels is required.
- 95% of tacrolimus is bound to erythrocytes, 5% bound to plasma proteins. Only the unbound fraction is pharmacologically active, and this is subject to considerable variability without changing of the concentration in whole blood. For example, the amount of unbound tacrolimus is increased in anaemia, hypalbuminaemia or uraemia. Caution: Toxic reactions are possible despite whole blood concentrations in the therapeutic range.
- Half-life approximately 16–43 hours depending on the amount of unbound fraction. Steady state is only reached after approx. 2–3 days, therefore no more than 2 dose changes per week.

Frequency of trough level monitoring:

There is some between centre variability here and clinician discretion is required, however, as a guide:

- First week post-transplant: once daily (in some cases twice daily)
- 2nd and 3rd week: every other day
- Months 2 to 6: once a week
- Beyond 6 months: every other week (or less often)

- Dose-related side effects respond to dose reduction only after a few days.
- Dose changes are usually in 25% increments of the initial dose.
- Tacrolimus clearance decreases in the first few months posttransplant, and dose reductions of up to 33% of the initial dose may be necessary.
- Hepatic metabolism and biliary excretion. With cholestasis, the proportion of pharmacologically predominantly inactive metabolites in the measured blood level is approximately 20%.
- Metabolism via the cytochrome P450 3A4 and 3A5 system in the liver. Decreased metabolism in severe hepatic impairment.

Possible mechanisms of drug interactions:
Induction or inhibition of the cytochrome P450 3A4/3A5 system by other drugs, thereby lowering or increasing blood levels (see Drug product information package insert).

- Drugs that increase tacrolimus blood levels include: Diltiazem, clotrimazole, fluconazole, ketoconazole, danazol, amoxicillin, macrolide antibiotics (erythromycin, clarithromycin, but not azithromycin or roxithromycin), imipenem, ibuprofen.
- Drugs that lower tacrolimus blood levels include: Rifampicin, carbamazepine, phenobarbital, phenytoin.

Prolonged-release and extended-release tacrolimus formulations
A prolonged-release tacrolimus formulation ((Advagraf™ in Europe, Astagraf™ in the United States) for older children and adolescents allows once daily dosing, which reduces the pill burden and may improve adherence. Comparative pharmacokinetic studies have shown that stable paediatric transplant recipients can be converted from immediate-release to prolonged-release-tacrolimus at the same total daily dose, using the same therapeutic drug monitoring method.

Extended-release, melt-dose tablets (LCP-Tac, Envarsus XR; Cary, NC: Veloxis USA, Inc.) is currently under investigation also in paediatric patients. LCP-Tac is a new formulation with improved bioavailability and lower maximum concentrations compared to immediate release tacrolimus. Preliminary data suggest that the daily dose of LCP tacrolimus should be 0.7 (70%) of the previous dose of immediate-release or extended-release tacrolimus.

3 Mycophenolate mofetil (MMF, CellCept®)

MMF dosage for co-medication with tacrolimus
Some centres use the same body surface-based dose of MMF for all paediatric patients, some centres stratify as follows:

Below 6 years of age:
Day 0–14: 800 mg/m² body surface area (BSA) per day in 2 divided doses p.o.;
After day 14: 600 (up to 900) mg/m² per day in 2 divided doses

Above 6 years of age:
Day 0–14: 1200 mg/m^2 per day in 2 divided doses;
After day 14: 600 (up to 900) mg/m^2 per day in 2 divided doses.

In the UK, MMF is given for all ages as part of an early steroid withdrawal regimen as follows (Dudley et al 2021):

Day 0–14: 1200 mg/m^2 per day in 2 divided doses;
After day 14: 600 mg/m^2 per day in 2 divided doses.

MMF dosage for co-medication with cyclosporine:
Below 6 years of age:
Day 0–14: 1200 mg/m^2 BSA per day in 2 doses p.o.
After day 14: 1200 mg/m^2 per day in 2 divided doses.

Above 6 years of age:
Day 0–14: 1800 mg/m^2 BSA per day in 2 doses p.o.
After day 14: 1200 mg/m^2 per day in 2 divided doses.

Living donor kidney transplantation: MMF may be started 5 days pre-transplant, MMF dose see above; reduce MMF dose by 50% for dialysed patients (poorer tolerability).

MMF suspension and i.v.-administration

- MMF suspension for young children who cannot swallow capsules and or tablets; the suspension also allows for more flexible dosing. If the MMF dose cannot be administered within ± 10% of the desired dose with 250 mg capsules, the use of MMF suspension should also be considered.
- If oral administration is not possible, MMF can be given intravenously on a temporary basis.

MMF-related side effects
Leukopenia: Reduce the MMF dose by 50% if leukopenia < 4000/µl or neutropenia < 1600/µl. If leukopenia < 2000/µl or neutropenia < 1300/µl, discontinue MMF treatment.

Diarrhoea: If diarrhoea persists for more than 3 days and is not due to another cause (e.g., infection), consider giving 3–4 times daily (same total daily dose).

If this is not successful consider reducing the MMF dose by 50% (consider increasing the (methyl)prednisolone dose at the same time). If the diarrhoea does not resolve, consider switching to everolimus, sirolimus or azathioprine, depending on the immunological risk.

If the MMF dose is reduced within the first 3 months after transplantation (e.g., due to diarrhoea), dual immunosuppression with CNI and steroids should be intensified (e.g., steroid dose doubled) to prevent rejection. If diarrhoea is severe, intravenous methylprednisolone should be considered.

Relative contraindications to MMF:

- Serological evidence of active HIV, hepatitis B or C infection
- Patients with severe systemic infection
- Leukopenia < 2500/µl or anaemia < 5 g/dL.

Absolute contraindication: If pregnancy is planned, MMF should be stopped at least 12 weeks before conception. Consider switching to azathioprine.

Therapeutic drug monitoring of MPA, the active moiety of MMF

Target pre-dose MPA plasma level (12 hours after oral intake of MMF): 1.5–4 mg/L (by mass spectrometry).

Pre-dose MPA plasma levels are a rather imprecise marker of MPA exposure (MPA-AUC_{0-12}); the determination of a mini-AUC of MPA by a limited sampling strategy (LSS) is preferable.

Mini-AUC of MPA using a limited sampling strategy (LSS)

Significance: MPA underexposure is associated with a higher incidence of acute rejection episode.

Time points: Day 7 post-transplant, day 14–21 post-transplant, months 3, year 1 (during the annual transplant follow-up visit), in the event of a relevant change in immunosuppressive co-medication

Blood sampling (via indwelling intravenous catheter): before MMF administration (C_0), at 0.5 ($C_{0,5}$) and at 2 hours (C_2) after oral MMF administration.

Algorithms for calculating the MPA-AUC:

MMF therapy in conjunction with tacrolimus: MPA-AUC =

$10.01391 + 3.94791 \times C_0 + 3.24253 \times C_{0.5} + 1.0108 \times C_2$; $r^2 = 0.81$

MMF therapy in conjunction with cyclosporine: MPA-AUC = 18.609 + 4.309 x C_0 + 0.536 x $C_{0.5}$ + 2.148 x C_2; r^2 = 0.72.

MMF therapy without calcineurin inhibitor co-medication: use the same algorithm as for tacrolimus co-medication.

Target MPA-AUC: > 40 mg*h/L (in conjunction with a calcineurin inhibitor)

Enteric-coated mycophenolate sodium (Myfortic®)
Mycophenolate mofetil (CellCept®) and enteric-coated (delayed-release) mycophenolate sodium (EC-MPS) (Myfortic®) are not equivalent. Mycophenolate mofetil 500 mg is considered equivalent to mycophenolate sodium 360 mg. In adolescent patient on MMF and marked upper gastrointestinal side effects, switch from MMF to EC-MPS at a molecularly equivalent dose is an option. The rate of lower gastrointestinal side effects (diarrhoea) of MMF and EC-MPS is comparable. Because of the delayed-release formulation of EC-MPS and the highly variable absorption of the drug and day-to-day fluctuation in enterohepatic cycling of MPA, therapeutic drug monitoring with a limited sampling strategy over the first 2 hours after dosing, as recommended for MMF, is not possible for EC-MPS; 3–4 or more concentration measures over the first 6 hours after dosing are necessary (Bergan et al 2021).

4 Methylprednisolone (Urbason®) or prednisolone (Solu-Decortin H®)

4 mg methylprednisolone is equivalent to 5 mg prednisolone. The dose information below refer to methylprednisolone.

Day 0: 300 mg/m² or 10 mg/kg b.w. as a short infusion over 30 minutes, at least 1 hour before reperfusion of the renal graft.
Day 1: 48 mg/m² p.o. in 2 doses
Days 2–7: 32 mg/m² p.o. in 2 doses
Week 2: 24 mg/m² p.o. in 1 dose in the morning
Week 3–4: 16 mg/m² p.o. in 1 dose in the morning
Week 5–6: 8 mg/m² p.o. in 1 dose in the morning
From week 7: 3–4 mg/m² p.o. in 1 ED, maximum 5 mg per day
(round doses up or down to a practical tablet size).

In the UK; prednisolone is prescribed as below (Dudley et al 2021):
Day 0: 600 mg/m^2 (maximum dose 500 mg) at induction or reperfusion of the renal graft.
Day 1–2: 60 mg/m^2 (maximum dose 60 mg) p.o. once daily
Days 3–7: 40 mg/m^2 (maximum dose 40 mg) p.o. once daily
Days 8–14: 30 mg/m^2 (maximum dose 30 mg) p.o. once daily
Days 15–21: 20 mg/m^2 (maximum dose 20 mg) p.o. once daily
Days 21–28: 10 mg/m^2 (maximum dose 10 mg) p.o. once daily
Days 29–90: 10 mg/m^2 (maximum dose 10 mg) p.o. on alternate days
Day 91 onwards: 5 mg/m^2 (maximum dose 5 mg) p.o. on alternate days

For early or late steroid withdrawal see Chapter 5.1.

5 Cyclosporin A (Sandimmun Optoral®)

Second-line calcineurin inhibitor, if tacrolimus is contraindicated or not tolerated.

Dosage:
Day 0: 400–500 mg/m^2 body surface area per day in 2 divided doses p.o., starting 6 hours after transplantation.
From day 1 onwards: 300 mg/m^2 BSA per day in 2 single doses p.o.
Dose adjustment according to whole blood trough levels (C_0) and 2 hour-blood levels (C_2).
If given intravenously, give 30% of the single oral dose over 4 hours (caution: nephrotoxicity).

Target whole blood trough level (by mass spectrometry):
Months 0–3: 120–200 ng/mL
Beyond month 4: 80–160 ng/mL

Target range 2 hour-level (C_2):
Weeks 0–4: 800–1400 ng/mL
Months 1–6: 800–1200 ng/mL
Months 7–12: 600–1000 ng/mL
Beyond month 12: 400–800 ng/mL

6 Azathioprine (Imurek®)

Indication
In case of intolerance or contraindication to MMF in patients at low immunological risk. Infants receiving MMF are particularly susceptible to MMF-related adverse events such as poor appetite or diarrhoea. In the UK, azathioprine is routinely prescribed as part of a steroid-maintenance regimen (Dudley et al 2021).

Dosage
2 mg azathioprine/kg per day as a single dose.
Approximately 10% of patients have reduced activity of the enzyme thiopurine methyltransferase (TPMT) due to genetic polymorphism. Azathioprine metabolism is impaired, particularly in homozygous carriers, and there is an increased risk of myelotoxic effects. Testing for a TPMT deficiency is recommended for those with evidence of myelotoxicity (Ma et al 2016) and may be considered before starting therapy.

Side effects
Myelosuppression (especially with concomitant drugs such as olsalazine, mesalazine and sulphasalazine, which inhibit the enzyme TPMT). Concomitant use of azathioprine and drugs with myelosuppressive properties such as penicillamine and cytostatics may increase myelotoxic effects and should be avoided. If allopurinol, oxipurinol or thiopurinol are taken concomitantly, the dose of azathioprine should be reduced to a quarter of the normal dose. Special care is needed when using azathioprine with tubocurarine and succinylcholine as the effect of depolarising muscle relaxants may be increased. There is an increased risk of myelosuppression when azathioprine is used with trimethoprim/sulfamethoxazole, cimetidine, indomethacin or the ACE inhibitor captopril.

7 Everolimus (Certican®)

mTOR inhibitor that inhibits activated T cells. Everolimus is usually given with low-dose CNI.
Half-life approx. 28 hours, steady state reached after approx. 4 days

Indication: MMF intolerance in patients with standard or high immunological risk, CNI toxicity, PTLD/malignancies, intolerance to primary immunosuppression. Some centres switch patients at high risk of CMV infection (donor CMV seropositive, recipient CMV seronegative) to low-dose CNI and everolimus at 4 weeks post-transplant, because everolimus has a direct anti-CMV effect.

Relative contraindications: High proteinuria, hyperlipidaemia, risk of impaired wound healing. Significantly impaired renal function (GFR < 35 ml/min/1.73 m^2).

Contraindication: If pregnancy is planned, everolimus therapy should be discontinued at least 12 weeks prior to conception.

Dosage:
If co-administered with *tacrolimus:*
Infants, children and adolescents: 2 x 2 mg/m^2 BSA per day p.o.

If co-administered with *cyclosporine:*
Infants and young children: 2 x 0.8 mg/m^2 BSA per day or 0.05 mg/kg per day p.o.
Adolescents: 2 x 0.75 mg absolute per day p.o.

Target trough levels:
If co-medicated with calcineurin inhibitor: Months 2–6: 3–8 ng/mL; from month 7: 2–5 ng/mL
Without calcineurin inhibitor: 6–8 ng/mL

Adverse reactions:
Leukopenia; reduce dose of everolimus by 50% if leukopenia < 4000/µl or neutropenia < 1600/µl. Discontinue everolimus if leukopenia < 2000/µl or neutropenia < 1300/µl. Hyperlipidaemia, impaired wound healing, proteinuria, myelosuppression, aphthae.

Cyclosporine dose and target trough levels in combination with everolimus:

Cyclosporine dose:
Weeks 1 and 2 posttransplant: 400 mg/m^2 BSA per day p.o. in 2 divided doses
Week 3 and beyond: 200 mg/m^2 BSA per day p.o. in 2 divided doses

Cyclosporine target trough level
Cyclosporine trough levels:
Weeks 1 and 2: 200–250 ng/mL
Week 3 to month 6: 50–100 ng/mL
Beyond month 6: 30–75 ng/mL

Tacrolimus dose and target trough levels in combination with everolimus:
Children < 40 kg: 0.3 mg/kg per day in 2 divided doses p.o.,
Children ≥ 40 kg: 0.2 mg/kg per day in 2 divided doses p.o.

Tacrolimus target trough levels:

Time post-transplant	Tacrolimus target trough level (ng/mL) in combination with everolimus	Tacrolimus trough level (ng/mL) in combination with MMF or azathioprine
Weeks 0–3	5–8	8–12
Week 4 – month 4	4–6	7–10
Months 4–6	4–6	7–10
Months 6–12	2–4	5–8
Beyond month 12	2–4	5–8

In patients at increased immunological risk, tacrolimus trough levels should be aimed at the upper target range. For standard or low immunological risk patients, the sum of the tacrolimus trough level and the everolimus trough level should be approximately 10 ng/mL in the first 6 months post-transplant.

References

1 Bergan S, Brunet M, Hesselink DA, et al. Personalized Therapy for Mycophenolate: Consensus Report by the International Association of Therapeutic Drug Monitoring and Clinical Toxicology. Therapeutic Drug Monitoring 43 (2), 150–200, 2021
2 Filler G, Feber J, Lepage N, Weiler G, Mai I. Universal approach to pharmacokinetic monitoring of immunosuppressive agents in children. Pediatr Transplant. 2002;6(5):411–8.
3 Dudley J, Christian M, Andrews A, et al Clinical practice guidelines standardisation of immunosuppressive and anti-infective drug regimens in UK paediatric renal transplantation: the harmonisation programme. BMC Nephrol. 2021 Sep 16;22(1):312.
4 Filler G, Webb NJ, Milford DV, et al. Four-year data after pediatric renal transplantation: a randomized trial of tacrolimus vs. cyclosporin microemulsion. Pediatr Transplant. 2005;9:498–503.
5 Lee MN, Butani L. Improved pharmacokinetic monitoring of tacrolimus exposure after pediatric renal transplantation. Pediatr Transplant. 2007;11(4):388–93.
6 Pape L. State-of-the-art immunosuppression protocols for pediatric renal transplant recipients. Pediatr Nephrol. 2019;34(2):187–194.
7 Scholten EM, Cremers SC, Schoemaker RC, Rowshani AT, van Kan EJ, den Hartigh J, Paul LC, de Fijter JW. AUC-guided dosing of tacrolimus prevents progressive systemic overexposure in renal transplant recipients. Kidney Int. 2005;67(6):2440–7.
8 Tönshoff B, David-Neto E, Ettenger R, Filler G, van Gelder T, Goebel J, Kuypers DRJ, Tsai E, Vinks AA, Weber LT, Zimmerhackl LB. Pediatric aspects of therapeutic drug monitoring of mycophenolic acid in renal transplantation. Transplantation Reviews 25: 78–89, 2011
9 Tönshoff B, Sarwal M, Marks SD, Moudgil A. Renal Transplantation: Immunosuppression and Managing Allograft Rejection, In: Pediatric Nephrology. S. 1927–58. Emma F, Goldstein S, Bagga A, Bates CM, Shroff R (Eds) Springer Berlin, 2022
10 Tönshoff B. Immunosuppressive therapy post-transplantation in children: what the clinician needs to know. Expert Rev of Clin Immunol 16: 139–154, 2020

11 Ma AL, Bale G, Aitkenhead H, Marks SD. Measuring Erythrocyte Thiopurine Methyltransferase Activity in Children – Is It Helpful? J Pediatr. 2016 Dec;179:216–218

12 Baghai Arassi M, Feißt M, Krupka K, Awan A, Benetti E, Düzova A, Guzzo I, Kim JJ, Kranz B, Litwin M, Oh J, Büscher A, Pape L, Peruzzi L, Shenoy M, Testa S, Weber LT, Zieg J, Höcker B, Fichtner A, Tönshoff B; Cooperative European Pediatric Renal Transplant Initiative Research Network. Age-Related Differences in Rejection Rates, Infections, and Tacrolimus Exposure in Pediatric Kidney Transplant Recipients in the CERTAIN Registry. Kidney Int Rep. 2024;9(11):3265–3277

CHAPTER 4.3 Therapeutic drug monitoring

Lutz T. Weber

Paediatric Nephrology, Children's and Adolescents' Hospital, University Hospital of Cologne, Faculty of Medicine, University of Cologne, Cologne, Germany

ORCID:
https://orcid.org/0000-0003-4116-598X

1 Introduction

Pharmacokinetic (PK) therapeutic drug monitoring (TDM) is defined as the measurement of drug concentrations in biological fluids to assess whether they correlate with the patients' clinical condition and whether the dosage or dosage intervals need to be changed. This is done to optimize the management of patients receiving drug therapy for the alleviation or prevention of disease [1]. Measurement of drug concentrations in whole blood, plasma or serum is the most obvious method [2].

PK TDM is the most commonly used form of drug monitoring in paediatric solid organ transplantation and stands for a concentration–time relationship. Within a dosing-interval one has to distinguish certain PK parameters (Figure 1), such as C_{max} (maximum concentration), T_{max} (time to maximum concentration) and C_0 (trough [predose] concentration). The area under the concentration–time curve (AUC) can be calculated by using the linear trapezoidal rule and reflects the total body drug exposure [3].

TDM is essential to optimise immunosuppressive therapy in paediatric kidney transplant patients. The main immunosuppressive agents, tacrolimus, cyclosporin A, mycophenolic acid (MPA), and everolimus have narrow therapeutic windows and significant variability in pharmacokinetics, especially when used together or with other drugs. TDM helps to achieve a good balance between efficacy and toxicity in this narrow therapeutic window (Figure 2). Drug-drug interactions (DDIs) between these agents and with other drugs can significantly affect their efficacy and safety, thereby affecting patient outcomes. This chapter provides an overview of TDM for these key immunosuppressants.

For the timing of TDM in children after kidney transplantation (KTx), see Chapter 4.2. In general, TDM is recommended early after initiation of therapy to rule out the possibility that a non-response is due to under-exposure. TDM may

Figure 1 Pharmacokinetic parameters during a dosing interval. C_{max} maximum concentration, Tmax time to maximum drug concentration, C_o trough (predose) concentration

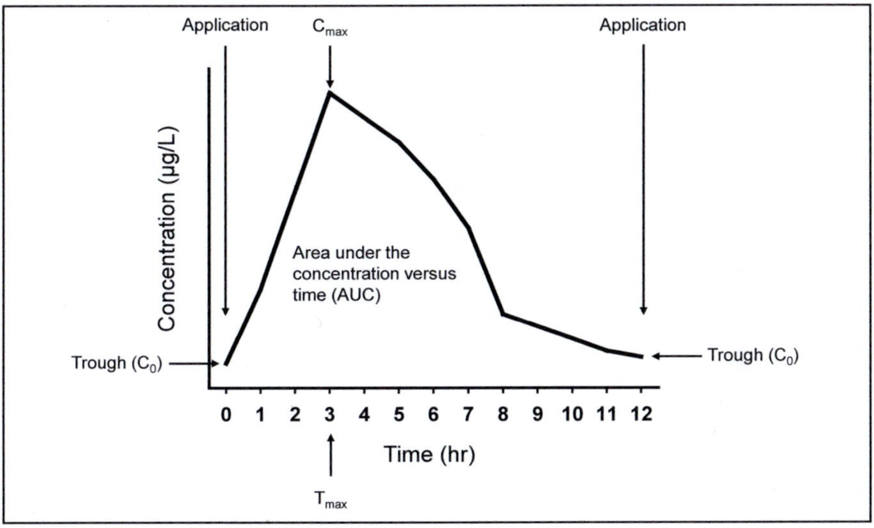

Figure 2 Balance between efficacy and toxicity showing the narrow therapeutic range. [Courtesy (and in honor of) V.W. Armstrong (†), Göttingen, Germany]

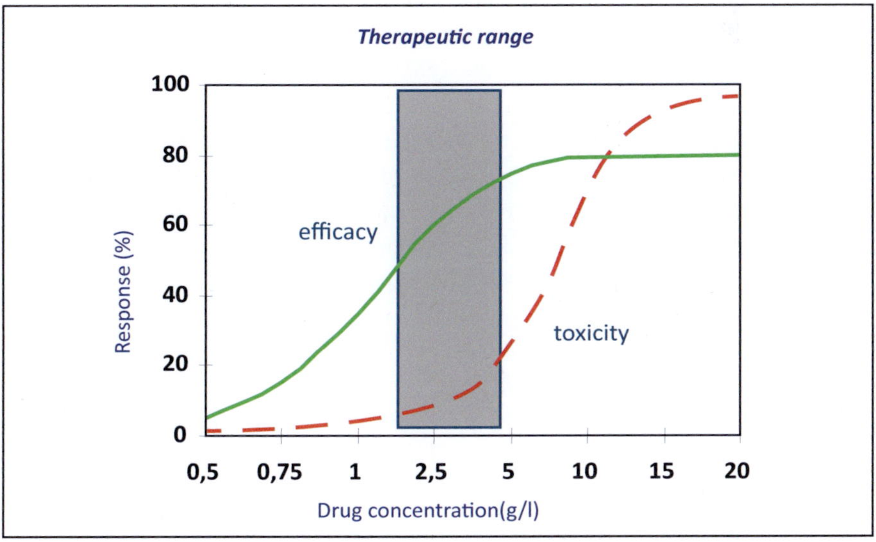

be useful in the setting of potential drug-related adverse events to verify an exposure that is well above the target range, which would allow dose reduction without the risk of loss of efficacy. TDM may also be useful after a change in therapy, especially with drugs that interact with the metabolism of the drug itself. In maintenance therapy, regular TDM at defined intervals can detect individual changes in the absorption and metabolism and thus facilitate dose adjustment.

2 Mycophenolic Acid (mycophenolate mofetil [MMF, CellCept©], mycophenolate sodium [EC-MPS, Myfortic©])

Mycophenolic acid (MPA) is the pharmacologically active moiety of MMF or EC-MPS formulations. Monitoring MPA exposure is complex due to high intra- and inter-individual variability. MPA underexposure is a serious concern as it increases the risk of graft rejection. Several factors influence MPA levels in children, including age, weight, albumin levels, and kidney function. The risk of underexposure is particularly high in young children due to their more rapid clearance and variable absorption of MMF. The MPA exposure that leads to overexposure is not well defined. Side effects may be more likely to correlate with free MPA exposure, which is difficult to measure.

Relying on predose level monitoring alone for MPA is less reliable than for other immunosuppressive agents (see below), because the predose level does not necessarily correlate with total body drug exposure (AUC). Therefore, calculation of an estimated MPA-AUC (eMPA-AUC) using a limited sampling strategy (LSS) is important to ensure adequate immunosuppressive efficacy.

To avoid underexposure, the following measures are recommended: (i) regular TDM (see also Chapter 4.2); (ii) dose adjustments: MMF doses should be individually adjusted based on TDM results. If necessary, an increase in the MMF dose may be considered; (iii) avoidance of drug interactions: The concomitant use of drugs that affect the pharmacokinetics of MPA should be closely monitored.

Algorithms for calculating MPA-AUC

MPA-AUC is considered the gold standard for monitoring MPA exposure, as it provides a reliable estimate of the immunosuppressive effect. However, in clinical practice, full AUC determination, which requires multiple blood samples over time, is rarely performed in clinical practise. Instead, abbreviated algorithms are used to estimate the AUC based on a limited number of samples (see also Chapter 4.2).

Common algorithms include:

i. Bayesian pharmacokinetic models: These models are based on population data and use a limited number of sampling points to estimate the full AUC. They take into account individual pharmacokinetic parameters to allow for more precise dose adjustments. However, these estimates are difficult to develop and use, because they require specialised PK modelling software.
ii. Linear algorithm: A simpler approach is to use a linear model, where the AUC is estimated based on two or three sampling points (see also Chapter 4.2). In the case of co-medication with cyclosporin A, a significant pharmacokinetic interaction with MPA must be considered: Cyclosporin A inhibits the multidrug resistance protein 2 (MRP-2), which is responsible for the excretion of MPA glucuronide (MPAG), an inactive metabolite of MPA, into the bile. Inhibition of this transporter reduces the conversion of MPAG back to MPA in the intestine, thereby reducing MPA reabsorption and, hence, MPA exposure. This DDI results in an overall decrease in MPA-AUC and C_{max} and an increase in T_{max}. Therefore, it is mandatory to use different LSSs and algorithms to estimate MPA-AUC with or without cyclosporin A co-administration (see also Chapter 4.2).
iii. Predose level-based AUC estimates: Due to enterohepatic recirculation, which causes a secondary peak in the plasma MPA concentration between 6 and 12 h after oral intake, the term predose level should be used instead of the term trough level. The predose level alone does not provide a reliable AUC estimate [4].

MPA can also be given mycophenolate sodium. Compared with MMF, EC-MPS has a delayed absorption and therefore has a different PK profile. An LSS for EC-MPS requires more concentration measurements, including later time points, than those for MMF (see also Chapter 4.2).

Key Drug-Drug Interactions

- Cyclosporin A: see above.
- Tacrolimus: Unlike cyclosporine, tacrolimus has a less pronounced effect on the pharmacokinetics of MPA. It does not significantly interfere with the enterohepatic recirculation of MPA. As a result, MPA exposure tends to be higher when used in combination with tacrolimus. However, careful moni-

toring of MPA levels is still required, especially in the early post-transplant period.
- Proton Pump Inhibitors (PPIs): PPIs such as omeprazole may reduce the bioavailability of mycophenolate mofetil by affecting gastric pH. This interaction can lead to lower MPA levels, however, these changes are regarded to be small and not likely to have clinically major effects.

3 Tacrolimus

Tacrolimus is a calcineurin inhibitor metabolized via the CYP3A4 and CYP3A5 pathways. In young children, tacrolimus clearance is faster due to higher enzyme activity compared to older children and adults. This results in lower tacrolimus blood levels at the same dosage. Therefore, this patient group often requires higher doses per kilogram of body weight to achieve therapeutic target levels (see also Chapter 7.2), resulting in a lower concentration-to-dose (C/D) ratio in smaller children [5]. TDM is crucial to regularly monitor trough levels, to avoid both underexposure, which increases the risk of rejection, and overexposure, which is associated with toxicity. Intrapatient variability of tacrolimus trough levels over time is associated with adverse graft outcomes and can help to assess potential underexposure [5].

Key Drug-Drug Interactions
- CYP3A4 Inhibitors/Inducers: Tacrolimus levels are highly susceptible to drugs that inhibit or induce CYP3A4. For instance:
  - CYP3A4 inhibitors such as ketoconazole, diltiazem, and macrolide antibiotics (e.g., erythromycin) increase tacrolimus levels, potentially leading to toxicity (e.g., nephrotoxicity, neurotoxicity).
  - CYP3A4 inducers like rifampin, carbamazepine, and phenytoin reduce tacrolimus levels, increasing the risk of graft rejection.
- Calcium Channel Blockers (CCBs): The CCBs diltiazem and verapamil increase tacrolimus concentrations by inhibiting its metabolism. These interactions require dose adjustments and close TDM to prevent toxicity.

Drug interactions, particularly with CYP3A4 modulators, necessitate frequent monitoring, especially when new medications are introduced or discontinued.

4 Cyclopsorine A (Sandimmun optoral©)

Cyclosporine A, a calcineurin inhibitor, inhibits T-cell activation by blocking the transcription of IL-2. Cyclosporine A has complex pharmacokinetics and numerous drug interactions, making TDM critical. Like tacrolimus cyclosporine A is metabolized via the CYP3A4 and CYP3A5 pathways and displays the same DDIs.

Key Drug-Drug Interactions

- Everolimus: Cyclosporine A can increase blood levels of mTOR inhibitors like everolimus by interacting with CYP3A4, the enzyme responsible for their metabolism. This can lead to increased risk of toxicity. TDM is essential to manage the delicate balance between effective immunosuppression and adverse effects when combining these drugs.
- Statins: Cyclosporine A also interacts with statins, which are increasingly used to manage post-transplant dyslipidemia in children (see also Chapter 11.5). It inhibits the metabolism of statins, potentially increasing the risk of myopathy and rhabdomyolysis. This interaction requires careful monitoring of statin doses and potential dose reductions.

Variations in drug absorption and metabolism, as well as interactions with medications like statins and mTOR inhibitors, require regular monitoring and dose adjustments.

5 Everolimus (Certican®)

Everolimus is a mammalian target of rapamycin (mTOR) inhibitor and is extensively metabolized by CYP3A4 in the gut and liver. Due to its narrow therapeutic index and significant pharmacokinetic variability, therapeutic drug monitoring (TDM) is essential to optimize dosing, reduce toxicity, and minimize the risk of graft rejection.

The PK of everolimus differs significantly between children and adults due to developmental differences in drug absorption, distribution, metabolism, and excretion. Infants and young children exhibit faster drug clearance and require higher doses to achieve therapeutic levels. Factors such as age, body weight, genetic polymorphisms in drug-metabolizing enzymes (e.g., CYP3A4 and

CYP3A5), and concurrent use of other medications can greatly influence blood levels of this mTOR inhibitor.

TDM for everolimus is usually based on trough levels, which are measured just before the next dose. Trough levels provide a reliable estimate of the drug's steady-state concentration and are easier to obtain in clinical practice compared to full pharmacokinetic profiles.

Key Drug-Drug Interactions

- Cyclosporine A: see above.
- Tacrolimus: Tacrolimus, being less of a CYP3A4 inhibitor than cyclosporin A, has a milder impact on everolimus levels. Nonetheless, the combination of tacrolimus and everolimus still requires careful monitoring due to the potential for nephrotoxicity and other side effects.
- CYP3A4 Inhibitors and Inducers: Similar to tacrolimus and cyclosporine A, everolimus levels are influenced by CYP3A4 inhibitors and inducers. Medications such as azole antifungals and macrolide antibiotics can increase everolimus concentrations, while rifampin and antiepileptic drugs can reduce its levels. Close TDM is essential when these agents are used concurrently with everolimus.

TDM should be performed regularly, especially when combined with other CYP3A4 substrates or inhibitors. Monitoring helps optimize immunosuppression while minimizing the risk of adverse events.

6 Conclusion

Therapeutic drug monitoring plays a critical role in managing immunosuppressive therapy in transplant patients, particularly when multiple agents with significant drug-drug interactions are used. Mycophenolic acid, cyclosporine A, tacrolimus, and everolimus all have narrow therapeutic windows and are subject to complex pharmacokinetic interactions. Effective TDM ensures appropriate drug exposure, minimizes toxicity, and reduces the risk of graft rejection, ultimately improving patient outcomes.

References

1 Soldin OP, Soldin SJ (2002) Review: therapeutic drug monitoring in pediatrics. Ther Drug Monit 24:1–8
2 Bergan S, Brunet M, Hesselink DA, et al. Personalized Therapy for Mycophenolate: Consensus Report by the International Association of Therapeutic Drug Monitoring and Clinical Toxicology. Therapeutic Drug Monitoring 43 (2), 150–200, 202
3 Weber LT. Therapeutic drug monitoring in pediatric renal transplantation. Pediatr Nephrol. 2015. 30:253–265
4 Ehren R, Schijvens AM, Hackl A, et al. Therapeutic drug monitoring of mycophenolate mofetil in pediatric patients: novel techniques and current opinion. Expert Opinion on Drug Metabolism & Toxicology. 2021:2:201–213
5 Baghai Arassi M, Feißt M, Krupka K, et al. Age-related differences in rejection rates, infections and tacrolimus exposure in pediatric kidney transplant recipients in the CERTAIN registry. KI Reports. 2024, accepted for publication

CHAPTER 4.4 Immune monitoring after kidney transplantation

Alexander Fichtner[1], Lien Pham[2] & Thuong Hien Tran[2]

[1] Heidelberg University, Medical Faculty Heidelberg, Department of Paediatrics I, University Children's Hospital Heidelberg, Germany
[2] Institute of Immunology, Heidelberg University Hospital, Heidelberg, Germany

ORCIDs:
Alexander Fichtner: https://orcid.org/0000-0002-9939-4059
Thuong Hien Tran: https://orcid.org/0000-0001-8587-5989

1 Introduction

Post-transplant immune monitoring is a critical component of patient management. It encompasses an array of laboratory assays primarily designed to detect graft rejection and optimise immunosuppressive therapy. In addition to conventional markers of graft function, such as serum creatinine, estimated glomerular filtration rate (eGFR) and proteinuria, both invasive and non-invasive approaches are employed. While graft biopsy remains the gold standard for diagnosing rejection, the risks involved, particularly bleeding, limit its repeated use in children. In recent years, numerous blood- and urine-based biomarkers have been investigated, with donor-specific anti-HLA antibodies (DSAs) now established as a key component of immune surveillance. Other promising candidates include donor-derived cell-free DNA (dd-cfDNA), urinary chemokines, and 'omics'-based signatures (transcriptomics, metabolomics, and proteomics). Immunosuppressive drug monitoring, traditionally based on trough levels, is being refined through emerging metrics such as tacrolimus intra-patient variability (TAC-IPV). Torque Teno Virus (TTV) load and virus-specific T-cell profiling may provide additional information about the recipient's actual immune status and help to refine immunosuppressive dosing strategies. Surveillance for opportunistic viral infections, including cytomegalovirus (CMV), Epstein–Barr virus (EBV) and polyomavirus, remains essential. While some of these approaches have entered routine practice, many are still investigational and require further validation, particularly in paediatric populations. Together, these evolving strategies hold significant promise for advancing personalised, precision-guided post-transplant care.

This chapter aims to provide an overview of the most well-established immune monitoring tools currently available, and how they are implemented in practice for kidney transplant recipients. For a more comprehensive and in-depth review, readers are referred to recent publications, including those by Peruzzi and Deaglio (2023) and Laroche and Engen (2024) [1, 2]. The post-transplant surveillance of DSAs is addressed in particular by expert consortia such as the "Sensitisation in Transplantation: Assessment of Risk (STAR)" Working Group and the European Society of Organ Transplantation (ESOT) Working Group on Subclinical DSA Monitoring [3, 4]. The "ESOT Working Group on Molecular Biomarkers of Kidney Transplant Rejection" has published recommendations on molecular biology testing for the non-invasive diagnosis of kidney allograft rejection [5]. However, it is important to note that the majority of the existing literature and evidence originates from adult cohorts, with comparatively limited data available for paediatric transplant populations.

2 Human Leukocyte Antigen (HLA) Antibodies

The impact of antibodies directed against donor HLA mismatches (DSAs) on the risk of rejection (particularly antibody-mediated rejection [AMR]) and subsequent graft loss is well established [6, 7]. In paediatric kidney transplantation, approximately 15–45% of patients develop de novo DSAs (dnDSAs) within the first five years post-transplant, depending on the definitions applied and the cohort studied [8, 9]. The current consensus is to use single-antigen bead (SAB) assays for DSA detection [10]. However, interpreting DSA positivity remains challenging in the absence of a universally accepted mean fluorescence intensity (MFI) threshold. Reported laboratory cut-offs vary widely, typically from 500 to 3,000. Based on analyses of inter-laboratory reproducibility and manufacturer-related variability, the STAR consortium recommends an MFI threshold of between 1,000 and 1,500 [3].

The DSA monitoring schedule should be tailored to the individual patient's risk profile, which is mainly constituted by the presence or absence of signs of graft dysfunction and immunological history (e.g. HLA antibody status, re-transplantation with repeated HLA mismatches, immunising events such as blood transfusions), the chosen immunosuppressive regimen (e.g., minimisation of immunosuppression, especially reduction or withdrawal of CNI, as well as non-tacrolimus-based regimens), non-adherence, and comorbidities [11].

Thus, the optimal scheme for routine monitoring of DSA in clinically stable kidney transplant recipients has not yet been established and remains debatable [12]. According to the ESOT consensus, this may include a baseline assessment prior to transplantation, followed by scheduled testing at three to six months post-transplant, and annually thereafter. Intensified monitoring in the first months after transplantation appears beneficial for patients with preformed DSAs due to the increased risk of early AMR [13]. With the emergence of advanced risk-stratification tools, such as molecular mismatch analysis, there is growing evidence that less intensive surveillance protocols may offer a favourable balance between cost-effectiveness and safety [14]. However, younger age within adult transplant cohorts has been associated with an increased risk of developing dnDSA. Together with the tendency towards a higher incidence of dnDSA in paediatric recipients, this observation may argue in favour of a more intensified monitoring schedule in paediatric recipients [9, 15]. The emergence of dnDSA, or a significant rise in MFI (defined as an MFI increase of 25–50% according to the STAR consortium), in combination with clinical and other laboratory parameters, may warrant consideration of a graft biopsy to assess for subclinical rejection [3]. DSA testing is recommended in conjunction with any biopsy, whether protocol-driven or indicated, to support diagnosis and management [16].

The clinical utility of additional assays that evaluate the complement-fixing capacity of DSAs (e.g., C1q, C3d or C4d binding tests) or that delineate IgG subclasses is still unclear. Complement binding assays, especially C1q positivity, are associated with high DSA MFI levels and DSA strength (titres), which increases the risk of rejection or graft loss [17, 18]. However, a recent meta-analysis examined the impact of C1q positivity beyond the mere association with high MFI levels, suggesting that C1q-positive DSAs could predict graft outcomes following therapy [19]. Patients who failed to clear C1q-binding antibodies had poorer outcomes. This suggests that, in certain clinical scenarios, these assays could provide additional information on the potential effectiveness of targeted therapeutic interventions [20, 21]. Nevertheless, these supplementary tests are not yet routinely incorporated into monitoring protocols [4, 22].

3 Non-HLA antibodies

The role of non-HLA antibodies in allograft injury is still being investigated. While several non-HLA targets have been suggested, the majority of existing studies have been limited by small sample sizes and single-centre designs, with notable exceptions including antibodies directed against the angiotensin II type 1 receptor (AT1R) and MHC class I chain-related gene A (MICA) [24–28]. Although there have been some observations of an association between non-HLA antibodies and poorer graft outcomes (graft survival and rejection), the current evidence is insufficient to justify routine screening for non-HLA antibodies in clinical practice [29]. Heterogeneity in antibody detection methods and threshold definitions further complicates the interpretation of test results [16]. However, as with testing for complement-binding HLA-DSAs, assessing non-HLA antibodies may be a useful diagnostic option in certain cases, such as AMR with incongruent HLA-DSAs [22].

4 Donor-derived cell-free DNA

Donor-derived cell-free DNA (dd-cfDNA) has emerged as a non-invasive biomarker for detecting allograft injury. Elevated dd-cfDNA levels have been consistently associated with biopsy-proven rejection in adult studies, and are quantified as the proportion or absolute amount of circulating donor-derived cell-free DNA in the recipient plasma that originates from the donor organ [30, 31]. When integrated with DSA testing, dd-cfDNA measurement has significant potential to enhance the early detection of alloimmune injury, particularly AMR [32–34]. However, thresholds in paediatric populations remain to be definitively established and prospectively validated. Reflecting this, paediatric-specific research is urgently needed to define the optimal cut-off values, timing and clinical application of dd-cfDNA in the context of long-term graft surveillance [35]. The European Society of Organ Transplantation recently made a 'weak but favourable recommendation' for serial dd-cfDNA monitoring in mainly adult patients with stable graft function as a strategy to exclude subclinical AMR [5]. However, a randomised clinical trial conducted at a single centre reported that dd-cfDNA-guided biopsy in patients with prevalent dnDSA can reduce the time to AMR diagnosis and thereby expedite therapy initiation. This suggests that testing for dd-cfDNA would probably be more meaningful and cost-efficient in a selected cohort of patients, i.e., those with dnDSA and therefore at higher risk of developing AMR [36].

5 Drug level monitoring

Recent studies have demonstrated that tacrolimus intrapatient variability (TacIPV) and the concentration-to-dose ratio (C/D) may be useful markers for predicting graft loss and rejection [37, 38]. In paediatric patients, TacIPV of more than 23% during months 6–12 post-transplant was associated with an increased risk of rejection after 12 months post-transplant. Similarly, a C/D ratio of less than 1.0 (i.e. rapid tacrolimus metabolism) was associated with a higher risk of rejection between months 6 and 12 [39]. Furthermore, high TacIPV has also been reported to be associated with an increased risk of dnDSA development, rejection episodes, and graft failure in both adult and paediatric patients [40–44]. These findings suggest that patients with these risk factors should be closely monitored and their immunosuppressive therapy adjusted accordingly.

6 Monitoring for viral infections and Torque Teno Virus

The reactivation of latent viral infections, particularly EBV, CMV and polyomaviruses (BKPyV and JC viruses), can provide valuable information about the immunological balance after a transplant, albeit indirectly. It is important to note that any reduction in immunosuppression, particularly in managing sustained viral replication, raises concerns about the development of dnDSA [45, 46]. Using virus-specific T cell assays could further improve the personalisation of immunosuppressive management [47]. However, their routine application is currently limited by technical complexity, restricting its use to specialist centres.

Another approach to assessing over- or under-immunosuppression, which is associated with an increased risk of infection or graft rejection, respectively, is Torque Teno Virus (TTV) load monitoring, which has emerged as a promising biomarker. TTV is a non-enveloped, circular, single-stranded DNA virus belonging to the Anellovirus family, and is not known to cause disease in humans. While it is detectable in approximately 90% of healthy individuals, it is present in almost all immunosuppressed transplant recipients [48]. Notably, TTV remains unaffected by conventional antivirals, and TTV plasma loads have been shown to inversely correlate with T-cell count and function, with higher viral loads observed in immunosuppressed patients compared to healthy controls. Conversely, patients experiencing allograft rejection tend to exhibit significantly lower TTV levels [49]. While the directionality of these associations is biologically plausible, the pooled diagnostic performance of TTV-DNA remains suboptimal for stand-alone clinical use, with a sensitivity of 72% and a specificity of 57% [50]. Despite these limitations, monitoring TTV load may provide a non-invasive adjunct to conventional markers of immune function. In paediatric transplantation, where balancing adequate immunosuppression with the risks of infection and long-term toxicity is particularly challenging, TTV represents a promising area for further research [51].

7 Gene expression profiling (transcriptomics) and protein biomarkers (proteomics)

Peripheral blood gene expression profiling and urinary chemokine assays have the potential to overcome the limitations of conventional monitoring tools. The combination of CXCL9 and CXCL10 in urine, for example, has shown promising results in ruling out subclinical rejection, encompassing both T cell-mediated rejection (TCMR) and AMR [52]. This approach may be particularly useful for paediatric recipients, for whom minimising invasive procedures is of heightened clinical importance [53]. As a 'weak but favourable recommendation' by ESOT, monitoring a combination of urine CXCL9 and CXCL10 can be used to exclude subclinical rejection in stable patients and acute rejection in patients with graft dysfunction. In contrast, the clinical applicability of peripheral blood gene expression profiling remains limited. Although initial studies suggested that such assays, such as the Kidney Solid Organ Response Test (kSORT), might offer a valuable adjunct in the early detection of rejection, most commercial platforms have been withdrawn from the market, primarily due to regulatory challenges and inconsistent performance [54]. Currently, there is no consensus on the implementation of blood gene expression profiling for diagnosing or excluding graft rejection.

8 Summary

In addition to traditional biomarkers, which have long been known to have low sensitivity and specificity, as well as an inability to detect subclinical kidney allograft rejection, a variety of new, non-invasive tests are now available. These tests have the potential to help monitor graft health, evaluate levels of immunosuppression, and reduce the need for biopsies in post-transplant care. However, key parameters for most of these novel biomarkers remain undefined, including standardised sampling protocols, defined post-transplantation timepoints and validated diagnostic thresholds. These knowledge gaps are particularly significant for paediatric kidney transplant cohorts. While these non-invasive biomarkers represent a promising frontier in transplant immunosurveillance, their translation into standard paediatric practice requires substantial refinement, harmonisation and regulatory clarity, as well as large and rigorous paediatric-specific studies.

References

1 Peruzzi, L. and S. Deaglio, Rejection markers in kidney transplantation: do new technologies help children? Pediatr Nephrol, 2023. 38(9): p. 2939–2955.
2 Laroche, C. and R.M. Engen, Immune monitoring in pediatric kidney transplant. Pediatr Transplant, 2024. 28(4): p. e14785.
3 Lefaucheur, C., et al., Clinical recommendations for posttransplant assessment of anti-HLA (Human Leukocyte Antigen) donor-specific antibodies: A Sensitization in Transplantation: Assessment of Risk consensus document. Am J Transplant, 2023. 23(1): p. 115–132.
4 van den Broek, D.A.J., et al., The Clinical Utility of Post-Transplant Monitoring of Donor-Specific Antibodies in Stable Renal Transplant Recipients: A Consensus Report With Guideline Statements for Clinical Practice. Transpl Int, 2023. 36: p. 11321.
5 Park, S., et al., European Society of Organ Transplantation Consensus Statement on Testing for Non-Invasive Diagnosis of Kidney Allograft Rejection. Transpl Int, 2023. 36: p. 12115.
6 Mohan, S., et al., Donor-specific antibodies adversely affect kidney allograft outcomes. J Am Soc Nephrol, 2012. 23(12): p. 2061–71.
7 Sharma, A., et al., Renal transplant outcomes and de novo donor-specific anti-human leukocyte antigen antibodies: a systematic review. Nephrol Dial Transplant, 2018. 33(8): p. 1472–1480.
8 Steinbach, E.J., et al., Donor specific antibody surveillance among pediatric kidney transplant programs: A report from the improving renal outcome collaborative. Pediatr Transplant, 2023. 27(3): p. e14498.
9 Fichtner, A., et al., Incidence, risk factors, management strategies, and outcomes of antibody-mediated rejection in pediatric kidney transplant recipients – a multicenter analysis of the Cooperative European Paediatric Renal

Transplant Initiative (CERTAIN). Pediatr Nephrol, 2025. 40(2): p. 491–503.
10 Tait, B.D., et al., Consensus guidelines on the testing and clinical management issues associated with HLA and non-HLA antibodies in transplantation. Transplantation, 2013. 95(1): p. 19–47.
11 Crespo, M., et al., Monitoring of Donor-specific Anti-HLA Antibodies and Management of Immunosuppression in Kidney Transplant Recipients: An Evidence-based Expert Paper. Transplantation, 2020. 104(8 Suppl 2): p. S1–S12.
12 Salhi, S., et al., Utility of Routine Post Kidney Transplant Anti-HLA Antibody Screening. Kidney Int Rep, 2024. 9(5): p. 1343–1353.
13 Senev, A., et al., Specificity, strength, and evolution of pretransplant donor-specific HLA antibodies determine outcome after kidney transplantation. Am J Transplant, 2019. 19(11): p. 3100–3113.
14 Wiebe, C., et al., A rational approach to guide cost-effective de novo donor-specific antibody surveillance with tacrolimus immunosuppression. Am J Transplant, 2023. 23(12): p. 1882–1892.
15 von Moos, S., et al., Age-associated decrease in de novo donor-specific antibodies in renal transplant recipients reflects changing humoral immunity. Immun Ageing, 2019. 16: p. 9.
16 Naesens, M., et al., The Banff 2022 Kidney Meeting Report: Reappraisal of microvascular inflammation and the role of biopsy-based transcript diagnostics. Am J Transplant, 2024. 24(3): p. 338–349.
17 Tambur, A.R., et al., Assessing Antibody Strength: Comparison of MFI, C1q, and Titer Information. Am J Transplant, 2015. 15(9): p. 2421–30.
18 Bouquegneau, A., et al., Complement-activating donor-specific anti-HLA antibodies and solid organ transplant survival: A systematic review and meta-analysis. PLoS Med, 2018. 15(5): p. e1002572.
19 Tasaki, M., et al., C1q-Fixing De Novo Donor Specific Antibodies in Therapeutic Management of Chronic Antibody-Mediated Rejection Postkidney Transplantation. Transplant Proc, 2024. 56(9): p. 1961–1966.
20 Al-Awadhi, S., et al., Complement-activating donor-specific anti-HLA antibodies in solid organ transplantation: systematic review, meta-analysis, and critical appraisal. Front Immunol, 2023. 14: p. 1265796.
21 Viglietti, D., et al., Complement-binding anti-HLA antibodies are independent predictors of response to treatment in kidney recipients with antibody-mediated rejection. Kidney Int, 2018. 94(4): p. 773–787.

22 Battle, R., et al., BSHI and BTS UK guideline on the detection of alloantibodies in solid organ (and islet) transplantation. Int J Immunogenet, 2023. 50 Suppl 2: p. 3–63.
23 Lefaucheur, C., et al., The emerging field of non-human leukocyte antigen antibodies in transplant medicine and beyond. Kidney Int, 2021. 100(4): p. 787–798.
24 Sorohan, B.M., et al., Angiotensin II type 1 receptor antibodies in kidney transplantation: An evidence-based comprehensive review. Transplant Rev (Orlando), 2020. 34(4): p. 100573.
25 Pearl, M.H., et al., Non-HLA Antibodies to G Protein-coupled Receptors in Pediatric Kidney Transplant Recipients: Short- and Long-term Clinical Outcomes. Transplantation, 2024. 108(1): p. 276–283.
26 Fichtner, A., et al., Association of angiotensin II type 1 receptor antibodies with graft histology, function and survival in paediatric renal transplant recipients. Nephrol Dial Transplant, 2018. 33(6): p. 1065–1072.
27 Lefaucheur, C., et al., Non-HLA agonistic anti-angiotensin II type 1 receptor antibodies induce a distinctive phenotype of antibody-mediated rejection in kidney transplant recipients. Kidney Int, 2019. 96(1): p. 189–201.
28 Carapito, R., et al., The MHC class I MICA gene is a histocompatibility antigen in kidney transplantation. Nat Med, 2022. 28(5): p. 989–998.
29 Tambur, A.R., et al., Sensitization in transplantation: Assessment of Risk 2022 Working Group Meeting Report. Am J Transplant, 2023. 23(1): p. 133–149.
30 Bloom, R.D., et al., Cell-Free DNA and Active Rejection in Kidney Allografts. J Am Soc Nephrol, 2017. 28(7): p. 2221–2232.
31 Bu, L., et al., Clinical outcomes from the Assessing Donor-derived cell-free DNA Monitoring Insights of kidney Allografts with Longitudinal surveillance (ADMIRAL) study. Kidney Int, 2022. 101(4): p. 793–803.
32 Kataria, A., D. Kumar, and G. Gupta, Donor-derived Cell-free DNA in SoUd-organ Transplant Diagnostics: Indications, Limitations, and Future Directions. Transplantation, 2021. 105(6): p. 1203–1211.
33 Halloran, P.F., et al., The Trifecta Study: Comparing Plasma Levels of Donor-derived Cell-Free DNA with the Molecular Phenotype of Kidney Transplant Biopsies. J Am Soc Nephrol, 2022. 33(2): p. 387–400.
34 Aubert, O., et al., Cell-free DNA for the detection of kidney allograft rejection. Nat Med, 2024. 30(8): p. 2320–2327.

35 Hogan, J., et al., Donor-derived Cell-free DNA as a Noninvasive Biomarker of Kidney Allograft Rejection in Pediatric Kidney Transplantation. Transplantation, 2025.
36 Akifova, A., et al., Donor-derived cell-free DNA monitoring for early diagnosis of antibody-mediated rejection after kidney transplantation: a randomized trial. Nephrol Dial Transplant, 2025. 40(7): p. 1384–1395.
37 Gonzales, H.M., et al., A comprehensive review of the impact of tacrolimus intrapatient variability on clinical outcomes in kidney transplantation. Am J Transplant, 2020. 20(8): p. 1969–1983.
38 Masset, C., et al., Early Determination of Tacrolimus Concentration-Dose Ratio Identifies Risk of Allograft Loss in Kidney Transplantation. Kidney Int Rep, 2025. 10(5): p. 1428–1440.
39 Baghai Arassi, M., et al., Association of intrapatient tacrolimus variability and concentration-to-dose ratio with outcomes in pediatric kidney transplantation. Pediatr Nephrol, 2025.
40 Baghai Arassi, M., et al., Association of intraindividual tacrolimus variability with de novo donor-specific HLA antibody development and allograft rejection in pediatric kidney transplant recipients with low immunological risk. Pediatr Nephrol, 2022. 37(10): p. 2503–2514.
41 Choi, J.S., et al., Effects of tacrolimus intrapatient variability and CYP3A5 polymorphism on the outcomes of pediatric kidney transplantation. Pediatr Transplant, 2022. 26(6): p. e14297.
42 Mendoza Rojas, A., et al., Impact of low tacrolimus exposure and high tacrolimus intra-patient variability on the development of de novo anti-HLA donor-specific antibodies in kidney transplant recipients. Expert Rev Clin Immunol, 2019. 15(12): p. 1323–1331.
43 Wiebe, C., et al., Class II Eplet Mismatch Modulates Tacrolimus Trough Levels Required to Prevent Donor-Specific Antibody Development. J Am Soc Nephrol, 2017. 28(11): p. 3353–3362.
44 Goodall, D.L., et al., High Intrapatient Variability of Tacrolimus Levels and Outpatient Clinic Nonattendance Are Associated With Inferior Outcomes in Renal Transplant Patients. Transplant Direct, 2017. 3(8): p. e192.
45 Hod-Dvorai, R., et al., Development of de novo donor-specific antibodies in renal transplant recipients with BK viremia managed with immunosuppression reduction. Transpl Infect Dis, 2023. 25(1): p. e13993.

46 Fichtner, A., et al., Risk of cellular or antibody-mediated rejection in pediatric kidney transplant recipients with BK polyomavirus replication – an international CERTAIN registry study. Pediatr Nephrol, 2025. 40(3): p. 835–848.
47 Ahlenstiel-Grunow, T. and L. Pape, Novel ways to monitor immunosuppression in pediatric kidney transplant recipients – underlying concepts and emerging data. Mol Cell Pediatr, 2021. 8(1): p. 8.
48 Focosi, D., et al., Torquetenovirus: the human virome from bench to bedside. Clin Microbiol Infect, 2016. 22(7): p. 589–93.
49 Gorzer, I., et al., Validation of plasma Torque Teno viral load applying a CE-certified PCR for risk stratification of rejection and infection post kidney transplantation. J Clin Virol, 2023. 158: p. 105348.
50 Zeng, J., et al., Torque-teno virus for the prediction of graft rejection and infection disease after kidney transplantation: A systematic review and meta-analysis. J Med Virol, 2023. 95(3): p. e28677.
51 Kelly, E., et al., Torque Teno Virus Loads as a Marker of Immunosuppression in Pediatric Kidney Transplant Recipients. Pediatr Transplant, 2024. 28(7): p. e14857.
52 Tinel, C., et al., Transforming kidney transplant monitoring with urine CXCL9 and CXCL10: practical clinical implementation. Sci Rep, 2024. 14(1): p. 20357.
53 Blydt-Hansen, T.D., et al., Validity and utility of urinary CXCL10/Cr immune monitoring in pediatric kidney transplant recipients. Am J Transplant, 2021. 21(4): p. 1545–1555.
54 Punukollu, R., et al., Genomic and Biomarker Innovations in Predicting Kidney Transplant Rejection. J Clin Med, 2025. 14(11).

CHAPTER 5
Specific immunosuppressive protocols

CHAPTER 5.1 Steroid minimisation strategies

Burkhard Tönshoff[1] & Lars Pape[2]

[1] Heidelberg University, Medical Faculty Heidelberg, Department of Paediatrics I, University Children's Hospital, Heidelberg, Germany
[2] Department of Paediatrics II, University Hospital of Essen, Essen, Germany.

ORCIDs:
Burkhard Tönshoff: https://orcid.org/0000-0002-6598-6910
Lars Pape: https://orcid.org/0000-0002-3635-6418

1 Introduction

Glucocorticoids, developed in the early 1950s, are one of the main agents used for both maintenance immunosuppression and treatment of acute rejection. Glucocorticoids have both anti-inflammatory and immunosuppressive effects. They also induce lymphopenia and monocytopenia that result from inhibition of lymphocyte proliferation, survival, activation, homing, and effector functions. The main glucocorticoids used are prednisone or prednisolone (given orally with comparable efficacy) and methylprednisolone (given orally or intravenously with 25% greater potency). These agents are rapidly absorbed and have short plasma half-lives (60–180 minutes), but long biological half-lives (18–36 hours).

In many transplant centres, the initial dose of glucocorticoids is usually given during surgery as intravenous methylprednisolone, at doses between 2 and 10 mg/kg body weight per day. The oral dose of glucocorticoids used for maintenance therapy varies between 15 and 60 mg/m^2 per day (0.5 to 2 mg/kg per day), which is gradually tapered over time to approximately 3 mg of prednisolone per m^2 of body surface area, usually taken as a single morning dose. Alternate day dosing is often used 6 to 12 months post-transplant to minimise the effect of glucocorticoids on growth.

2 Side effects of glucocorticoids

Glucocorticoids have numerous side effects in children, including impaired growth, susceptibility to infection, cushingoid appearance, body disfigurement, acne, cardiovascular complications, arterial hypertension, hyperglycaemia, lipid disorders, aseptic bone necrosis, osteopenia, cataracts, poor wound healing, and psychological effects. The negative effect of glucocorticoids on appearance may play a role in poor adherence, particularly in body image-conscious adolescents. The risk of infection is excessive with prolonged high-dose pulse therapy (typically > 3 g per 1.73 m^2). Glucocorticoid dosage should, therefore, be tapered during rejection treatment, even if kidney function does not improve. Interestingly, glucocorticoids are not associated with an increased risk of malignancy. One of the most important reasons for discontinuing glucocorticoids or switching to alternate day therapy is impaired longitudinal growth, which is often seen in those on continuous treatment. Steroids are the major cause of growth failure in paediatric kidney transplant recipients, in addition to suboptimal allograft function [Tönshoff 2023]. Pharmacological doses of steroids disrupt longitudinal growth by inhibiting growth hormone secretion and insulin-like growth factor activity, and by suppressing the local synthesis of growth factors and matrix proteins in the growth plate [Tönshoff et al. 2005].

3 Steroid minimisation strategies

Because of the many adverse effects of maintenance glucocorticoid therapy, attempts have been made to withdraw or minimise glucocorticoid (steroid) therapy in paediatric kidney transplant recipients [Benfield et al. 2010, Sutherland et al. 2009, Barletta et al. 2009, Höcker et al. 2009, Höcker et al. 2010, Sarwal et al. 2003, Chavers et al. 2009, Grenda et al. 2010, Webb et al. 2015, Sarwal et al 2012, Pape et al. 2010, Tönshoff et al. 2019, Tönshoff et al. 2021]. There are four main approaches to steroid minimisation: (i) complete steroid avoidance or early steroid withdrawal (< 7 days post-transplant), (ii) an intermediate approach combining elements of early and late withdrawal protocols that sometimes uses antibody induction, (iii) late steroid withdrawal (≥ 1 year post-transplant, and (iv) alternate day steroids.

Nevertheless, steroid withdrawal or avoidance following renal transplantation remains a controversial issue. Although the benefits of using steroid-free protocols in paediatric patients are promising, further studies are needed to determine the impact on long-term allograft function and to identify patients (e.g., low immunological risk) who can be successfully switched to steroid-free immunosuppression without increasing the risk of acute rejection.

The efficacy of steroid withdrawal may depend in part on adequate exposure to the remaining drugs, such as tacrolimus, MMF or mTOR inhibitors in order to sufficiently suppress the anti-allograft immune response. Thorough therapeutic drug monitoring of these immunosuppressants and targeting the appropriate therapeutic ranges to achieve sufficient immunosuppressive activity is therefore recommended (see Chapter 4.3). Unfortunately, there is currently no immunological test that can reliably predict the success or the risk of steroid withdrawal.

Complete steroid avoidance or early steroid withdrawal

Some centres in North America argue that complete steroid avoidance is a more promising approach than steroid withdrawal, because a completely steroid-free immunosuppressive milieu from the outset should not lead to steroid-dependent suppression of the immune response, which would make either steroid withdrawal or alternate day dosing hazardous for rebound rejection. However, an empirical or experimental support for this hypothesis is still lacking.

Steroid avoidance protocols have been used successfully and have been extensively evaluated in the United States. These protocols have selected low-risk individuals and used intensive induction therapy with thymoglobulin, tacrolimus, and MMF [Sarwal et al. 2012]. The results of the North American randomised controlled multicentre trial with a follow-up of 3 years post-transplant showed that the steroid-free group showed lower systolic blood pressure and lower cholesterol levels. The authors concluded that complete steroid avoidance is safe and effective in non-sensitised children undergoing primary kidney transplantation [Sarwal et al. 2012].

Regarding the efficacy and safety of early steroid withdrawal, a randomised controlled trial, the TWIST trial, in 196 paediatric kidney transplant recipients, showed that two doses of daclizumab in patients treated with a regimen of tacrolimus and MMF allowed early steroid withdrawal on day 5 post-transplant [Grenda et al. 2010]. There was a comparable rate of biopsy-proven acute rejection rates at six months in steroid-free patients compared with controls (10.2% vs. 7.1%). In addition, prepubertal patients with early steroid withdrawal showed improved growth and lipid and glucose metabolism profiles compared to controls, without an increase in graft rejection or loss. These beneficial effects were confirmed in a 2-year follow-up study [Webb et al. 2015]. The TWIST study has been criticised for reporting only biopsy-proven acute rejection episodes

≥ Banff I and not the rate of borderline rejection and/or treated rejection episodes in the two study arms, leaving some uncertainty about the immunosuppressive efficacy of this protocol.

Intermediate approach of steroid withdrawal at 6-9 months post-transplant

This intermediate approach combines elements of early and late withdrawal protocols, using antibody induction, but delaying the decision to withdraw steroids until 6–9 months post-transplant, when stable renal graft function (sometimes combined with a normal protocol biopsy) allows identification of suitable candidates (as in the late withdrawal approach) [Pape et al. 2010, Pape et al. 2019]. For example, the CRADLE study was a 36-month multicentre prospective randomised trial in paediatric kidney transplant recipients who were randomised at 4 to 6 weeks post-transplant to receive everolimus plus reduced-exposure tacrolimus with glucocorticoid withdrawal at 6 months post-transplant or to continue MMF and standard-exposure tacrolimus with glucocorticoids (Tönshoff et al. 2019, Tönshoff et al. 2021). The incidence of composite efficacy failure (biopsy-proven acute rejection, graft loss, or death) at month 36 was similar between groups (9.8% vs. 9.6%). Mean estimated glomerular filtration rate at month 36 was comparable between groups (68.1 vs. 67.3 mL/min/1.73 m^2). Growth was better in prepubertal patients on everolimus and reduced-exposure tacrolimus without glucocorticoids. The authors concluded that although the rate of study drug discontinuation due to adverse events was higher in the everolimus group, an everolimus plus reduced-exposure tacrolimus regimen is an alternative treatment option that allows the withdrawal of glucocorticoids and the reduction of calcineurin inhibitors.

Late steroid withdrawal

In the late steroid withdrawal approach, patients suitable for minimisation are identified by a stable post-transplant clinical course and renal function. Late steroid withdrawal does not require antibody induction in the perioperative period [Höcker et al. 2009, Höcker et al. 2010]. Steroid withdrawal has the advantage over steroid avoidance that immunologically high-risk patients and those with unstable graft function can be easily identified in advance and excluded from steroid-free immunosuppression. For example, in one study, 42 paediatric kidney transplant recipients at low or standard immunological risk were randomly assigned, at ≥ 1 year post-transplant, to continue taking or to withdraw steroids over 3 months. Two years after steroid withdrawal, longitudinal growth was superior to controls. The prevalence of the metabolic syndrome declined significantly. Steroid-free patients had less frequent arterial hypertension (50% versus 93%) and required less antihypertensive medication. They also had significantly improved carbohydrate and lipid metabolism with less hypercholesterolaemia and hypertriglyceridaemia. Patient and graft survival was 100%. Allograft function remained stable 2 years after steroid withdrawal. The incidence of acute rejection was similar in the steroid withdrawal group (4%) and controls (11%). The authors concluded that late steroid withdrawal in selected cyclosporine- and MMF-treated paediatric kidney transplant recipients improves growth, mitigates cardiovascular risk factors and reduces the prevalence of the metabolic syndrome without increasing the risk of acute rejection or graft dysfunction [Höcker et al. 2010].

Alternate-day steroids

One way to ameliorate or avoid steroid-specific side effects in paediatric kidney transplant recipients is to administer steroids on alternate days, as a cumulative dose of steroids has a significantly reduced inhibitory effect on growth velocity when administered on alternate days compared to a daily regimen without adversely affecting graft survival or long-term graft function [Broyer et al. 1992, Jabs et al. 1996]. However, the effect on longitudinal growth is only moderate and limited to the first 2 years post-transplant. For example, in a large study reported from the North American Pediatric Renal Transplant Cooperative Study (NAPRTCS) registry, relative height increased by 0.50 ± 0.06 SDS in the first 2 years post-transplant, but no additional height gain was observed in subsequent years [Jabs et al. 1996]. Therefore, it is thought that alternate-day steroid dosing may provide catch-up growth in young paediatric kidney transplant recipients with well-preserved graft function only in the first 2 years post-transplant.

References

1 Barletta GM, Kirk E, Gardner JJ, et al. Rapid discontinuation of corticosteroids in pediatric renal transplantation. Pediatr Transplant. 2009;13:571–578.

2 Benfield MR, Bartosh S, Ikle D, et al. A randomized double-blind, placebo controlled trial of steroid withdrawal after pediatric renal transplantation. Am J Transplant. 2010;10:81–88.

3 Broyer M, Guest G, Gagnadoux MF. Growth rate in children receiving alternate-day corticosteroid treatment after kidney transplantation. J Pediatr. 1992; 120:721–725
4 Chavers BM, Chang C, Gillingham KJ, et al. Pediatric kidney transplantation using a novel protocol of rapid (6-day) discontinuation of prednisolone: 2-year results. Transplantation. 2009; 88:237–241.
5 Grenda R, Watson A, Trompeter R, et al. A randomized trial to assess the impact of early steroid withdrawal on growth in pediatric renal transplantation: the TWIST Study. Am J Transplant. 2010;10:828–836.
6 Höcker B, Weber LT, Feneberg R, et al. Prospective, randomized trial on late steroid withdrawal in pediatric renal transplant recipients under cyclosporine microemulsion and mycophenolate mofetil. Transplantation. 2009;87:934–941.
7 Höcker B, Weber L, Feneberg R, et al. Improved growth and cardiovascular risk after late steroid withdrawal: 2-year results of a prospective, randomized trial in paediatric renal transplantation. Nephrol Dial Transplant. 2010;25:617–624.
8 Jabs K, Sullivan EK, Avner ED, Harmon WE. Alternate-day steroid dosing improves growth without adversely affecting graft survival or long-term graft function. A report of the North American Pediatric Renal Transplant Cooperative Study. Transplantation 1996;61:31–36
9 Pape L, Offner G, Kreuzer M, et al. De novo therapy with everolimus, low-dose cyclosporine A, basiliximab and steroid elimination in pediatric kidney transplantation. Am J Transplant. 2010;10:2349–2354.
10 Pape L. State-of-the-art immunosuppression protocols for pediatric renal transplant recipients. Pediatr Nephrol. 2019;34(2):187–194.
11 Sarwal MM, Vidhun JR, Alexander SR, et al. Continued superior outcomes with modification and lengthened follow-up of a steroid-avoidance pilot with extended daclizumab induction in pediatric renal transplantation. Transplantation. 2003;76:1331–1339.
12 Sarwal MM, Ettenger RB, Dharnidharka V, et al. Complete corticosteroid avoidance is effective and safe in children with renal transplants: a multicentre randomized trial with three year follow-up. Am J Transplant. 2012;12:2719–2729.
13 Sutherland S, Li L, Concepcion W, et al. Steroid-free immunosuppression in pediatric renal transplantation: rationale for and outcomes following conversion to steroid based therapy. Transplantation. 2009;87:1744–1748.

14 Tönshoff B, Höcker B, Weber LT. Steroid withdrawal in pediatric and adult renal transplant recipients. Pediatr Nephrol. 2005;20:409–417.
15 Tönshoff B, Ettenger R, Dello Strologo L, et al. Early conversion of pediatric kidney transplant patients to everolimus with reduced tacrolimus and steroid elimination: Results of a randomized trial. Am J Transplant 2019;19:811–822
16 Tönshoff B, Tedesco H, Ettenger R, et al. Three-year Outcomes from the CRADLE Study in De Novo Pediatric Kidney Transplant Recipients Receiving Everolimus With Reduced Tacrolimus and Early Steroid Withdrawal. Am J Transplant 2021;21:123–137.
17 Tönshoff B. Pathogenesis, evaluation and diagnosis of growth impairment in children with chronic kidney disease. In: UpToDate, Rose BD (Ed), UpToDate, Waltham, MA, 2023
18 Webb N, Douglas S, Rajai A, et al. Corticosteroid-free kidney transplantation improves growth: two-year follow-up of the TWIST randomized controlled trial. Transplantation. 2015;99:1178–1185.

CHAPTER 5.2 Kidney transplantation in highly sensitised patients

Burkhard Tönshoff[1], Thuong Hien Tran[2], Caner Süsal[2,3] & Christian Morath[4,5]

[1] Heidelberg University, Medical Faculty Heidelberg, Department of Paediatrics I, University Children's Hospital, Heidelberg, Germany
[2] Heidelberg University, Medical Faculty Heidelberg, Institute of Immunology, Transplantation Immunology, Heidelberg, Germany
[3] Transplant Immunology Research Centre of Excellence, Koç University School of Medicine, Istanbul, Turkey
[4] Department of Nephrology, University Hospital Heidelberg
[5] Clinic for Internal Medicine, Nephrology, Nuremberg Hospital, Germany

ORCIDs:
Burkhard Tönshoff: https://orcid.org/0000-0002-6598-6910
Thuong Hien Tran: https://orcid.org/0000-0001-8587-5989
Caner Süsal: https://orcid.org/0000-0003-2521-8201
Christian Morath: https://orcid.org/0000-0003-2218-7817

1 Introduction

Sensitisation against human leukocyte antigen (HLA) can be induced by pregnancy, blood transfusion, or a previous transplant. In the Eurotransplant (ET) allocation system, high sensitisation is defined by a panel-reactive antibody of at least 85% (traditionally in CDC-based tests; later extended to solid phase assays, provided that the HLA specificities can be attributed to an immunising event). Highly sensitised patients are disadvantaged because of their broad immunisation status that results in positive crossmatches with many kidney donors, precluding a transplantation in those cases of organ offer. There are several strategies that can help highly sensitised patients access to a more timely transplantation, including desensitisation to reduce the amount of pre-existing, circulating antibodies to a level that allows successful transplantation from a deceased or living kidney donor; participation in kidney paired donation (KPD) or transplantation within the ET Acceptable Mismatch (AM) programme.

2 Pre-transplant identification of high-risk patients

The HLA sensitisation of a potential transplant recipient is assessed prior to waitlisting, at regular time intervals thereafter, and after every immunising event. The objective is to measure the degree of HLA sensitisation and to identify HLA specificities that are targets of the patient's antibodies. Although transplant centres vary in their approach to measuring HLA sensitisation, all assess for the presence of HLA antibodies by testing patient sera in solid phase assays (using microbeads with attached HLA antigens) and in cellular assays (using a lymphocyte panel in a complement-dependent cytotoxicity (CDC) test). At our centre, in addition to CDC antibody screening, we perform mixed and single antigen bead assays (One Lambda) on a Luminex platform to screen for and characterisation of HLA antibodies, respectively [1]. Antigens against which antibody reactivities are detected either in CDC or in Luminex at a mean fluorescence intensity (MFI) of at least 5,000 (for patients without known history of allosensitisation) or 3,000 (for pre-sensitised patients) are designated as 'unacceptable antigens'. These unacceptable antigens are then entered into ENIS, the ET computer system used for organ allocation. If a patient has an unacceptable antigen listed in ENIS, kidneys from donors carrying that antigen will not be offered to the patient. A calculated panel-reactive antibody (cPRA), also called virtual PRA (vPRA) in the ET nomenclature, is then computed based on the patient's unacceptable antigens. Panel-reactive antibodies (PRA) estimate the percentage of the donor population against which the patient has antibodies and characterise the breadth of HLA sensitisation. Higher PRA is associated with lower chances of compatible transplantation and inversely correlates with the likelihood of an HLA compatible donor match. It should be noted that MFI levels can vary by approximately 20–25% between HLA laboratories and that the MFI threshold levels used to define an unacceptable antigen are not standardised across transplant centres. ET uses the term "non-sensitised" for patients with a vPRA of 0%. At our centre, patients with a vPRA of at least 30% are considered having an increased immunological risk and may be eligible for desensitisation treatment. We further stratify the immunological risk based on the number of transplant (first or retransplant), the presence of donor-specific antibodies (DSA) against the organ offer and the combination of other immunological test results (see section 3.1).

3 Assessment of the sensitised transplant candidate

The approach varies depending on whether the transplant candidate has a potential living donor. For sensitised patients with one or more potential living donors, we first perform antibody screenings and a virtual crossmatch to determine whether the patient has donor-specific anti-HLA antibodies (DSA). In addition, we perform a physical crossmatch (CDC crossmatch) with T, B and unseparated lymphocytes. The laboratory test results help us evaluate the potential risk of antibody-mediated rejection (AMR) and, if appropriate, consider desensitisation therapy, or advise against transplantation with the donor tested. All sensitised patients with a potential living donor are also listed for a deceased donor transplant.

Patients with a negative CDC crossmatch may be DSA negative or positive (that means, in the absence or presence of DSA in Luminex single antigen bead assays). This includes patients with a history of DSA that were not detectable at the time of testing above a defined MFI cut-off, which is a common scenario because DSAs can wane over time and/or fluctuate above and below the level of detection. Furthermore, patients may have memory B cells that can re-emerge upon antigen stimulation. For example, mothers may have been exposed to foreign HLA antigens in pregnancies and can mount a memory response when receiving a transplant from their child or their husband, although DSA were not detectable during antibody screening. Therefore, pre-sensitised patients with a negative CDC crossmatch are at risk of developing acute and/or chronic AMR, especially if low levels of DSA are present. We perform peri-operative desensitisation in these cases. For sensitised patients (vPRA ≥ 30%) without a potential living donor, we register them for the deceased-donor transplant list and offer pre-transplant desensitisation once an HLA incompatible, but otherwise acceptable organ offer is available (see section 4.2).

3.1 Assessment and classification of sensitised transplant candidates in Heidelberg

Patients are classified in four immunological risk categories based on their pre-transplant immunological work-up.

Risk category	Criteria (the presence of at least one criterion is sufficient)	Immunosuppressive therapy
High risk	• CDC PRA > 85% • Positive reactivity in the Luminex screening test for both class I and class II HLA antigens • In candidates for re-transplants, positive reactivity in the Luminex screening test for class I only • In candidates for re-transplants, positive reactivity in the Luminex screening test for class II only plus a positive B cell CDC crossmatch	See section 4.2
Intermediate high risk	Low level DSA that were not listed as unacceptable antigens (= DSA with MFI value < 3000 in patients with known allosensitising events; or < 5000 (in patients without previous allosensitisation)	Thymoglobulin, tacrolimus, MMF, steroids • pre-Tx: 1 x plasma exchange • post-Tx: 2 x plasma exchange
Intermediate low risk	vPRA > 30%, no detectable DSA (defined by using an MFI cutoff of 1,000)	Thymoglobulin, tacrolimus, MMF, steroids
Low risk	vPRA ≤ 30%, no detectable DSA (defined by using an MFI cutoff of 1,000)	IL2-receptor antagonists, Tacrolimus, MMF, steroids

The MFI values are measured with One Lambda Luminex test kits and may not be applicable to the Luminex kits from other vendors.

4 Pre-transplant desensitisation

The overall goal of HLA desensitisation is to increase the likelihood of a successful kidney transplant in patients with extensive HLA antibody sensitisation and to prevent post-transplant AMR in these patients. Desensitisation can be performed on patients awaiting either a living or deceased donor transplant. While the objectives are similar in both contexts, the approach may differ due to the unpredictable timing of deceased-donor transplantation in relation to the administration of desensitisation therapy. Although there is no universally accepted HLA desensitisation protocol, the most commonly used protocols employ a combination of the following strategies: (i) Immunomodulation of the recipient's immune system, typically with intravenous immunoglobulins (IVIG); (ii) B cell depletion, most commonly with the anti-CD20 monoclonal antibody rituximab; (iii) removal of circulating HLA antibodies, typically with extracorporeal methods such as plasmapheresis or immunoadsorption.

4.1 The Heidelberg approach to desensitisation

HLA desensitisation strategies vary between transplant centres, depending on clinical experience and preference. There is a lack of high-quality data in the form of randomised controlled trials comparing existing desensitisation approaches, and the optimal therapy remains undefined. The most critical components of an integrative approach are pre-transplant identification of high-risk patients on the waiting list (see Section 3.1) and risk-stratified organ allocation. For instance, patients with a high vPRA and/or positive results for both class I and II HLA antibodies in the Luminex antibody screening test are at an increased risk of graft loss. Such patients can be successfully and promptly transplanted if there are only a few HLA mismatches [2] or the transplantation is facilitated via the Eurotransplant Acceptable Mismatch Programme, which allocates organs to highly immunised patients with high priority [3].

All patients categorised as high risk receive apheresis treatment (one session pre-operatively and at least six sessions post-operatively until serum creatinine falls below 2 mg/dL and DSA become undetectable) during a deceased-donor organ offer process or in preparation for transplantation from a living donor. This treatment is used to reduce the level of potentially undetected antibodies and prevent an acute antibody-mediated allograft injury due to an early rebound of pre-existing DSA. To prevent the development of *de novo* DSA, apheresis is combined with the administration of the anti-B cell antibody rituximab. B cells are important antigen-presenting cells that are critical for T cell activation and the development of T cell memory during alloimmune responses. Despite having no effect on long-lived plasma cells, anti-CD20 therapy has been associated with a reduction in DSA reactivity in some reports. Rituximab may prevent antibody-producing cells from being generated from the naïve B cell pool and may target short-lived plasma cells that express CD20 on their surface. In addition, anti-CD20 therapy may deplete B cell aggregates within allografts. High-risk patients also receive T cell-depleting induction therapy with thymoglobulin, which targets an early T cell response that would support the development of *de novo* DSA. The Heidelberg Algorithm for diagnosing AMR in the early stages after successful kidney transplantation involves protocol biopsies on days 7 and 90, as well as post-transplant antibody monitoring.

Post-transplant antibody monitoring has been refined further with the introduction of the C1q assay. DSA with MFI greater than 3000 can be further tested for the presence of C1q-binding capacity. According to some reports, the appearance of C1q-binding DSA post-transplant can be considered a major risk factor for graft loss due to AMR [4, 5, 6].

4.2 Desensitization protocol for patients at high immunological risk on the *deceased donor* waiting list

See section 3.1 for definitions of high immunological risk.

1. A serum is taken before (and, optionally also after) plasmapheresis for a prospective CDC crossmatch.
2. Plasmapheresis (exchange volume = 2 times plasma volume; substitute with fresh frozen plasma [FFP] and citrate anticoagulation).
3. If the CDC crossmatch is negative (T lymphocytes, B lymphocytes, unseparated lymphocytes without and with DTT), administer Thymoglobulin® (dose: 1.5 mg/kg), followed by rituximab (dose: 375 mg/m^2). Kidney transplantation can then be performed. *Caution:* Since 200 mg/m^2 of methylprednisolone is administered for desensitisation prior to Thymoglobulin administration, only 100 mg/m^2 of methylprednisolone is given intraoperatively instead of the usual dose of 300 mg/m^2.
4. If the CDC crossmatch with either serum (pre- or post-plasmapheresis) is positive, kidney transplantation cannot be performed.
5. Tacrolimus, MMF and methylprednisolone are administered according to the standard regimen.
6. Following surgery, a further 2–3 doses of Thymoglobulin® are administered, with the dosage adjusted according to the total lymphocyte count (target: 100/µl).
7. Postoperatively, plasmapheresis or immunoadsorption is performed until transplant function stabilises, i.e. until serum creatinine falls below 2 mg/dL, GFR exceeds 30 mL/min/1.73 m^2 and DSA is less than 1,000 MFI. This process continues for at least six treatment sessions in the first two weeks post-transplant.

8. Prophylaxis against infection with cotrimoxazole for 12 months and valganciclovir as indicated.
9. Protocol biopsies are performed on days 7 and 90 post-transplant.
10. Perform an indication biopsy in the event of deterioration in graft function, an increase in pre-existing DSA and/or the development of *de novo* DSA.
11. Monitor DSA on days 0, 7, 30, 180, and then every six months, as well as on the intermediate days between plasmapheresis sessions initially.

4.3 Desensitisation protocol for patients at high immunological risk with a *living donor*

See section 3.1 for definition of high immunological risk.

1. At least six immunoadsorption sessions (Globaffin column, Fresenius) should be performed prior to transplantation. ACE inhibitor therapy should be discontinued one week beforehand. Immunoadsorption is performed on alternate days. Further postoperative immunoadsorption may be necessary until the serum creatinine level falls below 2 mg/dL, the GFR is greater than 30 mL/min/1.73 m^2, and the DSA is less than 1000 MFI.
2. DSA are determined on the days when no immunoadsorption takes place. If DSA reactivities are reduced below 1000 MFI, transplantation can be performed and has to be carried out as soon as possible due to potential DSA rebound.
3. Immunosuppressive therapy involving tacrolimus, mycophenolate mofetil (MMF) and methylprednisolone (24 mg/m^2 intravenously in the morning) should be started one week prior to transplant surgery.
4. Thymoglobulin® is administered preoperatively at a dose of 1.5 mg/kg.
5. Subsequently, rituximab is administered intravenously at a dose of 375 mg/m^2 pre-/intraoperatively.
6. Postoperatively, two to three further doses of Thymoglobulin® are administered, adjusted according to the total lymphocyte count (target: 100/µl). *Caution:* Since 200 mg/m^2 of methylprednisolone is administered prior to Thymoglobulin® administration, only 100 mg/m^2 is given intraoperatively.
7. Oral methylprednisolone is administered according to the standard regimen.
8. Prophylaxis against infection with cotrimoxazole (for 12 months) and valganciclovir (as indicated).

9. Protocol biopsies are performed on days 7 and 90 post-transplant.
10. Indications for biopsy include deterioration of graft function, an increase in pre-existing DSA and/or the development of *de novo* DSA.
11. Monitor DSA on days 0, 7, 30, 180 and then every six months. Initially, monitor on intermediate days when no immunoadsorption takes place.

5 Outcome

The decision to proceed with an HLA-incompatible kidney transplant rather than wait longer for a more suitable donor is often difficult, especially given the increased mortality observed among adult dialysis patients compared with transplant recipients [7]. In virtually all patient populations, the long-term risk of death is lower with a kidney transplant than with dialysis [8, 9]. A large multicentre study of 1,025 recipients of an HLA-incompatible living-donor kidney transplant found higher short- and long-term (up to eight years) patient survival rates among recipients of an HLA-incompatible transplant compared with matched controls on the waiting list [10]. Overall, however, a greater degree of HLA incompatibility is associated with a higher risk of graft loss and death. A positive flow or cytotoxic crossmatch was found to be associated with a 1.65- and 1.80-fold higher risk of graft loss, and a 1.32- and 1.51-fold higher risk of death, respectively, compared with HLA compatible recipients [11]. This study found that five-year unadjusted graft loss was 17%, 20%, 29%, and 40% for HLA compatible recipients, recipients with DSA but a negative flow crossmatch, recipients with a positive flow crossmatch but negative cytotoxic crossmatch and recipients with a positive cytotoxic crossmatch kidney transplant, respectively. The five-year unadjusted mortality rate was 9%, 10%, 13%, and 19% for HLA-compatible recipients, recipients with DSA but a negative flow crossmatch, recipients with a positive flow crossmatch but negative cytotoxic crossmatch, and recipients with a positive cytotoxic crossmatch kidney transplant, respectively.

In Heidelberg, we found that our approach can be used to transplant high-risk sensitised patients with graft survival rates similar to those of non-sensitised kidney recipients. In 28 adult recipients of deceased donor kidneys, the one-year graft survival rate, death-censored graft survival rate, and patient survival rate were 92%, 96%, and 96%, respectively. No graft loss or patient death was observed in the six living donor kidney recipients [12]. AMR occurred in one living and two deceased donor kidney transplant recipients during follow-up. This therapy was accompanied by rigorous infection prophylaxis with valganciclovir when the donor is CMV-positive and cotrimoxazole in all patients.

There are few published reports on the outcome of desensitisation protocols in paediatric kidney transplant recipients. One UK study reported that, of 711 living donor kidney transplants performed in the UK, six were HLA-incompatible [13]. At a median follow-up of 6.8 (3.6–14.0) years, patient survival was 100% and 96% in the HLA-incompatible and HLA-compatible groups, respectively. Death-censored kidney allograft survival was 100% in both groups at the final follow-up. There were no cases of primary non-function in the HLA-incompatible group, compared to 2% in the HLA-compatible group. The authors concluded that HLA-incompatible kidney transplantation is a feasible option for paediatric recipients when no compatible donors are available. However, an increasing degree of incompatibility is overall associated with a higher risk of graft loss. Data on infection-related complications in this population are limited, with some studies showing similar overall infection rates to those of average transplant recipients.

6 Investigational approaches

Several investigational therapies are being evaluated for use in desensitisation regimens. One such therapy is imlifidase, an IgG-degrading enzyme derived from Streptococcus pyogenes. This recombinant cysteine protease cleaves all four subclasses of human IgG into F(ab')2 and Fc fragments, thereby inhibiting complement-dependent cytotoxicity (CDC) and antibody-dependent cellular cytotoxicity. Imlifidase has received conditional approval from the European Medicines Agency (EMA) for use in desensitisation procedures for adult kidney transplantation within the European Union (so far not for paediatric patients). It is not yet approved by the US Food and Drug Administration (FDA) for use in the United States. Three-year outcomes were reported in an analysis that pooled adult patients from four open-label phase II studies [14]. Of the 39 patients who underwent a positive crossmatch kidney transplant, 15 (38%) experienced AMR. Overall three-year graft survival was 84%; among patients who experienced AMR, three-year graft survival was 93%, compared to 77% among those who did not. Among the 13 patients with vPRA of at least 99.9%, who were considered unlikely to have been transplanted under conventional protocols, three-year graft survival was comparable with that of the overall study population (92%) after receiving a positive crossmatch deceased-donor allograft.

However, seven of these patients (54%) experienced AMR within six months of the transplant, although none of the graft losses were attributed to AMR. Overall, the initial experience with imlifidase is encouraging, suggesting that it can facilitate HLA incompatible transplantation, although further research is required.

References

1 Süsal C, Fichtner A, Tönshoff B, Mehrabi A, Zeier M, Morath C. Clinical Relevance of HLA Antibodies in Kidney Transplantation: Recent Data from the Heidelberg Transplant Center and the Collaborative Transplant Study. J Immunol Res. 2017;2017:5619402.
2 Süsal C, Döhler B, Opelz G. Presensitized kidney graft recipients with HLA class I and II antibodies are at increased risk for graft failure: a Collaborative Transplant Study report. Human Immunology, 70: 569–573, 2009.
3 Claas FH, Rahmel A, Doxiadis II. Enhanced kidney allocation to highly sensitized patients by the acceptable mismatch program. Transplantation, 88: 447–452, 2009.
4 Loupy A, Lefaucheur C, Vernerey D et al. Complement-binding anti-HLA antibodies and kidney-allograft survival. N Engl J Med 369: 1215–1226, 2013.
5 Schaefer SM, Süsal C, Opelz G et al. Pre-transplant soluble CD30 in combination with total DSA but not pre-transplant C1q-DSA predicts antibody-mediated graft loss in presensitized high-risk kidney transplant recipients. HLA 87: 89–99, 2016.
6 Süsal C, Wettstein D, Döhler B et al. Association of kidney graft loss with de novo produced donor-specific and nondonor-specific HLA antibodies detected by single antigen testing. Transplantation, 99: 1976–1980, 2015.
7 Gill JS, Tonelli M, Johnson N, et al. The impact of waiting time and comorbid conditions on the survival benefit of kidney transplantation. Kidney Int 2005; 68:2345.
8 Merion RM, Ashby VB, Wolfe RA, et al. Deceased-donor characteristics and the survival benefit of kidney transplantation. JAMA 2005; 294:2726.
9 Massie AB, Luo X, Chow EK, et al. Survival benefit of primary deceased donor transplantation with high-KDPI kidneys. Am J Transplant 2014; 14:2310.

10 Orandi BJ, Luo X, Massie AB, et al. Survival Benefit with Kidney Transplants from HLA-Incompatible Live Donors. N Engl J Med 2016; 374:940.
11 Orandi BJ, Garonzik-Wang JM, Massie AB, et al. Quantifying the risk of incompatible kidney transplantation: a multicenter study. Am J Transplant 2014; 14:1573.
12 Morath C, Beimler J, Opelz G et al. An integrative approach for the transplantation of high-risk sensitized patients. Transplantation 90: 645–653, 2010.
13 Hew EY, Kessaris N, Stojanovic J, Jones H, Christian M, Edwards A, Milford DV, Ognjanovic M, Shenoy M, Baker RJ, Marks SD. Successful ABO and HLA incompatible kidney transplantation in children in the UK. Pediatr Nephrol. 2023 Feb;38(2):529–535.
14 Kjellman C, Maldonado AQ, Sjöholm K, et al. Outcomes at 3 years post-transplant in imlifidase-desensitized kidney transplant patients. Am J Transplant 2021; 21:3907.

CHAPTER 5.3 ABO-incompatible living donor kidney transplantation

Burkhard Tönshoff[1], Christian Morath[2, 3], Martin Zeier[2], Caner Süsal[4, 5] & Lars Pape[6]

[1] Heidelberg University, Medical Faculty Heidelberg, Department of Paediatrics I, University Children's Hospital, Heidelberg, Germany
[2] Department of Nephrology, University Hospital Heidelberg
[3] Clinic for Internal Medicine, Nephrology, Nuremberg Hospital, Germany
[4] Heidelberg University, Medical Faculty Heidelberg, Institute of Immunology, Transplantation Immunology, Heidelberg, Germany
[5] Transplant Immunology Research Center of Excellence, Koç University School of Medicine, Istanbul, Turkey
[6] Department of Paediatrics II, University Hospital of Essen, Essen, Germany

ORCIDs:
Burkhard Tönshoff: https://orcid.org/0000-0002-6598-6910
Christian Morath: https://orcid.org/0000-0003-2218-7817
Caner Süsal: https://orcid.org/0000-0003-2521-8201
Lars Pape: https://orcid.org/0000-0002-3635-6418

1 Introduction

Although kidney transplantation is still best performed in the absence of major ABO incompatibility, long waiting times for a deceased donor kidney transplant exceed eight years for adults in some countries, such as Germany, due to a large kidney failure population and an increasing organ shortage. One way to reduce waiting times is to perform transplants across ABO antibody barriers [1]. In theory, the number of kidney transplants from living donors could increase by up to 30% if patients were transplanted across the ABO antibody barrier. Using current protocols, up to 90% of patients with ABO incompatibility with their living donor can be effectively desensitised and transplanted. Desensitisation protocols aim to reduce and maintain anti-A/B antibodies (isoagglutinins) below a safe threshold (e.g., < 1:32 in the tube technique) during the first two weeks after transplantation. Thereafter, even when anti-A/B antibodies reappear at high levels, they will not harm the kidney transplant, a phenomenon known as accommodation. In recent years, graft survival rates after ABO-incompatible (ABOi) kidney transplantation have almost equalled those after ABO-compatible (ABOc) procedures. However, transplantation in the presence of major ABO incompatibility places the patient at a somewhat higher risk of early rejection, infection and infection-associated death. Therefore, ABOc procedures should be preferred wherever possible.

2 Blood group antigens and antibodies

The ABO antigen system consists of oligosaccharides that are predominantly found on red blood cells, as well as on endothelial cells, tubules and glomeruli. This makes the ABO antigen system important for kidney transplantation. Patients with different blood groups have different antigen densities on their erythrocytes. Compared to individuals with blood group A1 or B, individuals with blood group A2 (who make up 20% of all Caucasians with blood group A) have low expression (30–50%) of blood group antigen molecules on the surface of erythrocytes. This is believed to be responsible for the lower immunogenicity of organs from A2 donors [2, 3]. Due to the lower immunogenic risk posed by the A2 antigen, A2 donor kidneys can generally be successfully transplanted into non-A recipients with low pre-transplant anti-A titres without the need for desensitisation [4].

Anti-A/B antibodies are formed upon contact with gut bacteria in the early stages of infancy. Naturally occurring anti-A/B antibodies are predominantly of the IgM class, but in individuals with blood group O, they also consist of the IgG and IgA classes [5]. While the pathogenic importance of anti-A/B antibodies in solid organ transplantation is well known, the relative contribution of the different immunoglobulin isotypes and their subclasses to organ rejection remains to be elucidated. Individuals with blood group O tend to produce higher levels of anti-A and anti-B isoagglutinin antibodies than individuals with blood groups A or B, and recipients with blood group O have a higher incidence of antibody-mediated rejection (ABMR) following ABOi transplantation, although graft survival does not differ among blood groups.

The way in which institutions measure and report isoagglutinin antibody titres varies [8, 9], which makes it difficult to compare ABOi protocols and outcomes in the literature. The classic tube dilution method is most commonly used to report IgM isoagglutinin titres (saline test) and total isoagglutinin titres (indirect antiglobulin [Coombs] test), although direct IgG measurements can be obtained by treating plasma with dithiothreitol prior to testing to inactivate IgM. As the test depends on visual interpretation of the degree of agglutination, it should be considered semi-quantitative and may be subject to interobserver variability. Therefore, the reported result should be considered an approximation, meaning that a titre of 1:128 could represent values between 1:64 and 1:256. Although centre-specific protocols vary, the total isoagglutinin antibody titre is generally reduced to ≤ 1:8 before transplantation, as higher titres are associated with acute antibody-mediated rejection (ABMR) post-transplant [10].

3 Desensitisation for ABOi kidney transplantation

Despite the absence of a generally accepted desensitisation protocol for transplantation across the ABO antibody barrier, all currently proposed strategies share some common principles: (i) anti-A/B antibody depletion at the time of transplantation using plasmapheresis (PP), double-filtration PP/membrane filtration or selective/unselective immunoadsorption (IA); (ii) modulation of the recipient's immune system using intravenous immunoglobulins (IVIG); and (iii) reduction of the B lymphocyte pool using the anti-CD20 antibody rituximab. Figure 1 provides an overview of the Heidelberg desensitisation protocol for ABO-incompatible living donor kidney transplantation.

Figure 1 Desensitization protocol for ABOi living donor kidney transplantation at the University of Heidelberg. Anti-CD20 therapy is usually performed with rituximab 375 mg/m^2, anti-IL-2R therapy is performed with basiliximab. IA, immunoadsorption; PP, plasmapheresis (modified from ref. [1]).

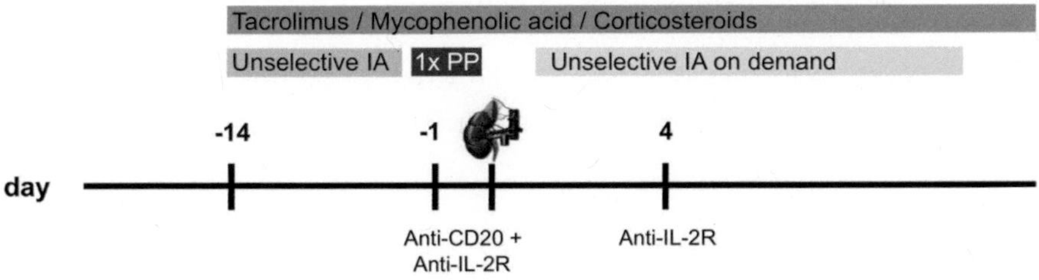

3.1 Antibody depletion by extracorporeal treatment

The patient's initial ABO isoagglutinin titres must be ≤1:256 for both IgG and IgM, as determined by the tube dilution method. Reducing circulating anti-A/B antibody levels to predetermined target titres is a key component of the ABO desensitisation protocol. The two most commonly used methods of antibody removal are plasmapheresis and immunoadsorption, with the aim of achieving titres of ≤ 1:8. In general, the titre can be expected to decrease by one dilution with each plasmapheresis session. This can be used to estimate the number of sessions necessary to achieve the target titre. For example, if the initial antibody level is 1:128, three plasmapheresis sessions are required to achieve a level of 1:16 (1:128 to 1:64, 1:64 to 1:32 and 1:32 to 1:16).

Antibody removal strategies can be categorised as methods that completely remove plasma proteins, such as plasmapheresis (PP); methods that remove a specific fraction of plasma proteins, including immunoglobulins, such as membrane separation; and more specific methods, such as unselective or selective immunoadsorption (IA). PP is the preferred antibody removal strategy in the United States, whereas membrane separation is popular in Japan and unselective and selective IAs are commonly used in Europe. Selective anti-A/B antibody removal is feasible using Glycosorb columns (Glykorex Transplantation AB, Lund, Sweden) containing a synthetic terminal tri-saccharide A or B blood group antigen linked to a sepharose matrix. These columns can also reduce total IgG, as well as IgG against polysaccharide antigens, such as anti-pneumococcus IgG [11]. Our centre in Heidelberg uses a desensitisation protocol for ABOi kidney transplant candidates that is very similar to the Swedish protocol [12, 13]. The main difference is the use of unselective instead of selective IA, which also allows desensitisation for HLA-incompatible living donor kidney transplantation. Other differences include the omission of IVIG application and the number of IA treatments varying depending on the strength of the anti-A/B antibodies. To more efficiently remove pathogenically relevant anti-A/B antibodies of the IgM class, at least one additional plasma purification (PP) treatment is performed in all patients the day before surgery [14].

3.2 Intravenous immunoglobulins

Many centres administer intravenous immunoglobulins before ABOi kidney transplantation to prevent anti-A/B antibody rebound in the early phase after transplantation. Additionally, IVIG infusion is believed to reduce infectious complications by replacing depleted immunoglobulins. However, it should be noted that IVIG preparations contain IgG antibodies directed against A/B antigens, which can increase anti-A/B antibody titres upon administration [12]. Some centres administer 0.5–2 g/kg of IVIG (maximum dose 140 g) immediately after the final plasmapheresis session. The optimal IVIG dose is uncertain.

3.3 B-cell depletion by splenectomy or rituximab

Prior to the introduction of pharmacological anti-B-cell therapies, splenectomy was an integral component of reducing the B-lymphocyte pool before ABOi kidney transplantation. However, due to the associated surgical risks and increased risk of sepsis, splenectomy has gradually been replaced by the anti-CD20 antibody rituximab. More recently, several groups have completely abandoned anti-B cell therapies in their protocols. However, the Collaborative Transplant Study (CTS) revealed a numerically higher rate of death-censored graft loss in ABOi kidney transplant recipients when rituximab was omitted (see below) [15].

3.4 Monitoring after transplantation

Following ABO desensitisation and transplantation, patients are monitored using an approach similar to that used for recipients of ABOc transplants. In addition, we monitor isoagglutinin titres daily while the patient is in hospital and twice weekly for the first month post-transplant. Pre-emptive plasmapheresis should be performed in patients with an isoagglutinin titre of ≥ 1:16 in the first week or ≥ 1:32 in the second week post-transplant, and a kidney biopsy should be performed if there is evidence of graft dysfunction (e.g., delayed/slow graft function or rising serum creatinine). We do not routinely perform protocol plasmapheresis post-transplant.

4 Outcome

The Heidelberg group reported CTS data on the three-year outcomes of 1,420 adult ABOi kidney transplant recipients who underwent transplantation at 101 different centres between 2005 and 2012 [15]. Patients were compared to a matched group of ABOc kidney transplant recipients, as well as to all ABOc kidney transplant recipients from centres that had performed at least five ABOi procedures. There were no statistically significant differences in overall graft survival, death-censored graft survival, or patient survival between the groups. However, early patient survival was reduced in ABOi kidney transplant recipients due to a higher rate of infection-associated death in the early stages. Specifically, an additional death per 100 patients occurred within the first year of

ABOi kidney transplantation due to an infectious complication. There was a trend towards a better 3-year death-censored graft survival in patients receiving anti-CD20 therapy, suggesting the need for anti-B cell therapies in cases of ABO incompatibility.

While studies initially focused on adult donors and recipients, evidence supporting this practice for paediatric recipients has increased in recent years. In 2018, an analysis of the Japanese Kidney Transplant Registry was published which described the results of 102 children who received ABOi kidney transplants from living donors. The outcomes of these recipients were compared with those of children on the registry who had undergone ABOc living donor transplantations. No difference was found in patient or allograft survival between the two groups [16]. The protocol involved the use of rituximab ± immunoadsorption and/or double filtration plasmapheresis if titres were ≥ 1:8. Several centres in the UK have reported on the outcomes of ABOi kidney transplantation in a cohort of 23 children, and have similarly found no statistically significant difference in patient or allograft survival, acute rejection, or graft function compared to ABO-compatible living donor transplants [17]. Other centres in Sweden [18] and Japan [19], which use a similar desensitisation approach, have also shared equally encouraging results. Some studies have even found that infants with low antibody titres prior to ABOi transplantation did not require pre-transplant desensitisation to achieve excellent results [18].

5 Complication and hurdles

5.1 Accommodation versus rejection

Unlike transplantation in HLA-sensitised patients, accommodation appears to be a frequent phenomenon after ABO incompatible (ABOi) kidney transplantation and is often associated with C4d deposition in the peritubular capillaries of allograft biopsies. The accommodation phenotype can be achieved through controlled exposure to anti-A/B antibodies in the early post-transplant phase. Approximately two weeks after successful transplantation, accommodation is established, rendering the kidney transplant resistant to even high anti-A/B antibody exposure. One possible mechanism is the local upregulation of complement regulatory proteins, such as CD45, CD55 and CD59, as a consequence of anti-A/B antibody-dependent inactivation of the ERK1/2 signalling pathway [20].

5.2 Infection and malignancy

The literature contains conflicting results regarding infectious complications after ABOi kidney transplantation. A higher frequency of viral infections, such as cytomegalovirus (CMV), herpes simplex virus (HSV), varicella zoster virus (VZV) and BK virus, as well as Pneumocystis jiroveci pneumonia, wound infections and severe urinary tract infections, has been reported in adults [1]. In the CTS and Heidelberg cohorts, an increased risk of severe early infections was observed, resulting in approximately one additional death per 100 ABOi kidney transplant recipients during the first year post-transplant [15]. We and others have also observed a higher incidence of BK virus replication and BK virus-associated nephropathy [1]. An increased risk of malignancy was, however, not found in an analysis of 1,420 ABOi transplants from the CTS study [15].

5.3 Risk of bleeding and surgical complications

A study from the US Renal Data System registry found an increased risk of early haemorrhage in 119 ABOi kidney transplant recipients compared to ABOc controls [21]. A higher bleeding risk was also observed in our cohort of three paediatric kidney transplant recipients, with two experiencing major bleeding episodes. This was attributed to the non-specific binding of coagulation factors during repeated IA [22]. This is supported by the findings of de Weerd et al., who found a significant correlation between the number of pre-transplant apheresis treatments and peri- and post-transplant bleeding risk [23]. Some authors have observed an increased rate of surgical complications following ABOi kidney transplantation. These complications have been attributed to the intensified immunosuppression involving mycophenolic acid, as well as the removal of coagulation factors through apheresis. The Freiburg group reported a significantly higher number of lymphoceles in ABOi patients than in ABOc controls (33% versus 15%; P = 0.003), with surgical revision required in 20% and 8% of patients, respectively (P = 0.013) [24]. Furthermore, the overall need for surgical revision was significantly higher in ABOi patients than in ABOc controls (38% vs. 24%; P = 0.032).

6 An ABOi transplant from a living donor or an ABOc transplant from a deceased donor?

In light of mounting evidence of favourable outcomes following ABOi kidney transplantation in children as well as evidence of improved allograft survival in kidneys from living donors, some centres are considering ABOi living donor kidney transplantation for children prior to listing them for deceased donor organs. However, to date, there has been no prospective study comparing the outcomes of patients receiving ABOi living donor transplants with those receiving ABO-compatible transplants from deceased donors. Some experts argue that ABOi transplants should be considered as an option for paediatric patients prior to proceeding with a transplant from a deceased donor, as this approach has the potential to lead to improved patient and allograft outcomes.

Other authors have argued that ABOi kidney transplantation carries a higher risk of rejection compared to ABO-compatible transplantation, particularly antibody-mediated rejection [25]. To overcome this, extensive pre-transplant conditioning and additional pre-transplant immunosuppressive therapy are required, including desensitisation techniques and intensified immunosuppression protocols. However, such complex treatments may expose children to a higher risk of bacterial and viral infections, post-transplant lymphoproliferative disease and other neoplasms. Apheresis techniques require central venous lines in the absence of an arteriovenous fistula, particularly in children undergoing peritoneal dialysis or pre-emptive transplantation. These procedures can be complicated by infection, thrombosis or bleeding, which can jeopardise future access to dialysis. Furthermore, these techniques may be impractical or risky in young children due to the volume of extracorporeal fluid required during immunoadsorption sessions. Therefore, ABOi kidney transplantation is rarely performed in children with a body weight below 20 kg. Furthermore, from an economic standpoint, ABOi transplantation is more expensive and resource-intensive than ABOc transplantation. The additional procedures, prolonged hospital stays and specialised therapies required for desensitisation significantly increase the overall cost of the transplant procedure. Additionally, some parents may wish to retain the option of donating a kidney for a second transplant in adulthood, when organ shortages may be even greater. Therefore, the advantages and disadvantages outlined above must be considered in the context of each child's specific medical condition and individual circumstances. The decision to pursue ABOi kidney transplantation should be made in consultation with the child's medical team, weighing up the potential benefits and risks.

References

1 Morath C, Zeier M, Döhler B, Opelz G, Süsal C. ABO-Incompatible Kidney Transplantation. Front Immunol. 2017 Mar 6;8:234. doi: 10.3389/fimmu.2017.00234. eCollection 2017
2 Alexandre GP, De Bruyere M, Squifflet JP, Moriau M, Latinne D, Pirson Y. Human ABO-incompatible living donor renal homografts. Neth J Med (1985) 28(6):231–4.
3 Squifflet JP, De Meyer M, Malaise J, Latinne D, Pirson Y, Alexandre GP. Lessons learned from ABO-incompatible living donor kidney transplantation: 20 years later. Exp Clin Transplant (2004) 2(1):208–13.
4 Forbes RC, Feurer ID, Shaffer D. A2 incompatible kidney transplantation does not adversely affect graft or patient survival. Clin Transplant (2016) 30(5):589–97. doi:10.1111/ctr.12724
5 Rieben R, Buchs JP, Fluckiger E, Nydegger UE. Antibodies to histo-blood group substances A and B: agglutination titers, Ig class, and IgG subclasses in healthy persons of different age categories. Transfusion (1991) 31(7):607–15.
6 Toki D, Ishida H, Horita S, et al. Blood group O recipients associated with early graft deterioration in living ABO-incompatible kidney transplantation. Transplantation 2009; 88:1186.
7 Montgomery JR, Berger JC, Warren DS, et al. Outcomes of ABO-incompatible kidney transplantation in the United States. Transplantation 2012; 93:603.
8 Kobayashi T, Saito K. A series of surveys on assay for anti-A/B antibody by Japanese ABO-incompatible Transplantation Committee. Xenotransplantation 2006; 13:136.
9 Kumlien G, Wilpert J, Säfwenberg J, Tydén G. Comparing the tube and gel techniques for ABO antibody titration, as performed in three European centers. Transplantation 2007; 84:S17.
10 Toki D, Ishida H, Setoguchi K, et al. Acute antibody-mediated rejection in living ABO-incompatible kidney transplantation: long-term impact and risk factors. Am J Transplant 2009; 9:567.
11 Valli PV, Puga Yung G, Fehr T, Schulz-Huotari C, Kaup N, Gungor T, et al. Changes of circulating antibody levels induced by ABO antibody adsorption for ABO-incompatible kidney transplantation. Am J Transplant (2009) 9(5):1072–80.

12 Morath C, Becker LE, Leo A, Beimler J, Klein K, Seckinger J, et al. ABO-incompatible kidney transplantation enabled by non-antigen-specific immunoadsorption. Transplantation (2012) 93(8):827–34.
13 Staley EM, Carruba SS, Manning M, Pham HP, Williams LA III, Marques MB, et al. Anti-blood group antibodies in intravenous immunoglobulin may complicate interpretation of antibody titers in ABO-incompatible transplantation. Am J Transplant (2016) 16(8):2483–6.
14 Becker LE, Siebert D, Susal C, Opelz G, Leo A, Waldherr R, et al. Outcomes following ABO-incompatible kidney transplantation performed after desensitization by nonantigen-specific immunoadsorption. Transplantation (2015) 99(11):2364–71.
15 Opelz G, Morath C, Süsal C, Tran TH, Zeier M, Döhler B. Three-year outcomes following 1420 ABO-incompatible living-donor kidney transplants performed after ABO antibody reduction: results from 101 centers. Transplantation. 2015 Feb;99(2):400–4.
16 Hattori M, Mieno M, Shishido S, Aikawa A, Ushigome H, Ohshima S, et al. Outcomes of Pediatric ABO-Incompatible Living Kidney Transplantations From 2002 to 2015: An Analysis of the Japanese Kidney Transplant Registry. Transplantation (2018) 102(11):1934–42.
17 Hew EY, Kessaris N, Stojanovic J, Jones H, Christian M, Edwards A, et al. Successful ABO and HLA Incompatible Kidney Transplantation in Children in the UK. Pediatr Nephrol (2023) 38(2):529–35.
18 Tydén G, Kumlien G, Berg UB. ABO-Incompatible Kidney Transplantation in Children. Pediatr Transpl (2011) 15(5):502–4.
19 Aikawa A, Kawamura T, Shishido S, Saito K, Takahashi K; ABO-Incompatible Transplantation Committee members. ABO-incompatible living-donor pediatric kidney transplantation in Japan. Clinics (Sao Paulo). 2014;69 Suppl 1(Suppl 1):22–7.
20 Iwasaki K, Miwa Y, Ogawa H, Yazaki S, Iwamoto M, Furusawa T, et al. Comparative study on signal transduction in endothelial cells after anti-a/b and human leukocyte antigen antibody reaction: implication of accommodation. Transplantation (2012) 93(4):390–7.
21 Lentine KL, Axelrod D, Klein C, Simpkins C, Xiao H, Schnitzler MA, et al. Early clinical complications after ABO-incompatible live-donor kidney transplantation: a national study of medicare-insured recipients. Transplantation (2014) 98(1):54–65.

22 Schäfer B, Tönshoff B, Schmidt J, Golriz M, Mehrabi A, Gombos P, Morath C, Wühl E, Schaefer F, Schmitt CP. Bleeding complications in pediatric ABO-incompatible kidney transplantation. Pediatr Nephrol. 2013 Feb;28(2):327–32.
23 de Weerd AE, van Agteren M, Leebeek FW, Ijzermans JN, Weimar W, Betjes MG. ABO-incompatible kidney transplant recipients have a higher bleeding risk after antigen-specific immunoadsorption. Transpl Int (2015) 28(1):25–33.
24 Zschiedrich S, Janigen B, Dimova D, Neumann A, Seidl M, Hils S, et al. One hundred ABO-incompatible kidney transplantations between 2004 and 2014: a single-centre experience. Nephrol Dial Transplant (2016) 31(4):663–71.
25 Boyer O, Pape L. Is ABO Incompatible Living Donor Kidney Transplantation in Children a Better Option than the Use of Optimal Grafts From Deceased Donors? A Plea for Better Prioritization of Deceased Kidney Grafts for Children. Transpl Int. 2023 Sep 18;36:11911.

CHAPTER 6
Rejection

CHAPTER 6.1 Diagnosis and treatment of acute and chronic cellular transplant rejection

Lars Pape[1], Nele Kanzelmeyer[2], Jan Ulrich Becker[3] & Jun Oh[4]

[1] Department of Paediatrics II, University Hospital of Essen, Essen, Germany
[2] Department of Paediatric Nephrology, Hepatology, Metabolic and Neurology Diseases, Hannover Medical School, Hannover, Germany
[3] Department of Pathology, University Hospital of Cologne, Cologne, Germany
[4] Department of Paediatric Nephrology and Hepatology, University Hospital Eppendorf, Hamburg, Germany

ORCIDs:
Lars Pape: https://orcid.org/0000-0002-3635-6418
Nele Kanzelmeyer: https://orcid.org/0000-0002-4865-4906
Jan Ulrich Becker: https://orcid.org/0000-0003-2929-8085
Jun Oh: https://orcid.org/0000-0003-1846-675X

1 Introduction

Acute rejection occurs in 10–30% of patients on current immunosuppressive regimens during the first post-transplant year with higher rates in adolescents than in younger children [1]. The incidence of acute rejection peaks in the first year post-transplant and then declines [2]. Accurate diagnosis is crucial, as the presence and severity of rejection have a significant impact on long-term graft outcomes. While experiencing one or even more episodes of acute rejection does not necessarily reduce 5-year graft survival, it is associated with a greater decline in graft function (eGFR) [1].

2 Definition

Acute rejection is usually defined by the identification of specific histopathological changes in a renal biopsy [3], making the biopsy a key diagnostic tool. However, also clinical parameters, mostly referred to as Additional Diagnostic Parameters (ADPs) must also be considered (https://banfffoundation.org/

central-repository-for-banff-classification-resources-3/; last accessed December 2024). The clinical presentation is often non-specific (e.g., swelling of the kidney on ultrasound, reduced urine output, possible weight gain; rarely fever, 'transplant pain', and increased blood pressure) or entirely absent. Therefore, the presumptive diagnosis is usually based on an elevated serum creatinine level. The presence or increase of albuminuria or haematuria may also indicate rejection or a recurrence of the underlying disease. Subclinical rejection may be detected in protocol biopsies [4], without any decrease of graft function.

3 Laboratory diagnostics

Blood tests: Creatinine (a 20% increase suggests rejection), urea, and donor-specific HLA antibodies (DD antibody-mediated rejection). If infection is suspected or to exclude it (depending on clinical focus): differential blood count, CRP, blood cultures, virology (CMV, BK polyomavirus), microbiology, and fungal testing.

Urine tests: U-protein/U-creatinine ratio, U-albumin/U-creatinine ratio, erythrocytes (for haematuria), leukocytes (to differentiate from urinary tract infection), urine culture (to differentiate from urinary tract infection).

4 Doppler ultrasound

Ultrasound should be performed routinely when acute rejection is suspected [5]. Key diagnostic issues include assessment of the size and echogenicity of the graft (swelling may indicate rejection, differential diagnosis [DD] could be pyelonephritis), detection of any urinary tract obstruction and measurement of vascular flow (DD arterial or venous thrombosis). Resistance indices (RIs) should be measured by ultrasound in at least two segmental arteries (an RI > 80% suggests rejection but with a low positive and negative predictive value).

5 Renal Biopsy

If acute rejection is suspected, a renal biopsy should always be performed within 24 hours (even at weekends). Histopathological examination of the light microscopic specimen should yield results within 8 hours (at least within 24 hours). The biopsy core should contain cortical, and medullary tissue to diagnose polyomavirus infection. At least one core should be obtained. The specimen should be transported in PBS-buffered 4% formalin, or if immunofluorescence is required, in Michel's fixative or fresh tissue, after consultation with the affiliated pathologist. The biopsy is graded according to the Banff Working Classification of Renal Allograft Pathology [3, Table 1], an international consensus revised every two years that provides criteria for diagnosis and biopsy quality. For example, a diagnostically valid renal biopsy requires the presence of at least 10 glomeruli and 2 arteries (or 7 glomeruli and 1 artery for a minimal sample).

Light and Electron Microscopy Diagnostics

Staining: Hematoxylin and eosin (HE), periodic acid-Schiff (PAS), and Jones silver, elastica staining.

Immunohistochemistry: C4d (as a diagnostic criterion for AMR), SV40 (to differentiate polyomavirus nephropathy), immunoglobulins and complement split products (routinely assessed one year post-transplant, to differentiate between relapse of the underlying disease or *de novo* glomerulonephritis).

If available, electron microscopy may be used to differentiate between relapse of the underlying disease, *de novo* graft glomerulonephritis, transplant glomerulopathy, or transplant peritubular capillaropathy. Diagnosis follows the Banff Classification (for the latest iteration see https://banfffoundation.org/central-repository-for-banff-classification-resources-3/; last accessed December 2024.

6 Treatment

Suspicious (borderline) for acute TCMR (Banff category 3)

Biopsy for cause: Give 4–6 intravenous boluses of (methyl)prednisolone at 300 mg/m^2 over 4–6 days (or methylprednisolone pulse therapy over 4 days (400 – 200 – 200 – 100 mg/m^2 body surface area per day as a short intravenous infusion over 15 minutes), followed by 1 mg/kg per day of intravenous furosemide if needed. At the end of the course, the dose of oral (methyl)prednisolone may be increased and then gradually tapered. A possible treatment regime is as follows:

Week 1: 16 mg methylprednisolone/m^2 per day;
Week 2: 12 mg methylprednisolone/m^2 per day;
Week 3: 8 mg methylprednisolone/m^2 per day;
from week 4: 3 mg/m^2 per day, usually no more than 5 mg methylprednisolone

In the case of steroid-free immunosuppression, consider reintroduction of oral steroid therapy.

Monitor trough levels of CNIs (and/or everolimus) and MPA-AUC and increase CNI and antimetabolites if trough levels and/or MPA-AUC values are below target.

Protocol biopsy: The therapeutic relevance still remains unclear. In many cases, an unnecessary increase in immunosuppression can be avoided.

T-cell mediated rejection (Banff category 4)

≥ Banff IA: Administer 4–6 intravenous boluses of (methyl)prednisolone at 300 mg/m^2 over 4–6 days (or methylprednisolone pulse therapy over 4 days (400 – 200 – 200 – 100 mg/m^2 body surface area per day as a short intravenous infusion over 15 minutes), followed by 1 mg/kg per day of intravenous furosemide as needed. At the end of the course, the dose of oral (methyl)prednisolone may be increased and then gradually tapered. A possible treatment regime is as follows:

Week 1: 16 mg methylprednisolone/m^2 per day;
Week 2: 12 mg methylprednisolone/m^2 per day;
Week 3: 8 mg methylprednisolone/m^2 per day;
from week 4: 3 mg/m^2 per day, usually

In the case of steroid-free immunosuppression, consider reintroduction of oral steroid therapy.

1. If trough levels of maintenance immunosuppressants (measured 12 hours after oral administration) are low, adjust the trough levels based on the time since transplantation:

Cyclosporin A target trough levels after rejection:
- < 12 months post-transplant: 200–250 μg/L
- ≥ 12 months post-transplant: 150–200 μg/L

Tacrolimus target trough levels:
- < 12 months post-transplant: 15 μg/L
- 12 months post-transplant: 10 μg/L
- Determine the MPA-AUC and increase the MMF dose if necessary (see Chapter 4.2 and 4.3).

2. If on cyclosporin A-based immunosuppression, switch to tacrolimus:
   - Start tacrolimus therapy 12 hours after the last dose of cyclosporin A. Refer to the target trough levels mentioned above.
   - Increase the dose of MMF to achieve an MPA-AUC of ≥ 60 mg x h/L.
3. In patients receiving concomitant mTOR inhibitors, increase the dose as needed:
   - Target trough levels: everolimus, 6–7 μg/L; sirolimus, 8–10 μg/L

In cases of steroid resistance, defined as no or insufficient reduction in serum creatinine levels by the 4th to 6th day after initiation of methylprednisolone therapy (creatinine remaining at 150% or more of the baseline value), repeat transplant biopsy should be performed and, in most cases, therapy with anti-thymocyte globulin (ATG) should be initiated: start with 1.5 mg/kg/d over 3–5 days; dose adoption according to lymphocyte count, a cumulative dose of 8 mg/kg should be the maximum [6].

There are no protocols for the treatment of chronic active T cell-mediated rejection in children. Therapy may be initiated with steroid pulses followed by an increase of the maintenance immunosuppressive therapy.

References

1 Baghai Arassi M, Feißt M, Krupka K, Awan A, Benetti E, Düzova A, Guzzo I, Kim JJ, Kranz B, Litwin M, Oh J, Büscher A, Pape L, Peruzzi L, Shenoy M, Testa S, Weber LT, Zieg J, Höcker B, Fichtner A, Tönshoff B; Cooperative European Pediatric Renal Transplant Initiative Research Network. Age-Related Differences in Rejection Rates, Infections, and Tacrolimus Exposure in Pediatric Kidney Transplant Recipients in the CERTAIN Registry. Kidney Int Rep. 2024 Sep 2;9(11):3265–3277. doi: 10.1016/j.ekir.2024.08.025. PMID: 39534206; PMCID: PMC11551099.

2 Verghese PS. Pediatric kidney transplantation: a historical review. Pediatr Res. 2017 Jan;81(1–2):259–264. doi: 10.1038/pr.2016.207. Epub 2016 Oct 12. PMID: 27732587.

3 Naesens M, Roufosse C, Haas M, Lefaucheur C, Mannon RB, Adam BA, Aubert O, Böhmig GA, Callemeyn J, Groningen MC, Cornell LD, Demetris AJ, Drachenberg CB, Einecke G, Fogo AB, Gibson IW, Halloran P, Hidalgo LG, Horsfield C, Huang E, Kikić Ž, Kozakowski N, Nankivell B, Rabant M, Randhawa P, Riella LV, Sapir-Pichhadze R, Schinstock C, Solez K, Tambur AR, Thaunat O, Wiebe C, Zielinski D, Colvin R, Loupy A, Mengel M. The Banff 2022 Kidney Meeting Report: Re-Appraisal of Microvascular Inflammation and the Role of Biopsy-Based Transcript Diagnostics. Am J Transplant. 2023 Oct 27:S1600–6135(23)00818-3. doi: 10.1016/j.ajt.2023.10.016. Epub ahead of print. PMID: 39491095.

4 Gordillo R, Munshi R, Monroe EJ, Shivaram GM, Smith JM. Benefits and risks of protocol biopsies in pediatric renal transplantation. Pediatr Nephrol. 2019 Apr;34(4):593–598. doi: 10.1007/s00467-018-3959-6. Epub 2018 May 3. PMID: 29725772.

5 Franke D. The diagnostic value of Doppler ultrasonography after pediatric kidney transplantation. Pediatr Nephrol. 2022 Jul;37(7):1511–1522. doi: 10.1007/s00467-021-05253-y. Epub 2021 Sep 3. PMID: 34477970; PMCID: PMC9192382.

6 Pape L, Becker JU, Immenschuh S, Ahlenstiel T. Acute and chronic antibody-mediated rejection in pediatric kidney transplantation. Pediatr Nephrol. 2015 Mar;30(3):417–24. doi: 10.1007/s00467-014-2851-2. Epub 2014 May 28. PMID: 24865478.

Table 1 BANFF 2022 diagnostic groups for diagnosis of acute rejection [3]

Category 1: Normal Biopsy or Nonspecific Change
Category 2: Antibody-mediated rejection and microvascular inflammation/injury (AMR/MVI)
- Active AMR
- Chronic active AMR
- Chronic AMR
- C4d staining without evidence of rejection
- Microvascular inflammation/injury (MVI), DSA-negative and C4d-negative
- Probable AMR
- C4d staining with acute tubular injury (ATI);

Category 3: Suspicious (Borderline) For Acute TCMR
Category 4: TCMR
- *Acute TCMR IA* Banff Lesion Score i ≥ 2 AND Banff Lesion Score t2
- *Acute TCMR IB* Banff Lesion Score i ≥ 2 AND Banff Lesion Score t3
- *Acute TCMR IIA* Banff Lesion Score v1 regardless of Banff Lesion Scores i or t
- *Acute TCMR IIB* Banff Lesion Score v2 regardless of Banff Lesion Scores i or t
- *Acute TCMR III* Banff Lesion Score v3 regardless of Banff Lesion Scores i or t
- *Chronic Active TCMR Grade IA* Banff Lesion Score ti ≥ 2 AND Banff Lesion Score i-IFTA ≥ 2, other known causes of i-IFTA (eg, pyelonephritis, BK-virus nephritis etc.) ruled out AND Banff Lesion Score t2
- *Chronic Active TCMR Grade IB* Banff Lesion Score ti ≥ 2 AND Banff Lesion Score i-IFTA ≥ 2, other known causes of i-IFTA ruled out AND Banff Lesion Score t3
- *Chronic Active TCMR Grade II* Arterial intimal fibrosis with mononuclear cell inflammation in fibrosis and formation of neointima

Category 5: IFTA (Interstitial Fibrosis and Tubular Atrophy)
- *Mild*
- *Moderate*
- *Severe*

Category 6: Other Changes Not Considered To Be Caused By Acute Or Chronic Rejection

Polyomavirus Nephropathy, Posttransplant Lymphoproliferative Disorder, Calcineurin Inhibitor Toxicity, Acute Tubular Injury, Recurrent Disease, De Novo Glomerulopathy (Other Than TG), Pyelonephritis, Drug-Induced Interstitial Nephritis

CHAPTER 6.2 Diagnosis and treatment of antibody-mediated transplant rejection

Burkhard Tönshoff[1], Alexander Fichtner[1], Caner Süsal[2, 3] & Christian Morath[4, 5]

[1] Heidelberg University, Medical Faculty Heidelberg, Department of Paediatrics I, University Children's Hospital, Heidelberg, Germany
[2] Heidelberg University, Medical Faculty Heidelberg, Institute of Immunology, Transplantation Immunology, Heidelberg, Germany
[3] Transplant Immunology Research Center of Excellence, Koç University School of Medicine, Istanbul, Turkey
[4] Department of Nephrology, University Hospital Heidelberg
[5] Clinic for Internal Medicine, Nephrology, Nuremberg Hospital, Germany

ORCIDs:
Burkhard Tönshoff: https://orcid.org/0000-0002-6598-6910
Alexander Fichtner: https://orcid.org/0000-0002-9939-4059
Caner Süsal: https://orcid.org/0000-0003-2521-8201
Christian Morath: https://orcid.org/0000-0003-2218-7817

1 Definitions

Active antibody-mediated rejection (AMR) is diagnosed based on specifically defined histopathologic and molecular lesions, primarily the presence of microvascular inflammation (MVI, defined by the lesions glomerulitis and peritubular capillaritis) or, alternatively, by biopsy-based transcript-analysis; secondly, on the presence of circulating donor-specific antibodies (DSAs); and thirdly, on the extend of C4d deposition. However, a diagnosis of AMR can be made without DSAs or C4d. AMR is caused by the binding of circulating antibodies to donor alloantigens on endothelial cells in the graft, resulting in inflammation, cell damage and, ultimately, graft dysfunction. These antigens include human leukocyte antigens (HLA) class I and class II antigens, and in recipients of ABO-incompatible transplants, ABO blood group antigens. Other non-major histocompatibility complex (MHC) antigens on the endothelium may also be targeted [1–4]. Acute TCMR and AMR may coexist in the allograft at the same time (i.e., mixed acute rejection). Acute rejection may also coexist with chronic rejection. Of note, from a molecular (transcriptomic) perspective, chronic AMR appears to share more similarities with TCMR than with active AMR.

Clinically, chronic rejection is characterised by the gradual deterioration of allograft function, accompanied by varying degrees of proteinuria and hypertension. It is a significant factor in the loss of grafts in the long term. It typically develops after the first year post-transplant and may occur with or without active inflammation (see Chapter 6.3) [5].

2 Incidence and risk factors

A recently published analysis of 337 paediatric kidney transplant recipients from the CERTAIN registry revealed that the cumulative incidence of *de novo* donor-specific class I HLA antibodies (HLA-DSAs) post-transplant was 4.5% in year 1, 8.3% in year 3 and 13% in year 5. The corresponding results for *de novo* class II HLA-DSAs were 10%, 22.5% and 30.6% respectively [6]. Five years post-transplant, the cumulative incidence of active AMR was 10%, and of chronic active AMR, 5.9%. HLA-DR mismatch and *de novo* HLA-DSA, particularly double positivity for class I and class II HLA-DSA, were significant risk factors for AMR. Other established risk factors for AMR are: (i) delayed onset of graft function, (ii) a previous episode of rejection, (iii) receiving a second or subsequent transplant, and (iv) not adhering to medication.

3 Clinical and laboratory findings

As most patients with AMR are asymptomatic, the condition is usually identified through abnormal laboratory testing. The most common laboratory finding among patients with acute allograft rejection is an acute or slow rise in serum creatinine. However, a rising serum creatinine level is not specific to acute rejection. It is a relatively late development in the course of a rejection episode and usually indicates significant histological damage. New or increasing proteinuria of more than 500 mg/m^2 per day may indicate active or chronic (active) AMR. However, post-transplant proteinuria may also be caused by glomerulosclerosis or interstitial fibrosis and tubular atrophy (IFTA) from chronic rejection, recurrent glomerular disease, and *de novo* glomerulopathies.

The development of *de novo* antibodies directed against the donor's HLA antigens (HLA-DSAs) or an increase in DSA reactivity in a patient with pre-existing DSAs has been associated with AMR. A systematic review and meta-analysis of seven retrospective cohort studies found that the presence of HLA-DSAs, as detected by a solid-phase assay, was associated with a risk of AMR that was almost double as high as that observed in the absence of HLA-DSAs [7]. DSAs to non-HLA antigens have also been observed in patients with AMR. These include the angiotensin II receptor [2, 3], MHC class I polypeptide-related sequence A (MICA) [4] and endothelial cell antigens [4]. However, a negative DSA test in serum does not rule out a diagnosis of AMR, as the DSAs could have been absorbed by the graft. Moreover, not all DSAs are equally pathogenic. A considerable number of studies have found that complement-binding antibodies (i.e., C1q-binding DSAs) are associated with a higher rate of AMR and poorer graft survival than non-complement-binding DSAs [8, 9]. However, testing for C1q-binding DSAs is not widely performed. In addition, it is likely that there are clinically relevant non-complement-binding DSAs that are not detected by this assay.

There is no consensus on when to test for DSAs in the absence of allograft dysfunction. The frequency of DSA monitoring varies between transplant centres and depends on the patient's immunological risk. Some centres perform annual HLA-DSA testing in stable recipients. Monitoring for the development of HLA-DSAs post-transplant may permit the early detection of AMR and allograft dysfunction, particularly in high-risk patients (see Chapter 4.4 and Chapter 5.2). However, routine monitoring of DSAs in low-risk patients may have a more limited impact in detecting early AMR [10]. The presence of circulating HLA-DSAs alone does not indicate active rejection, but it does indicate that a patient is at a higher risk of AMR. Other clinical and laboratory parameters must be assessed alongside DSA testing. In cases of an increasing or new HLA-DSA, but with no other signs of acute rejection and a normal kidney allograft biopsy, most transplant centres would only increase maintenance immunosuppressive therapy.

4 Histopathology

There are no specific laboratory findings that can accurately diagnose acute rejection. Acute rejection is currently diagnosed histologically using a kidney allograft biopsy (see Chapter 6.3). Histopathology differentiates between T cell-mediated rejection (TCMR) and AMR, grades the severity of rejection accurately, and determines the extent of irreversible kidney damage (interstitial fibrosis/tubular atrophy [IF/TA]). A biopsy of the allograft can also reveal other causes of kidney inflammation and injury, including cytomegalovirus disease, BK polyomavirus-associated nephropathy, interstitial nephritis, pyelonephritis, *de novo* or recurrent glomerular disease, and post-transplant lymphoproliferative disease (PTLD) (see Chapter 6.3). The Banff classification has been developed and revised by an expert panel of pathologists, immunologists, physicians, surgeons and immunogeneticists, with the aim of standardising the histological criteria for diagnosing and grading the severity of rejection [11]. Distinguishing between active AMR and severe acute TCMR can be difficult, and the two processes may coexist. In reality, AMR and TCMR diagnoses are part of a continuum representing different manifestations of the alloimmune response. In up to 25% of cases of allograft dysfunction attributed at least in part to AMR, the histological findings suggest only TCMR or acute tubular injury. It is important to identify AMR, if possible, since it is more resistant to treatment and often results in loss of the kidney allograft unless adequately treated [6].

DSA testing may produce a negative result among patients with AMR. Some of these patients may have antibodies against non-HLA antigens. If anti-HLA antibody testing is negative, but there is evidence of MVI (even below the threshold for AMR), testing for non-HLA antibodies may be advisable in selected scenarios [3, 4]. However, there are currently no universally established or validated clinical assays to detect these antibodies. Cases in which C4d staining is positive but DSA cannot be detected may result from DSA being below the level of detection due to immunoadsorption by the graft.

5 Chronic AMR

Chronic AMR refers to chronic microvascular injury that leads to remodelling of the glomerular or peritubular capillaries. Chronic AMR is further classified into chronic active and chronic inactive subtypes. *Chronic active AMR* generally develops more than six months after transplant and can occur in patients with or without a history of active AMR. The only difference in the diagnostic criteria between chronic active and active AMR is the presence or absence of chronic lesions (transplant glomerulopathy or severe multilayering of the peritubular capillary basement membrane [12].

Chronic inactive AMR is characterised by chronic lesions in conjunction with MVI below the threshold for AMR, DSA positivity and C4d negativity. In patients with chronic inactive AMR, prior diagnosis of active or chronic active AMR and/or documented evidence of post-transplant DSA count as DSA positivity.

6 Prevention

Preventing AMR depends on detecting HLA-DSAs before (pre-existing) or after *(de novo)* transplantation. Patients with pre-existing HLA-DSAs prior to transplantation are at greater risk of AMR and graft failure than non-sensitised patients [7]. The complement-fixing capacity of the DSA is a key factor in this risk, with patients who test positive for complement-dependent cytotoxicity (CDC) having a higher risk of AMR and graft loss than those who test positive for flow crossmatch. In turn, these patients have a higher risk than those who test positive for virtual crossmatch (antibodies detected by single antigen bead technology) [7]. For patients with a potential living donor, the approach depends on the results of the most recent crossmatch. For patients with a positive CDC crossmatch or strongly positive flow crossmatch, many transplant centres opt for kidney paired donation (KPD) programmes over desensitisation due to the high risk of AMR and graft loss in these patients [13]. Such KPD programmes enable sensitised patients with immunologically incompatible living donors to receive transplants from other living donors in similar situations who are willing to exchange organs. KPD could help participating centres avoid complex desensitisation protocols while improving long-term outcomes. KPD programmes will soon be available also in Germany.

Many centres employ HLA desensitisation strategies in patients with a positive virtual crossmatch (antibodies detected by single antigen bead technology) or a mild to moderate positive flow crossmatch (i.e., median channel shift of < 200). These strategies include treatment with plasmapheresis, rabbit antithymocyte globulin (rATG), rituximab and imlifidase (see Chapter 5.2). We employ HLA desensitisation strategies in patients without a potential living donor. For all patients with a pre-existing DSA before transplant who undergo kidney transplantation, we use induction and maintenance immunosuppression therapies appropriate for patients at high risk of developing acute rejection [14].

For patients with pre-existing DSAs, routine monitoring of DSA levels is recommended at months 1, 3, 6 and 12 post-transplant, followed by annual monitoring [14, 16]. Highly sensitized patients should be monitored more frequently, for example on post-transplant days 5, 10, 14 and 21. Many centres perform a kidney allograft biopsy in patients with a significant rise in HLA-DSA or who develop a *de novo* HLA-DSA within the first three months. This practice largely aligns with the Consensus Guidelines on Testing and Managing Clinical Issues Associated with HLA and Non-HLA Antibodies in Transplantation [14].

Kidney transplant recipients who develop *de novo* HLA-DSAs after transplantation can experience late-onset antibody-mediated rejection (AMR). AMR in patients with *de novo* HLA-DSAs has been associated with poorer outcomes than AMR in patients with a pre-existing HLA-DSA. The two most common causes of AMR due to *de novo* DSAs are non-adherence to medication and inadequate immunosuppression. The latter is often attributed to minimisation strategies. Additionally, acute T cell-mediated rejection, malignancy and opportunistic infections, such as BK polyomavirus (BKPyV) and cytomegalovirus (CMV) infections, which require a reduction in immunosuppression, may also influence the development of late-onset AMR [15]. Preventing AMR requires addressing non-adherence and under-immunosuppression, while ensuring the long-term safety and efficacy of immunosuppression.

7 Treatment

Active antibody-mediated rejection

The primary goal of treating AMR is to reduce the titres of existing pathogenic DSAs, eradicate the clonal population of B or plasma cells responsible for their production, prevent complement activation and reduce endothelial injury, and preserve graft function [16]. While previous trials primarily targeted the cause of AMR, recent data on the successful reversal of AMR activity by CD38 antibodies suggest that targeting the cellular inflammation with CD38-positive natural killer cells resulting from antibody binding to the endothelium could be an additional rational approach.

The following recommendations for treating AMR largely align with those set out in the 2009 Kidney Disease: Improving Global Outcomes (KDIGO) clinical practice guidelines and the 2019 Transplantation Society Working Group Expert Consensus [16, 17]. For patients diagnosed with active AMR within the first 6–12 months post-transplant (early onset), some authors recommend initial therapy comprising glucocorticoids (10 mg of methylprednisolone per kg of body weight daily for three to five days, followed by a rapid oral prednisone taper), whereas other experts recommend steroid pulse therapy only in patients with concomitant biopsy-proven TCMR (Figure 1) [18]. While DSA removal by plasmapheresis or immunoadsorption is supported by data from an RCT and recommended, the administration of IVIG is optional. Some experts also administer rituximab if the patient has better allograft function (e.g., eGFR of at least 20 ml/min/1.73 m^2 and lower chronicity scores on biopsy) and has

Figure 1 Proposed therapeutic algorithm for the management of AMR and DSA- and C4d-negative MVI. cg, transplant glomerulopathy; ci, interstitial fibrosis; ct, tubular atrophy; cv, vascular fibrous intimal thickening; g, glomerulitis; IA, immunoadsorption; PP, plasmapheresis; ptc, pertitubular capillaritis; TMA, thrombotic microangiopathy. Reproduced with permission from ref. [18].

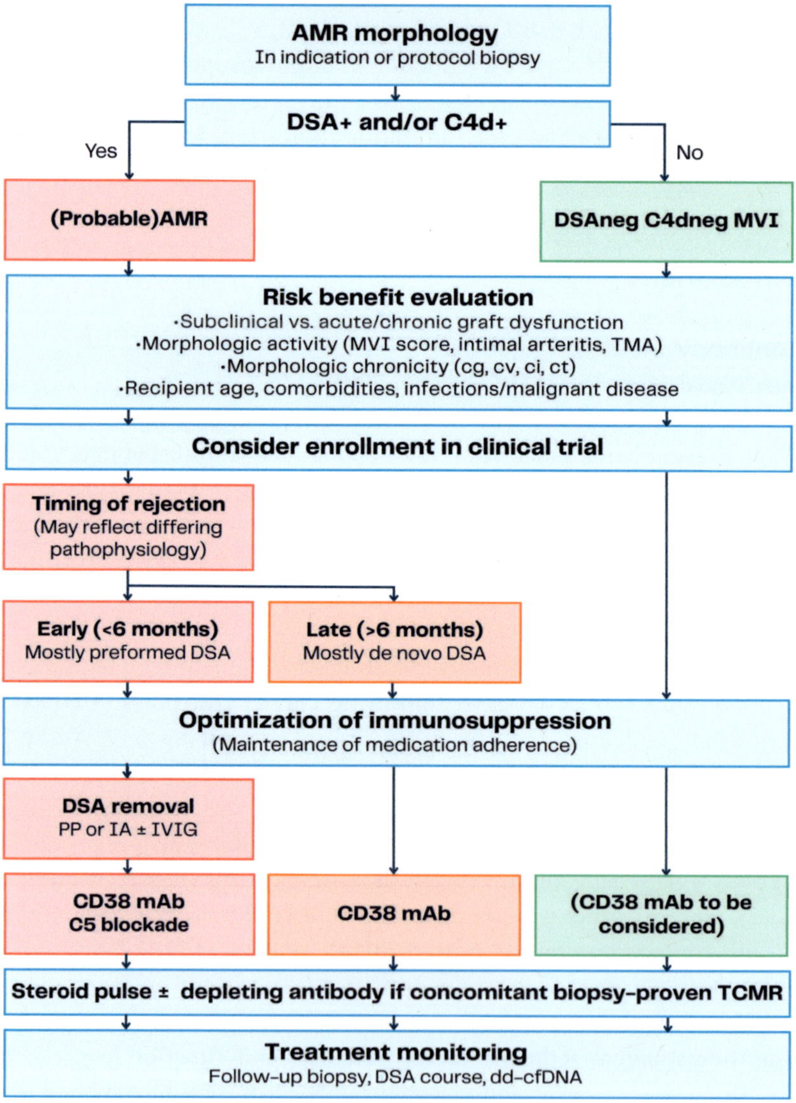

evidence of severe disease (e.g., higher DSA MFI levels or DSA-load measured by cumulative MFI, diffuse C4d staining or more extensive microvascular inflammation, i.e., a glomerulitis score and a peritubular capillary sum score of at least 4) on biopsy. For all patients, we augment maintenance immunosuppression as needed. For example, we increase the tacrolimus maintenance dose to achieve a trough level 20–25% above that at the time of rejection and/or above 5 μg/L, while maximising the antiproliferative agent dose (e.g., mycophenolate) and initiating steroid maintenance therapy in those off steroids, as well as evaluation and management of non-adherence.

Plasmapheresis is performed daily or every other day for up to six sessions, or until the serum creatinine level is within 20–30% of the baseline level. The initial treatment typically involves a 1.5-fold volume exchange with albumin, while subsequent treatments involve a one-volume exchange with albumin. We prefer an every-other-day plasmapheresis schedule, since albumin alone can often be administered for replacement, with the prothrombin time, partial thromboplastin time and fibrinogen recovering to acceptable levels within the interval, without the need to administer fresh frozen plasma. This avoids the risk of antigen sensitisation. However, one to two units of fresh frozen plasma may be used for replacement at the end of plasmapheresis to reduce the risk of bleeding in an appropriate clinical setting, such as on the same day as a kidney allograft biopsy. We administer IVIG at a dose of 2 g/kg body weight at the end of the apheresis course [18]. Rituximab is administered as a single 375 mg/m^2 dose after plasmapheresis and IVIG have been completed. Immunoadsorption, proteasome inhibitors, interleukin (IL)-6 blockade, or complement inhibitors may be considered for patients who do not respond to the initial treatment.

For patients diagnosed with active AMR after the first 6–12 months post-transplant (i.e., late-onset AMR), we recommend initial therapy comprising intravenous immunoglobulin (IVIG) at a dose of 200 mg/kg every two weeks for three doses, with no plasmapheresis due to a lack of evidence supporting its safety and efficacy in late-onset AMR. Some experts administer rituximab if the patient has better allograft function, lower chronicity scores on biopsy and evidence of severe disease, e.g., higher DSA, diffuse C4d staining or more extensive microvascular inflammation (i.e., a glomerulitis score and a peritubular capillary score of at least 4 on biopsy. For all patients, we also increase maintenance immunosuppression as outlined above.

Chronic active antibody-mediated rejection

Chronic AMR, the most common cause of graft failure, is more difficult to treat than active AMR since irreversible tissue damage to the kidney allograft has already occurred [19, 20]. While there is evidence to suggest that antibody-mediated injury requires a combination of strategies to inhibit B cell development, maturation and activity, it is unclear which combination of therapies is safe and effective for patients with chronic AMR. There is currently no high-quality evidence to inform optimal treatment for chronic active AMR, and the evidence supporting our treatment approach primarily comes from observational studies [21, 22]. The lack of strong evidence has resulted in substantial heterogeneity in clinical practice. A 2023 online survey in Europe [23] indicated that over half of adult patients with chronic active AMR receive no additional treatment beyond optimized immunosuppression. Common reasons highlighted in the survey to leave chronic active AMR untreated, despite the known association with impaired graft outcome, include appreciation of disease irreversibility, fear of costs and side effects, and the lack of robust trial data. When additional treatments are used, IVIG, steroid pulses, and apheresis are common, whereas rituximab or other biologics are used less frequently [23].

For paediatric patients with chronic active AMR, we recommend initial therapy involving IVIG and rituximab. In a prospective pilot study on antihumoral therapy consisting of high-dose IVIG (4 weekly doses of IVIG, 1 g/kg body weight per dose) and a single dose of rituximab (375 mg/m^2 body surface area 1 week after the last IVIG infusion) in 20 paediatric kidney transplant recipients, 14 patients (70%) responded: nine of nine patients (100%) without and five of 11 (45%) with transplant glomerulopathy [21]. C4d positivity in PTC decreased from 40 ± 18.5% in the index biopsy to 11.6 ± 12.2% in the follow-up biopsy. In four of nine biopsies (44%), C4d staining turned negative. During 2 years of follow-up, the median loss of eGFR in each of the four 6-month periods remained significantly lower compared with prior to therapy. Class I DSA declined in response to antihumoral therapy by 61%, class II DSA by 63% 12 months after intervention. IVIG and rituximab significantly reduced or stabilized the progressive loss of transplant function in paediatric patients with chronic AMR over an observation period of 2 years, apparently by lowering circulating DSA and reducing intrarenal complement activation [21]. All patients treated for active AMR should recommence antimicrobial and antiviral prophylaxis with a regimen identical to that administered in the immediate post-transplant period.

If the patient does not respond to initial therapy involving IVIG and rituximab, the anti-interleukin 6 receptor antibody tocilizumab could be considered, which is administered intravenously at a dose of 8 mg/kg once monthly. Limited data suggest that treatment with interleukin (IL)-6 blockade may benefit patients with chronic AMR [22]. Felzartamab, an investigational anti-CD38 monoclonal antibody that targets plasma cells and natural killer (NK) cells, was evaluated in a phase II pilot trial in which 22 adult kidney transplant recipients with AMR occurring after 180 days post-transplant (15 with chronic active AMR) were randomly assigned to receive nine infusions of felzartamab (16 mg/kg) or placebo [24]. At 24 weeks, mild to moderate adverse events (e.g., first-dose infusion-related reactions) occurred more frequently with felzartamab; however, the rate of serious adverse events was lower with felzartamab than with placebo (9% versus 36%). Patients receiving felzartamab had improved microvascular inflammation scores, lower molecular scores reflecting the probability of AMR and lower levels of donor-derived cell-free DNA (dd-cfDNA). A phase III trial with felzartamab is currently ongoing.

References

1 Süsal C, Fichtner A, Tönshoff B, Mehrabi A, Zeier M, Morath C. Clinical Relevance of HLA Antibodies in Kidney Transplantation: Recent Data from the Heidelberg Transplant Center and the Collaborative Transplant Study. J Immunol Res. 2017;2017:5619402.

2 Dragun D, Müller DN, Bräsen JH, et al. Angiotensin II type 1-receptor activating antibodies in renal-allograft rejection. N Engl J Med 2005; 352:558.

3 Fichtner A, Süsal C, Schröder C, Höcker B, Rieger S, Waldherr R, Westhoff JH, Sander A, Dragun D, Tönshoff B. Association of angiotensin II type 1 receptor antibodies with graft histology, function and survival in paediatric renal transplant recipients. Nephrol Dial Transplant. 2018;33: 1065–1072.

4 Fichtner A, Süsal C, Höcker B, Rieger S, Waldherr R, Westhoff JH, Sander A, Dragun D, Tönshoff B. Association of non-HLA antibodies against endothelial targets and donor-specific HLA antibodies with antibody-mediated rejection and graft function in pediatric kidney transplant recipients. Pediatr Nephrol. 2021;36:2473–2484.

5 Haas M, Loupy A, Lefaucheur C, et al. The Banff 2017 Kidney Meeting Report: Revised diagnostic criteria for chronic active T cell-mediated rejection, antibody-mediated rejection, and prospects for integrative endpoints for next-generation clinical trials. Am J Transplant 2018; 18:293.

6 Fichtner A, Gauché L, Süsal C, Tran TH, Waldherr R, Krupka K, Guzzo I, Carraro A, Oh J, Zirngibl M, Weitz M, König J, Büscher A, Berta L, Simon T, Awan A, Rusai K, Topaloglu R, Peruzzi L, Printza N, Kim JJ, Weber LT, Melk A, Pape L, Rieger S, Patry C, Höcker B, Tönshoff B; CERTAIN study group. Incidence, risk factors, management strategies, and outcomes of antibody-mediated rejection in pediatric kidney transplant recipients – a multicenter analysis of the Cooperative European Paediatric Renal Transplant Initiative (CERTAIN). Pediatr Nephrol. 2025;40:491–503.

7 Mohan S, Palanisamy A, Tsapepas D, et al. Donor-specific antibodies adversely affect kidney allograft outcomes. J Am Soc Nephrol 2012; 23:2061.

8 Fichtner A, Süsal C, Höcker B, Rieger S, Waldherr R, Westhoff JH, Sander A, Opelz G, Tönshoff B. Association of C1q-fixing DSA with late graft failure in pediatric renal transplant recipients. Pediatr Nephrol. 2016 Jul;31(7):1157–66.

9 Loupy A, Lefaucheur C, Vernerey D, et al. Complement-binding anti-HLA antibodies and kidney-allograft survival. N Engl J Med 2013; 369:1215.

10 Salhi S, Congy-Jolivet N, Hebral AL, et al. Utility of Routine Post Kidney Transplant Anti-HLA Antibody Screening. Kidney Int Rep 2024; 9:1343.

11 Loupy A, Mengel M, Haas M. Thirty years of the International Banff Classification for Allograft Pathology: the past, present, and future of kidney transplant diagnostics Kidney Int. 2022 Apr;101:678–691.

12 Naesens M, Roufosse C, Haas M, et al. The Banff 2022 Kidney Meeting Report: Reappraisal of microvascular inflammation and the role of biopsy-based transcript diagnostics. Am J Transplant. 2024;24:338–349. doi: 10.1016/j.ajt.2023.10.016. Pham TA, Lee JI, Melcher ML. Kidney paired exchange and desensitization: Strategies to transplant the difficult to match kidney patients with living donors. Transplant Rev (Orlando) 2017; 31:29.

13 Amrouche L, Aubert O, Suberbielle C, et al. Long-term Outcomes of Kidney Transplantation in Patients With High Levels of Preformed DSA: The Necker High-Risk Transplant Program. Transplantation 2017; 101:2440.

14 Tait BD, Süsal C, Gebel HM, et al. Consensus guidelines on the testing and clinical management issues associated with HLA and non-HLA antibodies in transplantation. Transplantation 2013; 95:19.

15 O'Leary JG, Samaniego M, Barrio MC, et al. The Influence of Immunosuppressive Agents on the Risk of De Novo Donor-Specific HLA Antibody Production in Solid Organ Transplant Recipients. Transplantation 2016; 100:39.
16 Schinstock CA, Mannon RB, Budde K, et al. Recommended Treatment for Antibody-mediated Rejection After Kidney Transplantation: The 2019 Expert Consensus From the Transplantion Society Working Group. Transplantation 2020; 104:911.
17 Kidney Disease: Improving Global Outcomes (KDIGO) Transplant Work Group. KDIGO clinical practice guideline for the care of kidney transplant recipients. Am J Transplant 2009; 9 Suppl 3:S1.
18 Böhmig GA, Naesens M, Viklicky O, Thaunat O, Diebold M, Rostaing L, Budde K. Antibody-mediated rejection-treatment standard. Nephrol Dial Transplant. 2025 Aug 1;40(8):1615–1627.
19 Redfield RR, Ellis TM, Zhong W, et al. Current outcomes of chronic active antibody mediated rejection – A large single center retrospective review using the updated BANFF 2013 criteria. Hum Immunol 2016; 77:346.
20 Parajuli S, Mandelbrot DA, Muth B, et al. Rituximab and Monitoring Strategies for Late Antibody-Mediated Rejection After Kidney Transplantation. Transplant Direct 2017; 3:e227.
21 Billing H, Rieger S, Süsal C, Waldherr R, Opelz G, Wühl E, Tönshoff B. IVIG and rituximab for treatment of chronic antibody-mediated rejection: a prospective study in paediatric renal transplantation with a 2-year follow-up. Transpl Int. 2012;25:1165–73.
22 Choi J, Aubert O, Vo A, et al. Assessment of Tocilizumab (Anti-Interleukin-6 Receptor Monoclonal) as a Potential Treatment for Chronic Antibody-Mediated Rejection and Transplant Glomerulopathy in HLA-Sensitized Renal Allograft Recipients. Am J Transplant 2017; 17:2381.
23 Rostaing LPE, Böhmig GA, Gibbons B et al. Post-transplant surveillance and management of chronic active antibody-mediated rejection in renal transplant patients in Europe. Transpl Int 2023; 36:11381.
24 Mayer KA, Schrezenmeier E, Diebold M, et al. A randomized phase 2 trial of felzartamab in antibody-mediated rejection. N Engl J Med 2024; 391:122.

CHAPTER 6.3 Histopathological classification of transplant rejection according to Banff

Jan Ulrich Becker

Institute of Pathology, University Hospital of Cologne, Cologne, Germany

ORCID:
https://orcid.org/0000-0003-2929-8085

1 Introduction

The Banff Classification of Renal Allograft Nephropathy is the result of a consensus process managed by the Banff Foundation (www.banfffoundation.org; last accessed December 2024). This started in 1991 with an expert meeting in Banff, Canada; the results of these biannual meetings have been published in more than a dozen manuscripts. The latest iteration is based on the 2022 meeting held in Banff again [1]. As the only such project after termination of the Cooperative Clinical Trials in Transplantation (CCTT) Classification [2], the Banff Classification has become the dominant classification scheme for kidney allograft pathology for clinical practice, scientific and pharmaceutical trials. Unfortunately, the high expectations for such a classification regarding transparency, clarity and practical applicability have not always been met. Currently, the entire up-to-date content of the Banff Classification can be found on the Banff Foundation's website (https://banfffoundation.org/central-repository-for-banff-classification-resources-3/; last accessed December 2024). The following sections provide a guide to the general principles and implementation of the Banff Classification in its most recent form. We refrain from copying the most recent iteration, as this would quickly become outdated. Instead, we encourage the users of this manual to consult the Banff website. The Banff Classification in their most recent iteration should be implemented by transplant centres in a consensus between clinicians, nephropathologists and immunogeneticists under consideration of local resources. Individual patients and their biopsies are not always best served by rigorous adherence to the Banff Classification. Instead other available evidence and reason will provide additional guidance in the interdisciplinary diagnostic process.

2 General principles of the Banff Classification of renal allograft pathology

The content of the Banff Classification can be divided into four parts: Banff Definitions, Banff Lesion Scores, Additional Diagnostic Parameters (ADPs) and Banff Diagnostic Categories and Subcategories. Throughout this text, all official Banff terms will be given in capitals. The best-known parts of the Banff Classification are the Banff Lesion Scores, e.g., Banff t for tubulitis, g for glomerulitis. These are all histopathological decriptors on an ordinal scale of 0, 1, 2, 3, where 0 is usually denoting absence and 3 a severe finding. Note that severity can be graded in an individual tissue compartment, as in t for tubulitis or cg for transplant glomerulopathy, where the most severely affected tubule or glomerulus would dictate the score. For other Lesion Scores it is graded as the extent of involvement, as in the Banff Lesion Score g for transplant glomerulitis. Again, the reader is referred to the Banff website for the most recent overview of these Lesion Scores.

Overlooked until the review published in 2018 were the Additional Diagnostic Parameters (ADPs). ADPs have been around since the beginning. They are, with the exception of "C4d Staining On Fresh-Frozen Or Paraffin-Embedded Tissue", binary (yes or no, absent or present) defined by the non-Lesion Score nodes in the Banff Classification decision tree to reach all Diagnostic Categories. They refer not only to histopathology, as in "Absence Of Recurrent Or De Novo Glomerulonephritis", but also to other diagnostic disciplines, as in "Prior Evidence Of Donor-Specific Antibody". The Banff definitions underpin the other components of the Banff Classification. To define endarteritis for the Banff Lesion Score v, Banff provides a definition of "artery" as opposed to arterioles. Finally, the Banff Classification provides diagnostic categories and subcategories. With some minor changes in Banff 2019 that were quickly reversed, these categories are the following for the 2022 iteration [1]:

Table 1 Banff Diagnostic Categories

Banff Diagnostic Categories	**Banff Diagnostic Subcategories**
1. Normal biopsy or nonspecific changes	None
2. Antibody-mediated rejection and microvascular inflammation/injury (AMR/MVI)	Active AMR, chronic AMR, chronic-active AMR, C4d-staining without evidence of rejection, microvascular inflammation/injury (MVI), DSA-negative and C4d-negative, probable AMR; C4d staining with acute tubular injury (ATI)
3. Suspicious (borderline) for acute T cell-mediated rejection (TCMR)	None
4. T cell-mediated rejection (TCMR)	Acute TCMR IA, IB, IIA, IIB, III Chronic-active TCMR IA, IB, II
5. Interstitial fibrosis and tubular atrophy	Grade I (mild), grade II (moderate), grade III (severe)
6. Other changes not considered to be caused by acute or chronic rejection	Polyomavirus nephropathy, post-transplant lymphoproliferative disorder, calcineurin inhibitor toxicity, acute tubular injury, recurrent disease, de novo glomerulopathy (other than transplant glomerulopathy), pyelonephritis, drug-induced interstitial nephritis

Modified from (https://banfffoundation.org/central-repository-for-banff-classification-resources-3/; last accessed December 2022)

Obviously, Category 5 is not a diagnosis *per se.* It grades interstitial fibrosis and tubular atrophy of the cortex (as codified in the Banff Lesion Scores ci and ct) into the usual ordinal scale of absent, mild (Grade I), moderate (Grade II) and severe (Grade III). While Category 1 is mutually exclusive with Categories 2, 3, 4 and 6, and Category 3 is mutually exclusive with Category 4, all other Categories may coexist in a summary Banff diagnosis. For example, a biopsy could show chronic-active antibody-mediated rejection (caAMR) from Category 2, acute T cell-mediated rejection IIA from Category 4, moderate IFTA from Category 5 and a diagnosis of recurrent IgA glomerulonephritis from Category 6. Indeed, several diagnoses from Category 6 may co-exist.

3 Banff Diagnostic Category 2: Antibody-mediated rejection and microvascular inflammation/injury (AMR/MVI)

In line with the rapidly accumulating and evolving understanding of AMR over the years, Category 2 has undergone by far the most changes of all diagnostic categories in the Banff Classification. A concise review of these changes prior to 2017 can be found elsewhere [3, 4]. Considering the new subcategories added in 2022 Microvascular Inflammation/Injury (MVI), DSA-Negative And C4d-Negative, Probable AMR, C4d Staining With Acute Tubular Injury (ATI), it is important not to interpret them as *bona fide,* true AMR. Rather, they should be considered as provisional subcategories with unknown clinical implications. Similarly, at the time of writing, "Probable AMR" should not AMR proper or a mild form of AMR, but rather a subcategory of unknown diagnostic and therapeutic significance. It is clear that the focus of the Banff Classification is not to be a tool for clinical practice and pharmaceutical trials, but rather to drive research that may or may not provide the evidence for such novel diagnostic subcategories. This ignores the needs of both clinicians and pharmaceutical researchers who require internationally recognised, evidence-based diagnostic definitions. This gap has been filled by a critical review of the evidence base of AMR-relevant Banff Lesion Scores, ADPs and Category 2 diagnoses on behalf of the European Society of Organ Transplantation and the European Medicines Agency, which consolidates the evidence-based core consensus definitions of AMR diagnostic categories and may also serve as a useful reference point for daily clinical practice [4].

4 Banff Diagnostic Category 3: Suspicious (Borderline) For Acute T cell-Mediated Rjection (TCMR) and Category 4 TCMR

Categories 3 and 4 can be considered as a continuum of increasingly severe manifestations of TCMR in the cortical tubulointerstitial compartment (borderline and acute TCMR IA, IB) and in the arterial compartment (acute TCMR IIA,

IIB, III, chronic-active TCMR II). Frequently, Category 2 diagnoses of AMR also include Category 3 or Category 4 diagnoses as mixed AMR plus TCMR.

5 Banff Diagnostic Category 6: Other changes not considered to be caused by acute or chronic rejection

The 8 officially recognised subcategories in 6 should be considered as examples rather than an exhaustive list. A number of other kidney transplant diseases can mimic rejection histologically, such as adenovirus nephropathy. To accurately and reliably diagnose these subcategories and other diseases and other *de novo* or recurrent nephropathies, a full triple diagnostic work-up as for native kidney biopsies is required. This includes standard paraffin histology with haematoxylin-eosin, periodic acid-Schiff, silver and trichrome stains, immunostaining for immunoglobulin heavy and light chains and complement factor 1 and 3 split products (usually C1q and C3c). This must be left to experienced nephropathologists.

6 Molecular diagnostics

Molecular diagnostics, specifically RNA expression studies have been part of the Banff Classification for several iterations. In the Banff 2022 update, they are listed under ADPs as "Biopsy-Based Transcript Diagnostics For AMR/MVI Above A Defined Threshold, *If Thoroughly Validated For Use As A Substitute For AMR/MVI And Available*". They have been used as evidence of antibody interaction with transplant tissue and as a surrogate parameter for the presence of donor-specific antibodies and even for a microscopy-based diagnosis of AMR. However, no assay has yet been officially recognised by the Banff Foundation as "thoroughly validated". Frankly, it is not clear why the well-established [5, 6] commercial hybridisation assay is not considered "validated ... and available", given the certainly inferior evidence for some other diagnostic criteria for AMR. Meanwhile, the Banff Foundation appears to have started the development cycle all over again on a different assay platform. This means that, although early results look promising [7, 8], the transplant community will have to wait for an officially recognised histomolecular platform.

7 Practical considerations and outlook

Routine diagnostics of renal transplant biopsies should be evidence-based, clinically relevant, economically feasible and follow international standards which are set by the Banff Classification. Centres should strive to achieve these goals as a multidisciplinary effort to the best of their ability. Ideally, all involved clinics and diagnostic institutes in a given transplant centre should agree on an evidence-based consensus definition for their daily routine diagnostics, taking into account their centre's resources, their experiences and emerging evidence.

It is increasingly recognised that alloreactive processes may not fit into the diagnostic boxes of the Banff Classification, but may be better defined by mechanism (TCMR vs. AMR), activity and chronicity, very similar to the biopsy assessment in lupus nephritis. Such novel concepts, the advent of digital nephropathology, computer vision and machine learning, and transcriptomics could lead to more reproducible and accurate diagnoses and pave the way for prognostic and theranostic classifiers.

References

1 M. Naesens et al., The Banff 2022 Kidney Meeting Report: Reappraisal of microvascular inflammation and the role of biopsy-based transcript diagnostics. American journal of transplantation: official journal of the American Society of Transplantation and the American Society of Transplant Surgeons 10.1016/j.ajt.2023.10.016 (2023).
2 R.B. Colvin et al., Evaluation of pathologic criteria for acute renal allograft rejection: reproducibility, sensitivity, and clinical correlation. Journal of the American Society of Nephrology: JASN 8, 1930–1941 (1997).
3 C. Roufosse et al., A 2018 Reference Guide to the Banff Classification of Renal Allograft Pathology. Transplantation 10.1097/TP.0000000000002366 (2018).
4 C. Roufosse et al., Proposed Definitions of Antibody-Mediated Rejection for Use as a Clinical Trial Endpoint in Kidney Transplantation. Transplant international: official journal of the European Society for Organ Transplantation 35, 10140 (2022).

5 P.F. Halloran et al., Real Time Central Assessment of Kidney Transplant Indication Biopsies by Microarrays: The INTERCOMEX Study. American journal of transplantation: official journal of the American Society of Transplantation and the American Society of Transplant Surgeons 10.1111/ajt.14329 (2017).
6 A. Loupy et al., Molecular Microscope Strategy to Improve Risk Stratification in Early Antibody-Mediated Kidney Allograft Rejection. Journal of the American Society of Nephrology: JASN 10.1681/ASN.2013111149 (2014).
7 H. Varol et al., Feasibility and Potential of Transcriptomic Analysis Using the NanoString nCounter Technology to Aid the Classification of Rejection in Kidney Transplant Biopsies. Transplantation 10.1097/tp.0000000000004372 (2022).
8 I.A. Rosales et al., Banff Human Organ Transplant Transcripts Correlate with Renal Allograft Pathology and Outcome: Importance of Capillaritis and Subpathologic Rejection. Journal of the American Society of Nephrology: JASN 33, 2306–2319 (2022).

CHAPTER 7
Infectious complications and prevention

CHAPTER 7.1 Cytomegalovirus infection

Christian Patry[1], Burkhard Tönshoff[1], Lutz T. Weber[2] & Britta Höcker[1]

[1] Heidelberg University, Medical Faculty Heidelberg, Department of Paediatrics I, University Children's Hospital Heidelberg, Germany
[2] Pediatric Nephrology, Children's and Adolescents' Hospital, University Hospital Cologne, Medical Faculty University of Cologne, Germany

ORCIDs:
Christian Patry: https://orcid.org/0000-0002-1270-6508
Burkhard Tönshoff: https://orcid.org/0000-0002-6598-6910
Lutz T. Weber: https://orcid.org/000-003-4116-598X
Britta Höcker: https://orcid.org/0000-0003-4131-2273

1 Cytomegalovirus and kidney transplantation

Despite recent advances, cytomegalovirus (CMV) infection remains one of the most common complications in solid organ transplant recipients, with an increased risk of complications, graft loss, morbidity, and mortality [1]. While adult and paediatric transplant recipients share common risk factors for CMV disease, children face unique challenges that increase their risk of exposure and infection. Because they are likely to be CMV-naïve at the time of transplantation, they are more likely to acquire primary CMV infection post-transplant. In addition, CMV donor (D)-negative and recipient (R)-negative paediatric kidney transplant recipients are at increased risk of de novo infection from community sources, such as day care. Prior to the introduction of prophylactic and preemptive therapy, CMV disease occurred in approximately 15% of paediatric kidney transplant recipients [2]. Antiviral prophylaxis and preemptive treatment strategies have reduced the burden of CMV disease, while standardized quantitative nucleic acid testing has allowed more effective monitoring [3]. In the current era, CMV DNAemia affects approximately 20% of paediatric kidney transplant patients, with 1–10% developing CMV disease and 14% experiencing late-onset disease [1, 4, 5]. In addition to established therapeutic agents such as valganciclovir and ganciclovir, novel antiviral agents and adjunctive treatments such as virus-specific T cells offer promising options for safer and more effective prevention and treatment [3].

2 Definitions

CMV DNAemia: Detection of CMV DNA in the blood in the absence of clinical symptoms [3].

CMV infection: Evidence of CMV replication regardless of symptoms, defined as isolation of virus or detection of viral proteins (antigens) or nucleic acid in any body fluid or tissue specimen [6], e.g., positive PCR, positive pp65 antigen, positive cell culture, and/or histopathological evidence.

CMV disease: Evidence of CMV infection accompanied by attributable symptoms. CMV disease can be further categorized as a CMV syndrome or as tissue invasive disease [1]

CMV syndrome: CMV replication plus one or more of the following criteria: Fever, malaise, leukocytopenia, thrombocytopenia.

Tissue invasive disease: CMV replication plus one or more of the following criteria: Gastrointestinal disease, pneumonia, hepatitis, central nervous system disease, retinitis, others (nephritis, cystitis, myocarditis, pancreatitis, etc.).

3 Pre-transplant CMV diagnostics

As in adults, the risk of CMV disease in paediatric transplant recipients depends on the donor and recipient serostatus (D/R). Pre-transplant CMV serostatus defines the risk of CMV after transplantation and guides decisions about either antiviral prophylaxis or active surveillance (with preemptive therapy) [1]. However, in infants younger than 12 months, interpretation of serostatus is complicated by maternal CMV antibodies transferred across the placenta and the intermittent shedding of CMV in saliva and urine [1]. Prior to the introduction of routine CMV prevention strategies, CMV-related disease in solid organ transplant (SOT) recipients typically occurred within the first three months (early-onset). After discontinuation of early-onset post-transplant prophylaxis, complications are more likely to occur as late-onset CMV disease, particularly in high-risk CMV-positive donor/CMV-negative recipient (D+/R–) cases [7].

Risk categories are generally defined and treated as (exceptions, see further below):

- (D+/R–) High risk
- (D+/R+) Intermediate risk
- (D–/R–) Low risk
- (D–/R+) The risk associated with (D–/R+) serostatus and its management both depend whether or not the recipient has received induction therapy with lymphocyte-depleting antibodies.

We also recommend:
- Pre-transplant serological testing of all donors and recipients: Ideally prior to any necessary blood transfusion to avoid transmission of CMV antibodies. (Sample usually required: 1 mL of serum (or 2 mL of whole-blood) for CMV IgG serostatus determination)
- If the donor has received multiple transfusions prior to organ retrieval, consider possible CMV transmission and classify the donor as CMV IgG positive.
- For donors and recipients younger than 12 months of age, assume the highest possible CMV risk for the recipient due to possible maternal antibody transmission [1].

Donor < 12 months	**Recipient < 12 months**	**Highest risk categorization**
+	+ or –	D+/R–*
–	+	D–/R+
–	–	D–/R–

** If the recipient is confirmed positive by CMV culture or nucleic acid testing, assign D+/R+.*

4 Post-transplant CMV decisions: Prophylaxis vs. pre-emptive strategy

Given the high incidence of primary CMV infection and reactivation in paediatric solid organ transplantation, preventive strategies play a crucial role in enhancing transplant success and improving clinical outcomes. The choice between prophylaxis and pre-emptive strategies depends on the CMV risk profile of the patient and the level of immunosuppression administered [1]. These strategies help to mitigate the risk of CMV infection and disease, while also reducing the associated indirect effects of CMV infection [1, 6, 7]. Similar to adults, paediatric evidence supports the use of serostatus-guided antiviral prophylaxis in paediatric kidney transplant recipients. However, its use in young children is limited due to the risk of bone marrow suppression and the lack of comprehensive pharmacokinetic data for valganciclovir. Universal prophylaxis involves the administration of antiviral medication to all patients or a selected group of high-risk patients, starting within the first 10 days post-transplant and continuing for a defined period, typically 3 to 6 months [1].

On the other hand, preemptive therapy reduces antiviral-related toxicity but requires frequent viral load monitoring [1]. Effective preemptive therapy (PET) relies on routine blood monitoring for CMV at regular intervals (e.g., weekly CMV viral load testing) to detect viral replication at an early stage. Once a predefined assay threshold is reached – ideally before clinical symptoms emerge – antiviral treatment is initiated to prevent progression to clinical disease. Advances in assay availability and standardization have made this approach increasingly feasible. However, due to differences in diagnostic specimen types (whole-blood vs. plasma) and variability in assay platforms, a universally applicable threshold for initiating therapy has yet to be established [1, 8, 9].

Definitions:

- Prophylaxis: Administration of valganciclovir (or ganciclovir) for 3–6 months post-transplant.
- Preemptive strategy: Regular CMV PCR surveillance post-transplant and initiation of antiviral therapy (double prophylactic dose) if CMV DNAemia is detected by PCR, irrespective of clinical symptoms.

We recommend:

- Patients at high CMV risk (CMV D+/R–) or intermediate risk (CMV D+/R+) receive valganciclovir prophylaxis.

- CMV S−/E+ patients receiving ATG/Thymoglobulin®: treat as high CMV risk (valganciclovir prophylaxis)
- CMV S−/E+ patients without ATG/Thymoglobulin® therapy follow a pre-emptive strategy approach (CMV PCR surveillance, initiation of antiviral therapy at relevant CMV DNAemia).
- Low risk patients (CMV S−/E−) are followed clinically; if CMV infection is suspected, PCR testing is performed.

Duration of prophylaxis:
The duration of prophylaxis depends on the intensity of immunosuppressive therapy.

- For patients receiving standard immunosuppression (dual/triple therapy), we recommend 3 months of prophylaxis.
- For patients receiving ATG/Thymoglobulin® induction or treatment, we recommend 6 months of prophylaxis.
- Patients on methylprednisolone pulse therapy: 3 months prophylaxis, if high or intermediate risk category.

Valganciclovir prophylactic dosage
- Single daily dose (mg/day) = 7 × BSA (m^2) × eGFR ($ml/min/1.73\ m^2$)[a]
- Maximum eGFR value to use in formula: 150 mL/min/1.73 m^2 (to avoid overdosing)[b]
- Maximum prophylactic daily dose: 900 mg
- Valganciclovir available as: 450 mg tablets or 50 mg/ml suspension
- For persistent anuria post-transplant: Start intravenous ganciclovir (0.625 mg/kg 3 × weekly after haemodialysis) or valganciclovir suspension according to product guidelines at 48 h post-transplant.

[a] *Calculation of eGFR using k = 0.413 [10].*

[b] *Other centers have adopted lower age-dependent upper eGFR limits in children to avoid over-exposure to valganciclovir [11]*

5 Post-transplant CMV diagnostics

In immunosuppressed patients, seroconversion during primary infection may be delayed or absent. Therefore, antibody detection is only useful for determining pre-transplant CMV serostatus, but not for diagnosing active CMV infection after transplantation [7]. As CMV DNA concentrations may vary between whole blood and plasma, surveillance should be performed consistently using the same sample type for each patient [7].

We recommend:

- 10 days post-transplant (except for D–/R– patients and those under prophylaxis): 2 ml EDTA-treated blood for CMV quantitative PCR testing.
- In cases of clinical suspicion or unexplained leukocytopenia/neutropenia, CMV PCR testing should also be considered during ongoing prophylaxis.

Post-transplant, quantitative nucleic acid amplification testing is the preferred method for diagnosing CMV infection, guiding preemptive strategies, and monitoring response to therapy [1, 12]. Although there is no universally accepted threshold for initiation of therapy, a clinically significant increase in CMV DNA viral load is currently defined as at least a threefold increase ($\geq 0.5 \log_{10}$ copies/mL) in viremia within one week [7]. Another issue that remains controversial is routine surveillance for breakthrough CMV DNAemia during antiviral prophylaxis. While studies in paediatric SOT recipients have reported breakthrough CMV DNAemia during valganciclovir prophylaxis, its clinical significance remains uncertain [3]. It has been associated with adverse outcomes such as graft rejection, secondary infections, and potential valganciclovir/ganciclovir resistance. However, the respective paediatric data are inconclusive and causality has not been firmly established. Furthermore, progression from breakthrough CMV DNAemia to CMV disease is rare [3]. In accordance with the German guideline on S2k guideline on the management of viral infections in organ transplantation, we currently do not recommend routine screening for CMV DNAemia during prophylaxis unless there is clinical suspicion of CMV replication [7].

We recommend the following monitoring schedule:

- For patients after 3 months of prophylaxis, we recommend the following schedule:
  - Months 3–6: twice a month
  - Months 6–12: once a month
  - After 12 months: twice per year and if clinical symptoms or graft dysfunction occur.
- For patients after 6 months of prophylaxis, we recommend the following schedule:
  - Months 6–9: twice a month

  - Months 9–12: once a month
  - After 12 months: twice a year and if clinical symptoms or graft dysfunction occur.
- For patients following a preemptive strategy, we recommend the following schedule:
  - Months 0–4: once a week
  - Months 4–12: once a month
  - After 12 months: twice a year and if graft dysfunction occurs.

Regarding the diagnostic workup after solid organ transplantation, it has to be mentioned that a negative CMV DNA test does not necessarily rule out tissue invasive CMV disease [13, 14]. Higher CMV DNA levels in tissue compared to peripheral blood suggest tissue invasion, which is particularly relevant in pulmonary or intestinal involvement. In such cases, histological and immunohistochemical analyses are essential for diagnosis [14–17].

6 Treatment of CMV replication and CMV disease after paediatric kidney transplantation

Both oral valganciclovir and intravenous ganciclovir can be used for non-life-threatening CMV disease; valganciclovir is generally preferred if feasible because of its oral formulation, which can help to reduce or avoid hospital stays and reduce the risk of infectious and vascular complications associated with intravenous therapy. Conversely, intravenous ganciclovir is the preferred option for the initial treatment of life-threatening CMV disease, as it ensures optimal drug exposure when immediate and effective antiviral activity is critical [1, 18]. Antiviral treatment should be given for at least two weeks and continued until both clinical symptoms have resolved and CMV DNAemia falls below a defined threshold (lower limit of quantification < 200 IU/mL) in two consecutive weekly tests [1, 7]. Once clinical improvement is achieved, intravenous ganciclovir can be switched to valganciclovir in patients who can tolerate oral therapy. In cases of leukopenia, it is not recommended to discontinue or substitute (val) ganciclovir before considering the use of granulocyte colony-stimulating factor and/or discontinuing other myelosuppressive medications [1].

For the treatment of asymptomatic CMV replication and CMV syndrome we recommend:

- Therapeutic dose of valganciclovir: The prophylactic dose given two times a day.
- Maximum therapeutic daily dose: 900 mg twice daily (total 1800 mg/d).
- Reduce maintenance immunosuppressive therapy if possible.
- Frequent clinical monitoring and weekly CMV DNAemia testing by PCR
- If CMV DNAemia recurs, consider switching to an everolimus-based immunosuppressive therapy
- During CMV replication, pneumocystis jirovecii pneumonia prophylaxis should be maintained for the duration of viremia.

For the treatment of tissue invasive CMV disease we recommend:

- IV ganciclovir: 10 mg/kg/day divided into two doses as a short infusion for 14 days. Followed by 5 mg/kg/day once daily as a short infusion until clinical resolution and two consecutive negative CMV PCR results. Minimum treatment duration: 3 weeks. Caution: Dose adjustments required for GFR < 70 mL/min/1.73 m^2 (see Table 1).
- For CMV pneumonitis or enterocolitis, consider adding 100 mg/kg b.w. of hyperimmune globulin, depending on the patient's condition.
- CMV DNAemia testing by PCR: Twice weekly.
- Reduce maintenance immunosuppressive therapy if possible.
- Depending on immunosuppressive regimen, secondary prophylaxis with valganciclovir for 1–3 months may be considered.

Ensuring the correct dose of antiviral medication is critical to the effective management of CMV disease (Table 1). Inadequate dosing may lead to treatment failure and increase the risk of resistance development, while excessive doses may increase the risk of toxicity. To optimize therapy, renal function should be closely monitored by regular assessment of serum creatinine levels [1, 19, 20]. We recommend the following adjustments to the dose and dosing interval of i.v. ganciclovir in relation to kidney function.

Table 1 Dosage of i.v. ganciclovir in relation to kidney function

	Initial therapy		Maintenance therapy	
Creatinine clearance (according to Schwartz) (mL/min·1.73 m²)	**Dose (mg/kg BW[1])**	**Dosing interval (h)**	**Dose (mg/kg BW[1])**	**Dosing Interval (h)**
≥ 70	5.0	12	5.0	24
50–69	2.5	12	2.5	24
25–49	2.5	24	1.25	24
10–24	1.25	24	0.625	24
< 10	1.25	3 × per week[2]	0.625	3 × per week[2]

[1] body weight; [2] after haemodialysis

Regarding dosing of oral valganciclovir please refer to section 4.

7 Management of treatment-resistant CMV disease

Drug resistance is characterized by viral genetic mutations that reduce susceptibility to one or more antiviral drugs, often resulting in persistent or increasing viral load or symptomatic disease despite adequate treatment. It can manifest in varying degrees, from asymptomatic cases that resolve without intervention to severe or even fatal organ disease [21, 22]. The development of resistance is strongly associated with increased morbidity and mortality, highlighting the importance of early detection and treatment [1, 23, 24].

We recommend:

- If the CMV viral load is not reduced by 50% after 2 weeks of therapy, resistance testing by RT-PCR genotyping (UL97 and UL54 mutations) should be performed.
- If necessary, biopsy material or bronchoalveolar lavage (BAL) fluid should also be tested for CMV mutation.
- After consultation with virology/infectious disease specialists, alternative agents such as foscarnet may be used (caution: nephrotoxicity).

In paediatric kidney transplantation, the use of everolimus in combination with low-dose cyclosporine A has been associated with a significantly lower incidence of CMV disease compared with mycophenolate mofetil (MMF) with standard-dose calcineurin inhibitors. Although data on switching to mTOR inhibitors during active CMV infection are lacking, an mTOR-based immunosuppressive regimen may be considered in cases of recurrent CMV viremia [7, 25].

8 Exposure prophylaxis and hospital hygiene

- Patient isolation: not generally required.
- Precautions: Avoid contact with pregnant women, neonates and immunosuppressed patients (see hospital hygiene guidelines).

References

1 Kotton CN, Kumar D, Caliendo AM, Huprikar S, Chou S, Danziger-Isakov L, et al. The Third International Consensus Guidelines on the Management of Cytomegalovirus in Solid-organ Transplantation. Transplantation. 2018;102(6).
2 Iragorri S, Pillay D, Scrine M, Trompeter RS, Rees L, Griffiths PD. Prospective cytomegalovirus surveillance in paediatric renal transplant patients. Pediatric Nephrology. 1993;7(1).
3 Downes K, Danziger-Isakov L, Varela-Fascinetto G, Herold B, Green M, L'Huillier AG. Debates in management and treatment of CMV in pediatric solid organ transplant recipients: a case-based discussion. Pediatric Transplantation. 2025; in press.
4 Hashim F, A. Gregg J, R. Dharnidharka V. Efficacy of Extended Valganciclovir Prophylaxis in Preventing Cytomegalovirus Infection in Pediatric Kidney Transplantation. Open Urol Nephrol J. 2014;7(1).
5 Höcker B, Zencke S, Krupka K, Fichtner A, Pape L, Strologo L Dello, et al. Cytomegalovirus infection in pediatric renal transplantation and the impact of chemoprophylaxis with (val-)ganciclovir. Transplantation. 2016;100(4).
6 Ljungman P, Boeckh M, Hirsch HH, Josephson F, Lundgren J, Nichols G, et al. Definitions of cytomegalovirus infection and disease in transplant patients for use in clinical trials. Clinical Infectious Diseases. 2017;64(1).

7 Virusinfektionen bei Organ- und allogen Stammzell-Transplantierten: Diagnostik, Prävention und Therapie (Version 2.0, aktualisiert August 2024) S2k-Leitlinie AWMF Registernummer 093-002.
8 Preiksaitis JK, Hayden RT, Tong Y, Pang XL, Fryer JF, Heath AB, et al. Are We There Yet? Impact of the First International Standard for Cytomegalovirus DNA on the Harmonization of Results Reported on Plasma Samples. Clinical Infectious Diseases. 2016;63(5).
9 Pang XL, Fox JD, Fenton JM, Miller GG, Caliendo AM, Preiksaitis JK. Interlaboratory comparison of cytomegalovirus viral load assays. American Journal of Transplantation. 2009;9(2).
10 Schwartz GJ, Muñoz A, Schneider MF, Mak RH, Kaskel F, Warady BA, et al. New equations to estimate GFR in children with CKD. Journal of the American Society of Nephrology. 2009;20(3):629–37.
11 Gerthoffer E, Pozderac A, Darland L, Yasechko S, Crooker A, Hambrick HR, et al. Association of neutropenia with valganciclovir prophylaxis dosing practices within pediatric solid organ transplant recipients. Pediatric Transplantation. 2025; in press.
12 Caliendo AM, St. George K, Allega J, Bullotta AC, Gilbane L, Rinaldo CR. Distinguishing cytomegalovirus (CMV) infection and disease with CMV nucleic acid assays. J Clin Microbiol. 2002;40(5).
13 Eid AJ, Arthurs SK, Deziel PJ, Wilhelm MP, Razonable RR. Clinical predictors of relapse after treatment of primary gastrointestinal cytomegalovirus disease in solid organ transplant recipients. American Journal of Transplantation. 2010;10(1).
14 Westall GP, Michaelides A, Williams TJ, Snell GI, Kotsimbos TC. Human cytomegalovirus load in plasma and bronchoalveolar lavage fluid: A longitudinal study of lung transplant recipients. Journal of Infectious Diseases. 2004;190(6).
15 Lautenschlager I, Halme L, Höckerstedt K, Krogerus L, Taskinen E. Cytomegalovirus infection of the liver transplant: Virological, histological, immunological, and clinical observations. Transplant Infectious Disease. 2006;8(1).
16 Chemaly RF, Yen-Lieberman B, Castilla EA, Reilly A, Arrigain S, Farver C, et al. Correlation between Viral Loads of Cytomegalovirus in Blood and Bronchoalveolar Lavage Specimens from Lung Transplant Recipients Determined by Histology and Immunohistochemistry. J Clin Microbiol. 2004;42(5).

17 Solans EP, Yong S, Husain AN, Eichorst M, Gattuso P. Bronchioloalveolar lavage in the diagnosis of CMV pneumonitis in lung transplant recipients: An immunocytochemical study. Diagn Cytopathol. 1997;16(4).
18 Åsberg A, Humar A, Jardine AG, Rollag H, Pescovitz MD, Mouas H, et al. Long-term outcomes of CMV disease treatment with valganciclovir versus IV ganciclovir in solid organ transplant recipients. American Journal of Transplantation. 2009;9(5).
19 McGavin JK, Goa KL. Ganciclovir: An update of its use in the prevention of cytomegalovirus infection and disease in transplant recipients. Vol. 61, Drugs. 2001.
20 Emery VC, Griffiths PD. Prediction of cytomegalovirus load and resistance patterns after antiviral chemotherapy. Proc Natl Acad Sci U S A. 2000;97(14).
21 Boivin G, Goyette N, Farhan M, Ives J, Elston R. Incidence of cytomegalovirus UL97 and UL54 amino acid substitutions detected after 100 or 200 days of valganciclovir prophylaxis. Journal of Clinical Virology. 2012; 53(3).
22 Eid AJ, Arthurs SK, Deziel PJ, Wilhelm MP, Razonable RR. Emergence of drug-resistant cytomegalovirus in the era of valganciclovir prophylaxis: Therapeutic implications and outcomes. Clin Transplant. 2008;22(2).
23 Avery RK, Arav-Boger R, Marr KA, Kraus E, Shoham S, Lees L, et al. Outcomes in Transplant Recipients Treated with Foscarnet for Ganciclovir-Resistant or Refractory Cytomegalovirus Infection. Transplantation. 2016; 100(10).
24 Bonatti H, Sifri CD, Larcher C, Schneeberger S, Kotton C, Geltner C. Use of cidofovir for cytomegalovirus disease refractory to ganciclovir in solid organ recipients. Surg Infect. 2017;18(2).
25 Höcker B, Zencke S, Pape L, Krupka K, Köster L, Fichtner A, et al. Impact of Everolimus and Low-Dose Cyclosporin on Cytomegalovirus Replication and Disease in Pediatric Renal Transplantation. American Journal of Transplantation. 2016;16(3).

CHAPTER 7.2 Epstein-Barr virus infection and post-transplant lymphoproliferative disorder (PTLD)

Britta Höcker[1] & Britta Maecker-Kolhoff[2]

[1] Heidelberg University, Medical Faculty Heidelberg, Department of Paediatrics I, University Children's Hospital Heidelberg, Germany
[2] Hannover Medical School, Pediatric Haematology and Oncology, Hannover, Germany

ORCIDs:
Britta Höcker: https://orcid.org/0000-0003-4131-2273
Britta Maecker-Kolhoff: https://orcid.org/0000-0001-8164-514X

1 Epstein-Barr virus

Epstein-Barr virus (EBV) infection is typically caused by salivary transmission ("kissing disease"). After productive infection of epithelial cells and B cells of the oropharynx (lytic phase), naïve circulating B cells are infected and progress from latently infected proliferating blasts to long-lived memory B cells (latent phase). In the context of solid organ transplantation (SOT), EBV is also transmissible through the transplant, and reactivation of virus-producing cells is possible at any time, especially under immunosuppressive medication [1]. Primary EBV infection and viral reactivation in the course of subsequent latent virus persistence may be asymptomatic, oligosymptomatic or cause severe systemic disease, including infectious mononucleosis and post-transplant lymphoproliferative disorder (PLTD, see below).

In paediatric kidney transplant (KTx) recipients, the 5-year incidence of EBV-associated PTLD is 1–10%. Risk factors for the development of PTLD include the recipient's EBV seronegativity prior to KTx, which is found in approximately 41% of paediatric KTx patients, and the type and intensity of immunosuppression [2, 3]. As EBV-specific antiviral drugs and effective EBV vaccines are lacking, early diagnosis of EBV infection or reactivation and surveillance are necessary in paediatric KTx patients.

2 EBV diagnostics

Prior to kidney transplantation, both donor and recipient should be serologically tested for EBV. Patients with an EBV D+/R– serostatus are at highest risk of primary EBV infection. After transplantation, EBV infection/reactivation is diagnosed by determining the virus load in whole blood, plasma or serum by quantitative PCR (qPCR) [4]. Viral load in cell-containing material reflects the abundance of virus-infected cells, whereas in plasma or serum it reflects free viral nucleic acid from productively infected or dead cells. Quantitative EBV DNA testing can also be performed on cerebrospinal fluid, biopsy material, bronchoalveolar lavage (BAL), etc., where the viral load of all non-liquid materials should be related to a cellular genome. Where possible, virus concentrations should be reported in international units/ml, using the WHO EBV standard (www.nibsc.org/documents/ifu/09-260.pdf).

Because there is no absolute viral load threshold for predicting EBV-associated PTLD, longitudinal monitoring of EBV viral loads should be performed using the same specimen and laboratory [4, 1]. This helps to distinguish patients with increasing viral loads from those with elevated but stable viral loads. Transplanted patients can have persistent high viral loads without developing PTLD. In contrast, an undetectable or low viral load does not rule out the development of PTLD, including EBV-associated PTLD. An increasing viral load should prompt a physical examination with imaging, tissue biopsy, immunophenotyping, and preemptive therapy as appropriate. Where possible, mutational analysis may also be helpful in estimating the risk of PTLD, as mutations in the EBV LMP1 gene (positions 212 and 366) have been associated with an almost 12-fold increased risk of EBV-positive PTLD [1].

Table 1 Viral diagnostics

	EBV VC IgG[1]	EBV qPCR[2]	LMP1 mutation analysis[3]
Donor	Before Tx[4]		
All KTx recipients	Before Tx[5]	In case of clinical signs of EBV disease (e.g. infectious mononucleosis, PTLD) or transplant dysfunction	Consider in case of chronic high EBV viral load
D+/R– recipients		Month 0, 1, 2, 3, 4, 5, 6, 9, 12 post-transplant	
D–/R– recipients		Surveillance until primary EBV infection (community-acquired infection)	
R+ recipients		Surveillance in case of additional risk factors (e.g. T-cell depletion, recent EBV primary infection, re-transplantation, etc.)	

[1] in serum

[2] usually in whole blood (if necessary, in plasma or serum). Use same specimen type and laboratory, assay calibrated according to WHO standard. In case of PTLD, additional monitoring in other specimens (e.g. cerebrospinal fluid, BAL, biopsy specimens, etc.) is recommended.

[3] specific LMP1 mutations associated with increased risk of PTLD

[4] consider donors < 3 months of age EBV-positive in the case of positive EBV VC IgM result

[5] consider recipients < 12 months of age EBV-negative (regardless of EBV VC IgG result) due to maternal antibodies

3 Prophylaxis and treatment of EBV infection

Despite many efforts, the development of a vaccine to provide reliable, long-term protection against EBV infection has not been successful. There are no specific antiviral drugs. Acyclovir and ganciclovir inhibit EBV in the lytic phase *in vitro* and *in vivo,* and therefore theoretically have prophylactic potential to prevent primary EBV infection. However, in a systematic review with meta-analysis, their benefit could not be proven. Therefore, their use is not recommended, but at the same time the available data are not sufficient to reject their use [5].

Although rituximab is often used to pre-emptively treat EBV replication in haematopoietic stem cell transplant (HSCT) patients, its beneficial effect as a preemptive therapy to prevent manifest PTLD in SOT recipients has not been proven. It is therefore not generally recommended for paediatric KTx recipients, but may be considered on a case-by-case basis.

For prophylaxis and treatment of EBV infection, immunosuppressive medication can be reduced in order to strengthen the patient's cellular defence against EBV. However, the patient's individual risk-benefit ratio needs always be taken into account to avoid transplant rejection [1, 5, 6].

4 Diagnosis of PTLD

Symptoms of PTLD can be variable with either classic symptoms (lymphadenopathy, hepato-/splenomegaly, blood count abnormalities, fever, night sweats, weight loss) or atypical symptoms (failure to thrive, abdominal pain, diarrhoea, chronic fatigue, unexplained cough). Biopsy is mandatory to confirm the diagnosis, and pathological workup should include immunohistochemistry (CD20, CD30), evaluation of c-myc translocations and EBV association (EBER in situ hybridisation; staining for LMP or EBNA). PTLD is classified according to the WHO classification with polymorphic or monomorphic B-cell disease being the most frequent subtypes [7].

Table 2 The WHO classification of PTLD (2017)

Category	Examples
Non-destructive PTLD	Reactive plasmacytic hyperplasia Infectious mononucleosis Florid follicular hyperplasia
Polymorphic PTLD	
Monomorphic PTLD	Diffuse large B-cell lymphoma Burkitt lymphoma Plasma cell myeloma, plasmacytoma EBV-positive Marginal Zone lymphoma Peripheral T-cell lymphoma, not otherwise specified Hepatosplenic T cell lymphoma
Classical Hodgkin lymphoma PTLD	

5 Diagnostic workup and staging

Diagnosis and treatment should be carried out by an interdisciplinary team of paediatric oncologists and transplant physicians. Except for non-destructive PTLD of the tonsils or adenoid tissue all other patients require complete staging. Imaging should include ultrasound and/or MRI of the abdomen and cervical lymph nodes, and chest CT. A ^{18}FDG-PET CT/MRI should be performed to secure all active lesions. Bone marrow histology and lumbar puncture are performed to evaluate bone marrow or central nervous system (CNS) involvement. Peripheral blood EBV qPCR and measurement of lactate dehydrogenase should be performed as baseline for follow-up investigations.

Staging is performed according to the International Paediatric Non-Hodgkin Lymphoma staging system [8] or the St. Jude staging system [9]. Both systems identify 4 stages based on the number and location of lymph node regions involved, extralymphatic disease, and bone marrow or CNS involvement. Stages I to IV are associated with the absence (a) or presence (b) of general symptoms such as fever, night sweats and weight loss.

6 Treatment of PTLD

Treatment of PTLD has been extensively reviewed in a recent IPTA report and should be carried out in multi-disciplinary teams [6]. Reduction of immunosuppressive medication without risk of graft rejection is the cornerstone of PTLD treatment. Preclinical data suggest that cessation of calcineurin inhibitors and/or a switching to an mTOR inhibitor-based regimen may be beneficial, but clinical evidence is lacking. In CD20+ PTLD, rituximab is the first-line treatment of choice. In the Ped-PTLD trial, 3-weekly doses of rituximab (375 mg/m^2) were administered and, if a complete or partial remission was achieved, were followed by 3 further rituximab infusions on a 3-weekly schedule. In patients who do not respond to rituximab alone, low-dose chemotherapy (modified COMP, cyclophosphamide, vincristine, methotrexate, prednisolone) should be added [7]. Alternatively, 6 cycles of rituximab + low-dose chemotherapy (cyclophosphamide + prednisolone) resulted in similar survival rates [10]. In patients who progress on this regimen, more intensive chemotherapy regimens have been used according to NHL-BFM, DA-EPOCH, FAB/LMB or COG schemes. Supportive measures should include antifungal and *Pneumocystis jirovecii* prophylaxis. Recently, EBV-specific T cells have been approved by the EMA for second-line treatment of relapsed or refractory EBV+ PTLD (tabelecleucel, Ebvallo® [11]). Alternatively, EBV+ T cells freshly isolated from partially HLA-matched donors have been used with similar success rates [12]. These cells have also been used successfully in patients with CNS involvement, who otherwise have a poor prognosis [13].

In a retrospective analysis of Hodgkin-like PTLD treated with conventional Hodgkin's disease chemotherapy, 81% of patients achieved and maintained complete remission at 5 years [14]; therefore, Hodgkin-like PTLDs should be treated according to protocols developed for *de novo* Hodgkin's disease. For rare types of PTLD (e.g. monomorphic T-cell PTLD, plasmacytoma-like PTLD), no standardised recommendations have been evaluated and treatment should be individualised.

References

1 S2k-Leitlinie Virusinfektionen bei Organ- und allogen Stammzell-Transplantierten: Diagnostik, Prävention und Therapie. https://register.awmf.org/de/leitlinien/detail/093-002

2 Höcker B, Fickenscher H, Delecluse HJ, et al. Epidemiology and morbidity of Epstein-Barr virus infection in pediatric renal transplant recipients: a multicenter, prospective study. Clin Infect Dis. 2013;56(1):84–92.

3 Höcker B, Böhm S, Fickenscher H, et al. (Val-)Ganciclovir prophylaxis reduces Epstein-Barr virus primary infection in pediatric renal transplantation. Transpl Int. 2012;25(7):723–31.

4 Preiksaitis J, Allen U, Bollard CM, et al. The IPTA Nashville Consensus Conference on Post-Transplant lymphoproliferative disorders after solid organ transplantation in children: III – Consensus guidelines for Epstein-Barr virus load and other biomarker monitoring. Pediatr Transplant. 2024; 28(1):e14471.

5 Green M, Squires JE, Chinnock RE, Comoli P, et al. The IPTA Nashville consensus conference on Post-Transplant lymphoproliferative disorders after solid organ transplantation in children: II – consensus guidelines for prevention. Pediatr Transplant. 2024;28(1):e14350.

6 Allen UD, L-Huillier AG, Bollard CM, et al. The IPTA Nashville consensus conference on post-transplant lymphoproliferative disorders after solid organ transplantation in children: IV – consensus guidelines for the management of post-transplant lymphoproliferative disorders in children and adolescents. Pediatr Transplant. 2024;28(5):e14781.

7 Swerdlow SH, Campo E, Pileri SA, et al. The 2016 revision of the World Health Organization classification of lymphoid neoplasms. R, Watson A, Vondrak K, et al. A prospective, randomized, multicenter trial of tacrolimus-based therapy with or without basiliximab in pediatric renal transplantation. Blood. 2016;127(20):2375–90.

8 Rosolen A, Perkins SL, Pinkerton CR, et al. Revised International Pediatric Non-Hodgkin Lymphoma Staging System. J Clin Oncol. 2015;33(18): 2112–8.

9 Murphy SB. Classification, staging and end results of treatment of childhood non-Hodgkin's lymphomas: dissimilarities from lymphomas in adults. Semin Oncol. 1980;7(3):332–9.

10 Gross TG, Orjuela MA, Perkins SL, et al. Low-dose chemotherapy and rituximab for posttransplant lymphoproliferative disease (PTLD): a Children's Oncology Group Report. Am J Transplant. 2012;12(11):3069–75.
11 Mahadeo KM, Baiocchi R, Beitinjaneh A, et al. Tabelecleucel for allogeneic haematopoietic stem-cell or solid organ transplant recipients with Epstein-Barr virus-positive post-transplant lymphoproliferative disease after failure of rituximab or rituximab and chemotherapy (ALLELE): a phase 3, multicentre, open-label trial. Lancet Oncol. 2024;25(3):376–387.
12 Bonifacius A, Lamottke B, Tischer-Zimmermann S, et al. Patient-tailored adoptive immunotherapy with EBV-specific T cells from related and unrelated donors. J Clin Invest. 2023;133(12):e163548.
13 Taj MM, Maecker-Kolhoff B, Ling R, et al. Primary post-transplant lymphoproliferative disorder of the central nervous system: characteristics, management and outcome in 25 paediatric patients. Br J Haematol. 2021;193(6):1178–84.
14 Kampers J, Orjuela-Grimm M, Schober T. Classical Hodgkin lymphoma-type PTLD after solid organ transplantation in children: a report on 17 patients treated according to subsequent GPOH-HD treatment schedules. Leuk Lymphoma. 2017;58(3):633–8.

CHAPTER 7.3 BK Polyomavirus and JC Polyomavirus infection

Lars Pape[1] & Burkhard Tönshoff[2]

[1] Department of Paediatrics II, University Hospital of Essen, Essen, Germany
[2] Heidelberg University, Medical Faculty Heidelberg, Department of Paediatrics I, University Children's Hospital, Heidelberg, Germany

ORCIDs:
Lars Pape: https://orcid.org/0000-0002-3635-6418
Burkhard Tönshoff: https://orcid.org/0000-0002-6598-6910

1 Introduction

After kidney transplantation, immunosuppressive treatment disturbs the individual balance between virus replication and cellular immune response, resulting in an increased incidence of severe viral complications. After primary infection mainly during childhood, BK polyomavirus (BKPyV) persists in the renourinary tract. While BKPyV infection occurs without apparent signs or symptoms in healthy individuals, BKPyV causes BKPyV-associated nephropathy (BKPyVAN) in 1% to 10% of all kidney transplant recipients, leading to premature graft failure in 10–80% [1–7]. Recently, new guidelines for the management of BKPyV after kidney transplantations have been published [8]. This text summarises the most important paediatric aspects of this guideline.

2 Definition of BKPyV nephropathy

- *Probable* BKPyV nephropathy – plasma BKPyV DNAaemia > 1000 c/mL (or equivalent) persisting for > 2 weeks
- *Presumptive* BKPyV nephropathy – plasma BKPyV DNAaemia > 10,000 c/mL (or equivalent)
- *Proven* BKPyV nephropathy – detection of compatible cytopathic effects in a graft biopsy plus immunohistochemistry and a specific diagnostic test that identifies BKPyV as opposed to JC polyomavirus (JCPyV)

3 Risk factors for BKPyV DNAaemia

- Younger recipient age
- Obstructive uropathy
- Zero HLA-DR match
- Lymphocyte depleting induction therapy
- Tacrolimus-based immunosuppressive therapy

4 Diagnostic recommendations

- For paediatric kidney transplant recipients, we recommend monthly screening for plasma BKPyV DNAaemia until month 9, then every 3 months until month 36
- In paediatric kidney transplant recipients with BKPyV DNAaemia, we recommend that a kidney biopsy be performed if clinically indicated (e.g., increase in serum creatinine, proteinuria, haematuria).
- In paediatric kidney transplant recipients with stable kidney function and persistent BKPyV DNAaemia > 10,000 c/mL (*or equivalent*) despite reducing immunosuppression, we suggest performing a renal allograft biopsy.
- In paediatric kidney transplant recipients with stable kidney function, persistent BKPyV DNAaemia and increased immunological risk (e.g. ABO incompatible kidney transplantation, HLA-DSA, re-transplantation, poor adherence, multi-organ transplant, history of previous rejection) or virological risk (e.g. graft loss due to BKPyV nephropathy), we suggest performing a renal allograft biopsy to exclude subclinical rejection before reducing immunosuppression.

5 Treatment recommendations

- Start treatment if of BKPyV DNA 1000–10.000 c/mL twice or > 10.000 c/mL
- We recommend reduction of maintenance immunosuppression as the primary treatment of persistent BKPyV DNAaemia, presumptive or proven BKPyV nephropathy in paediatric kidney transplant patients without concurrent acute rejection. See below for details:

- We suggest measurement of plasma creatinine and BKPyV DNA aemia every 1–2 weeks during taper of immunosuppression.
- We suggest re-increasing of immunosuppression after sustained clearance of BKPyV DNAaemia.
- We suggest monthly monitoring of BKPyV DNAemia for 3 months in the event of re-increasing immunosuppression because of rejection therapy.
- We do not recommend adjunctive therapies including leflunomide, cidofovir and fluoroquinolones due to the lack of well-designed studies that were confounded by concomitant reduction in immunosuppression.

Reduction of immunosuppression in case of (presumptive) BKPyVAN

- We suggest first confirming that all immunosuppressive drug doses and concentrations are within the institutional target range.
- We recommend monitoring for BKPyV DNAaemia every 2–4 weeks until clearance.

Strategy 1: Antimetabolite is reduced first

I. Reduce the antimetabolite dose by at least 50%.
   We suggest further reduction of immunosuppression if BKPyV DNAaemia does *not* decrease by 10-fold or does *not* clear below the lower limit of detection (weak, low) after 4 weeks, as follows:
II. Discontinue the antimetabolite and taper the corticosteroid dose to 5–10 mg/1.73 m^2 per day of prednisone or equivalent, if applicable.
   For patients not on corticosteroids, we suggest a maintenance dose of 5–10 mg/1.73 m^2 per day of prednisone or equivalent to avoid CNI monotherapy.
III. If further reduction in immunosuppression is required, we suggest a stepwise reduction of the calcineurin inhibitor dose (tacrolimus trough target 5 ng/mL; cyclosporine trough target 100 ng/mL)
   Target concentrations for further reductions are not well described and need to be individualised. Expert opinion and case reports discuss a tacrolimus target trough concentration of 3 ng/mL and a cyclosporine target trough concentration of 75 ng/mL, followed by a tacrolimus target trough of 1.5 ng/mL and a cyclosporine target trough of 50 ng/mL.

Strategy 2: Calcineurin inhibitor is reduced first

I. Reduce calcineurin inhibitor dose by 25–50% in one or two steps to target trough concentrations of tacrolimus of 3–5 ng/mL and cyclosporine trough concentrations of 75–125 ng/mL)
We suggest further reduction of immunosuppression if BKPyV DNAaemia does *not* decrease by 10-fold or fall below the lower limit of detection after 4 weeks as follows:

II. Reduce the antimetabolite by 50% and taper the corticosteroid dose to 5–10 mg/1.73 m^2 per day of prednisone or equivalent, if applicable.

III. Antimetabolite discontinuation
We suggest a maintenance dose of 5–10 mg/1.73 m^2 per day of prednisone or equivalent for patients who are not on corticosteroids to avoid CNI monotherapy.
Target concentrations for further reduction are poorly described and need to be individualised. Expert opinion and case reports suggest target concentrations of 3 ng/mL for tacrolimus and target concentrations of 75 ng/mL for cyclosporine, followed by nest steps of 1.5 ng/mL and 50 ng/mL, respectively.

6 JC Polyomavirus nephropathy

As JC polyomavirus (JCPyV) nephropathy is very rare, universal screening as for BKPyV is not recommended. The diagnosis of JCPyV nephropathy should be suspected in biopsies detecting LTag expression using the cross-reacting SV40-LTag antibody in a kidney transplant recipient without detectable BKPyV DNAaemia or high-level BKPyV DNAuria [12]. Morphologically, BKPyV and JCPyV nephropathy are indistinguishable. The specific diagnosis of JCPyV nephropathy requires immunohistochemistry staining with JCPyV-specific antibodies, such as those raised against the JCPyV major capsid Vp1 protein or in situ hybridisation with JCPyV-specific probes. Another approach is to determine the tissue viral load of JCPyV-DNA in biopsy material by (semi-)quantitative molecular testing, whereby BKPyV DNA should not be detectable. Kidney transplant patients with JCPyV nephropathy are characterised by high urinary JCPyV loads of >10 million c/mL (or equivalent), while urinary BKPyV loads are low or undetectable. In contrast to BKPyV screening, plasma JCPyV loads are not a reliable marker for screening, diagnosis, or monitoring of JCPyV nephropathy, as they are usually undetectable or low.

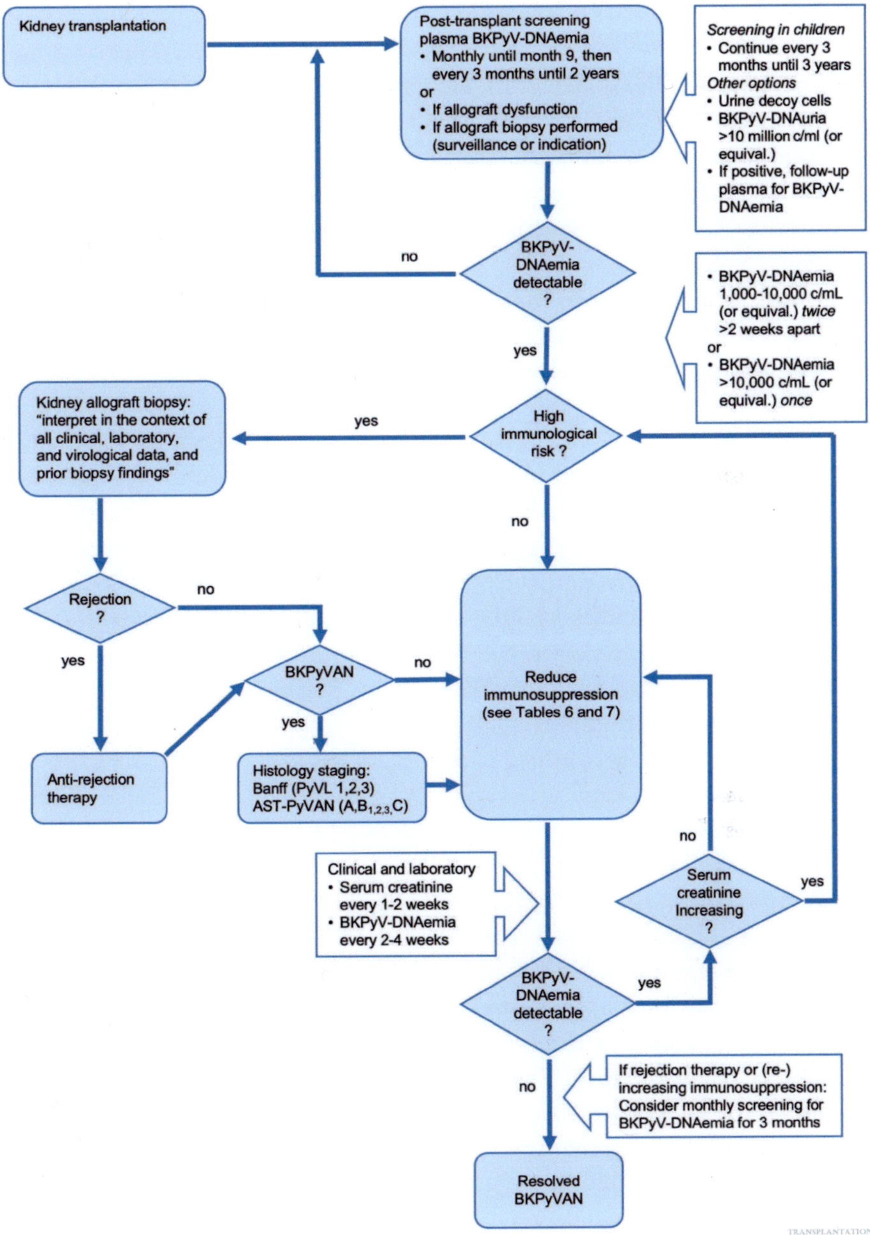
Kidney transplantation
Post-transplant screening plasma BKPyV-DNAemia
• Monthly until month 9, then every 3 months until 2 years
or
• If allograft dysfunction
• If allograft biopsy performed (surveillance or indication)
Screening in children
• Continue every 3 months until 3 years
Other options
• Urine decoy cells
• BKPyV-DNAuria >10 million c/ml (or equival.)
• If positive, follow-up plasma for BKPyV-DNAemia
BKPyV-DNAemia detectable ?
no
yes
• BKPyV-DNAemia 1,000-10,000 c/mL (or equival.) twice >2 weeks apart
or
• BKPyV-DNAemia >10,000 c/mL (or equival.) once
High immunological risk ?
yes
no
Kidney allograft biopsy: "interpret in the context of all clinical, laboratory, and virological data, and prior biopsy findings"
Rejection ?
no
yes
BKPyVAN ?
no
yes
Anti-rejection therapy
Histology staging: Banff (PyVL 1,2,3) AST-PyVAN (A,B1,2,3,C)
Reduce immunosuppression (see Tables 6 and 7)
Clinical and laboratory
• Serum creatinine every 1-2 weeks
• BKPyV-DNAemia every 2-4 weeks
Serum creatinine Increasing ?
no
yes
BKPyV-DNAemia detectable ?
yes
no
If rejection therapy or (re-) increasing immunosuppression: Consider monthly screening for BKPyV-DNAemia for 3 months
Resolved BKPyVAN

References

1 Leuzinger K, Hirsch HH. 2023. Human polyomaviruses, p 2093–2130. In Carroll KC, Pfaller MA (ed), Manual of Clinical Microbiology, 13th ed. ASM Press, Washington, DC.
2 Hirsch HH. 2023. Polyomaviruses, p 2227–2233. In Goldman L, Cooney KA (ed), Goldman-Cecil Medicine, 27th ed, vol 2. Elsevier, Philadelphia, PA.
3 Hirsch HH, Knowles W, Dickenmann M, Passweg J, Klimkait T, Mihatsch MJ, Steiger J. 2002. Prospective study of polyomavirus type BK replication and nephropathy in renal-transplant recipients. N Engl J Med 347:488–496.
4 Jiang D, Mantas A, Studier-Fischer A, Fuchs J, Uluk D, Loos M, Mieth M, Zeier M, Husen P, Golriz M, Kahlert C, Ryschich E, Mehrabi A, Pratschke J, Michalski CW, Czigany Z. 2024. Clinical Research in Renal Transplantation: A Bibliometric Perspective on a Half-century of Innovation and Progress. Transplantation doi:10.1097/TP.0000000000004887.
5 Kaminski MM, Abudayyeh OO, Gootenberg JS, Zhang F, Collins JJ. 2021. CRISPR-based diagnostics. Nat Biomed Eng 5:643–656.
6 Hirsch HH, Mengel M, Kamar N. 2022. BK Polyomavirus Consensus. Clin Infect Dis 75:2046–2047.
7 Höcker B, Schneble L, Murer L, et al. Epidemiology of and Risk Factors for BK Polyomavirus Replication and Nephropathy in Pediatric Renal Transplant Recipients: An International CERTAIN Registry Study. Transplantation. 2019;103(6):1224–1233
8 Kotton CN, Kamar N, Wojciechowski D, Eder M, Hopfer H, Randhawa P, Sester M, Comoli P, Tedesco Silva H, Knoll G, Brennan DC, Trofe-Clark J, Pape L, Axelrod D, Kiberd B, Wong G, Hirsch HH, Transplantation Society International BK Polyomavirus Consensus Group. 2024. The Second International Consensus Guidelines on the Management of BK Polyomavirus in Kidney Transplantation. Transplantation 2024;108(9):1834–1866
9 Ahlenstiel-Grunow T, Pape L. Diagnostics, treatment, and immune response in BK polyomavirus infection after pediatric kidney transplantation. Pediatr Nephrol. 2020 Mar;35(3):375–382.
10 Ahlenstiel-Grunow T, Pape L. Immunosuppression, BK polyomavirus infections, and BK polyomavirus-specific T cells after pediatric kidney transplantation. Pediatr Nephrol. 2020 Apr;35(4):625–631.

11 Fichtner A, Schmidt J, Süsal C, et al. Risk of cellular or antibody-mediated rejection in pediatric kidney transplant recipients with BK polyomavirus replication – an international CERTAIN registry study. Pediatr Nephrol. 2024 Oct 11. doi: 10.1007/s00467-024-06501-7. Online ahead of print.
12 Höcker B, Tabatabai J, Schneble L, et al. JC polyomavirus replication and associated disease in pediatric renal transplantation: an international CERTAIN Registry study. Pediatr Nephrol. 201833(12):2343–2352.

CHAPTER 7.4 Pneumocystis jirovecii

Burkhard Tönshoff & Britta Höcker

Heidelberg University, Medical Faculty Heidelberg, Department of Paediatrics I, University Children's Hospital, Heidelberg, Germany

ORCIDs:
Burkhard Tönshoff: https://orcid.org/0000-0002-6598-6910
Britta Höcker: https://orcid.org/0000-0003-4131-2273

1 Epidemiology

Pneumocystis jirovecii (PJP) is a potentially life-threatening infection in immunocompromised individuals [1]. Pneumocystis is transmitted via the airborne route. New infections in humans are most likely acquired through person-to-person spread [2]. Individuals with normal immune systems may be asymptomatically colonised in the lungs and serve as a reservoir for the spread of Pneumocystis to immunocompromised hosts [3].

2 Risk factors

Patients with human immunodeficiency virus (HIV) and a low CD4 count are at the highest risk of PJP. For patients without HIV, the most significant risk factors are glucocorticoid treatment and defects in cell-mediated immunity [4]. Glucocorticoids increase the risk of developing PJP by suppressing cell-mediated immunity and altering lung surfactant. Other specific risk factors include taking other immunosuppressive medications, having had a solid organ transplant, undergoing treatment for organ rejection or certain inflammatory conditions (particularly rheumatological diseases), having a primary immunodeficiency (e.g., severe combined immunodeficiency) and being severely malnourished.

In the absence of prophylaxis, approximately 5 to 15% of patients who undergo solid organ transplantation develop PJP [5]. Rates are lowest among renal transplant recipients and highest among lung and heart-lung transplant recipients. The period of highest risk for PJP following solid organ transplantation is one to six months post-transplant if prophylaxis is not administered.

Several clusters or outbreaks of PJP in solid organ transplant recipients, primarily kidney transplant recipients, have been reported [2, 6]. Hospitalised patients with PJP should be cared for using standard precautions; however, they should not share a room with other immunocompromised individuals due to the potential for person-to-person transmission.

3 Clinical manifestations

Patients with PJP may present with fulminant respiratory failure, accompanied by fever and a dry cough. However, as clinical awareness of PJP has increased and laboratory diagnosis has improved, patients more commonly present with mild to moderate PJP, experiencing less severe and more indolent dyspnoea and cough. Almost all patients with PJP will experience either hypoxaemia at rest or during exertion, or an increased alveolar–arterial oxygen tension gradient.

The typical *radiographic features* of PJP are diffuse, bilateral interstitial infiltrates. If the chest radiograph is normal, high-resolution computed tomography scanning may reveal extensive ground-glass opacities or cystic lesions.

4 Diagnosis

A diagnosis of PJP should be considered for patients with risk factors for PJP who present with pneumonia and radiographic findings that are suggestive of the condition. Prompt evaluation is warranted. Diagnosis includes microbiological identification of the organism in a sample of induced sputum or bronchoalveolar lavage (BAL) fluid, when possible. The most rapid and least invasive method of diagnosing PJP is analysis of sputum induced by inhaling hypertonic saline [1]. If PJP is not identified using this method, bronchoscopy with BAL should be performed. Detection of the organism in respiratory specimens is most commonly achieved by microscopy with staining of an induced sputum specimen or BAL fluid. Staining is necessary because Pneumocystis cannot be cultured. Several PCR assays have been developed to detect Pneumocystis in induced sputum, bronchoalveolar lavage (BAL) fluid, blood or nasopharyngeal aspirates. These assays are particularly useful for patients without HIV, as the sensitivity of microscopy with staining is substantially lower in this group. BAL and induced sputum samples demonstrate the highest sensitivity and specificity. However, when BAL or induced sputum samples are unavailable, PCR can be performed on upper respiratory tract samples (e.g., nasopharyngeal aspirates or oral washes), although false positives and negatives can occur [7]. When PCR is used to diagnose lower respiratory tract infection in samples from the upper respiratory tract, it is important to distinguish between a positive result due to colonisation or infection.

5 Treatment

Trimethoprim-sulfamethoxazole (TMP-SMX) is the recommended medication for treating PJP in patients without HIV [8, 9]. For patients with normal renal function, the recommended dose of TMP-SMX is 15 to 20 mg/kg body weight per day, administered intravenously or orally in three or four divided doses. However, several studies have suggested low-dose TMP-SMX (7.5 mg/kg to 15 mg/kg) may be safer and just as effective at treatment of PJP [9]. The dosage is based on the TMP component. The dose may need to be adjusted if creatinine clearance changes during therapy. Patients should receive intravenous therapy until they are clinically stable and have a functioning gastrointestinal tract. The usual duration of therapy is 21 days. After completing the course of treatment, patients should be considered for secondary prophylaxis with a reduced dose of the same antimicrobial therapy to prevent recurrent infection. The antimicrobial regimens used for secondary prophylaxis are the same as those used to prevent the initial infection (see below). When TMP-SMX cannot be used for the treatment of PJP, alternative drugs include clindamycin plus primaquine, trimethoprim plus dapsone, atovaquone and pentamidine administered intravenously (IV).

Adjunctive glucocorticoids are recommended for patients with severe disease, for example an arterial blood gas measurement showing a partial pressure of oxygen of less than 70 mmHg, an alveolar-arterial oxygen gradient of at least 35 mmHg, or hypoxaemia on pulse oximetry, while breathing room air. The recommended dosing algorithm is as follows: 40 mg of prednisolone per 1.73 m^2 body surface area orally twice daily for five days, followed by 40 mg per 1.73 m^2 orally once daily for five days, then 20 mg per 1.73 m^2 orally once daily for 11 days.

6 Prophylaxis

PJP is a potentially life-threatening infection that is difficult to treat. PJP prophylaxis is therefore recommended for all paediatric kidney transplant recipients during the first 6–12 months post-transplant, as this almost completely prevents PJP. TMP-SMX is the recommended first-line agent for PJP prophylaxis due to its proven efficacy. TMP-SMX is generally well tolerated in patients without HIV infection, as a meta-analysis found that adverse events necessitating cessation of therapy (leukopenia, thrombocytopenia, or severe dermatologic reactions) occurred in only 3.1 % of adults [10].

Indications for prophylaxis:

- Universal prophylaxis for all paediatric kidney transplant recipients for the first 6 months post-transplant
- Following treatment for an acute rejection episode by glucocorticoid pulse therapy or a lymphocyte-depleting antibody (e.g., thymoglobulin or ATG, especially in cases where the CD4+ T cell count is below 150/µL); administer TMP-SMX prophylaxis for 6 months
- After rituximab therapy, administer TMP-SMX prophylaxis for the duration of B-cell depletion, typically for 12 months.
- All patients with CMV viremia, for as long as CMV viremia persists.

Recommended dosing for prophylactic TMP-SMX:

- Children up to 13 years: 150 mg of trimethoprim per m^2 of body surface area per day and 750 mg of sulfamethoxazole per m^2 per day, taken orally in two daily doses three times per week on alternating days, e.g., on Monday, Wednesday, and Friday. The maximum absolute dose is 160 mg of trimethoprim and 800 mg of sulfamethoxazole.
- Adolescents aged over 13 years: 160 mg of trimethoprim and 800 mg of sulfamethoxazole in one dose, three times per week on alternate days (e.g., Monday, Wednesday, and Friday).

Reducing the dose of TMP-SMX in cases of renal insufficiency:
eGFR 15–30 mL/min/1.73 m^2: reduce the dose by 50%.
For eGFR < 15 mL/min/1.73 m^2, administration is not recommended.

For patients who cannot take TMP-SMX (e.g., those with a history of severe allergic reactions such as Stevens–Johnson syndrome or toxic epidermal necrolysis), we recommend either dapsone (with pyrimethamine if Toxoplasma prophylaxis is required) or atovaquone. For patients for whom haematological toxicity is not a concern, we prefer dapsone as it is cheaper than atovaquone. Patients should undergo testing for glucose-6-phosphate dehydrogenase deficiency prior to taking dapsone.

Another option for PJP prophylaxis is *aerosolised pentamidine,* for example for patients with an eGFR of less than 15 ml/min/1.73 m^2. However, this method is less effective than other regimens, requires specialised equipment and has been associated with the transmission of Mycobacterium tuberculosis. Furthermore, it only has a local effect; if the aerosol does not reach all areas of the lungs, untreated areas remain at risk of PJP.

References

1 Thomas CF Jr, Limper AH. Current insights into the biology and pathogenesis of Pneumocystis pneumonia. Nat Rev Microbiol 2007; 5:298.
2 Höcker B, Wendt C, Nahimana A, Tönshoff B, Hauser PM. Molecular evidence of Pneumocystis transmission in pediatric transplant unit. Emerg Infect Dis. 2005;11(2):330–2.
3 Ponce CA, Gallo M, Bustamante R, Vargas SL. Pneumocystis colonization is highly prevalent in the autopsied lungs of the general population. Clin Infect Dis 2010; 50:347.
4 Rodriguez M, Fishman JA. Prevention of infection due to Pneumocystis spp. in human immunodeficiency virus-negative immunocompromised patients. Clin Microbiol Rev 2004; 17:770.
5 Radisic M, Lattes R, Chapman JF, et al. Risk factors for Pneumocystis carinii pneumonia in kidney transplant recipients: a case-control study. Transpl Infect Dis 2003; 5:84.
6 Le Gal S, Toubas D, Totet A, et al. Pneumocystis Infection Outbreaks in Organ Transplantation Units in France: A Nation-Wide Survey. Clin Infect Dis 2020; 70:2216.
7 Brown L, Rautemaa-Richardson R, Mengoli C, et al. Polymerase Chain Reaction on Respiratory Tract Specimens of Immunocompromised Patients to Diagnose Pneumocystis Pneumonia: A Systematic Review and Meta-analysis. Clin Infect Dis 2024; 79:161.

8 Limper AH, Knox KS, Sarosi GA, et al. An official American Thoracic Society statement: Treatment of fungal infections in adult pulmonary and critical care patients. Am J Respir Crit Care Med 2011; 183:96.
9 Fishman JA, Gans H; AST Infectious Diseases Community of Practice. Pneumocystis jiroveci in solid organ transplantation: Guidelines from the American Society of Transplantation Infectious Diseases Community of Practice. Clin Transplant. 2019 Sep;33(9):e13587.
10 Stern A, Green H, Paul M, et al. Prophylaxis for Pneumocystis pneumonia (PCP) in non-HIV immunocompromised patients. Cochrane Database Syst Rev 2014; CD005590.

CHAPTER 7.5 Urinary tract infections

Markus J. Kemper[1] & Ulrike John-Kroegel[2]

[1] Asklepios Medical School Hamburg, Department of Paediatrics, AK Hospital Hamburg-North, Germany
[2] Department of Pediatric Nephrology, University Children's Hospital of Jena, Germany

ORCIDs:
Markus J. Kemper: https://orcid.org/0000-0002-9205-7906
Ulrike John-Kroegel: https://orcid.org/0009-0007-3575-7256

1 Definition

Urinary tract infection (UTI) is a relevant and frequent complication after paediatric kidney transplantation (KTx); febrile UTI must be distinguished from afebrile UTI. Bacteria growth in excess of 10^5 colony forming units/ml in freshly voided urine is abnormal. The method of bladder urine collection is important (invasive, non-invasive) and has been discussed elsewhere; it mainly depends on the age of the patient and the clinical presentation [1]. Other typical additional urinary abnormalities in UTI include leukocyturia, haematuria and nitrituria, often detected by dipstick testing. Testing for inflammatory markers (leukocytosis, CRP, procalcitonin) is important [2].

2 Risk factors

Risk factors for UTI *before kidney transplantation* include anatomical factors (hydronephrosis, posterior urethral valves, vesicoureteral reflux [VUR] and others) and lower urinary tract dysfunction (e.g. neurogenic bladder). Urinary tract malformations are a common cause of end-stage kidney failure in children. This has implications for the diagnostic work-up prior to KTx: in addition to renal ultrasound, MCUG/CEUS (contrast enhanced ultrasonography) and uroflowmetry should be performed and in more complex patients (posterior urethral valves, neurogenic bladder, Prune Belly syndrome and others) urodynamic studies are necessary [2].

After kidney transplantation, secondary VUR into the transplanted kidney in a previously normal urinary tract must be considered a significant risk factor for febrile UTI. Ranchin et al. [3] demonstrated a 58% prevalence of VUR and an increased rate of UTI. Whether strict anti-reflux surgery can reduce the risk of febrile UTI after renal transplantation has not been studied. Surgical correction of VUR into the kidney graft was shown to reduce the incidence of UTI in a small series, but was associated with obstructive complications [4], particularly in the cohort with associated abnormal bladder anatomy. More recently, Deflux® injection has been performed also in children after KTx, although this appears to be more challenging than in native VUR [5]. Foreign material such as stents, urinary catheters and suture material can cause UTI due to bacterial (and fungal) colonization. Therefore, these devices should only be used for a short time or avoided if possible.

Sex: The rate of UTI in girls is much higher than in boys [6]. Anatomical reasons (e.g. shortened urethra) may be relevant, and sexual activity must be taken into account in female adolescents. *Immunosuppressive therapy* has an impact on defence mechanisms; one study suggested an increased risk in patients on mycophenolate-based regimens [7]. An accumulation of risk factors (e.g. unnecessary catheterisation or manipulation of the urinary tract) should be avoided or at least limited in immunocompromised patients.

3 Clinical presentation

Fever and renal dysfunction are the typical features of febrile UTI after KTX. Some patients may develop symptoms and signs of urosepsis. An acute, concomitant decline in renal function is common during UTI [8], reflecting the inflammatory parenchymal response and the risk of tissue damage to the transplanted kidney (scarring). Acute rejection episodes may be triggered by febrile UTI [9], and also the development of an intrarenal abscess in the graft following UTI has also been described [10].

4 Prevalence

A high prevalence of febrile UTI in children after KTx has been reported in several retrospective studies [2, 7]. They are not limited to the immediate post-transplant period but also occur later, especially in girls [9]. In paediatric studies, the prevalence ranged from 15% to 33%. A higher prevalence of up to 61% has been reported in adults, but some studies have used less stringent inclusion criteria and for instance included patients with (asymptomatic) afebrile bacteriuria. Pelle et al. demonstrated a prevalence of UTI of 75.1%; 18.7% of these patients developed transplant pyelonephritis [11]. This leads to a higher hospitalisation rate especially in children.

5 Epidemiology

Although *Escherichia coli* remained the most commonly isolated microorganism, as in other studies, it was isolated less frequently than in the general paediatric population, where it is found in up to 80% of UTIs [12]. This may be due to the underlying immunosuppression and colonisation of the urinary tract. Therefore, from a practical point of view, it is important that surveillance urine cultures are performed in every patient at risk to increase awareness of local antibiotic resistance. Particular attention should be paid to patients with lower urinary tract abnormalities and neurogenic bladder requires attention, in order to identify bacteria with multiple resistances (Pseudomonas species and Enterobacter). In recent years, there has been an increase in UTI with drug-resistant pathogens such as vancomycin-resistant Enterococcus, -extended-spectrum beta-lactamase-producing Enterobacteriaceae (ESBL-E), carbapenem-resistant Enterobacteriaceae and carbapenem-resistant Enterobacteriaceae, and carbapenem-resistant Pseudomonas species [13, 14].

6 Treatment

Febrile UTI post-transplant on immunosuppressive therapy should be considered as complicated pyelonephritis and be treated aggressively with parenteral antibiotics, at least until clinical improvement and culture results are available. The optimal duration of treatment has not been studied, but most would favour a total (i.e. parenteral followed by oral treatment) of 10–14 days in transplant pyelonephritis [2, 7]. As Enterococci and Pseudomonas species are more common, we currently use an initial combination of ceftazidime and ampicillin/sulbactam or clavulanate to cover E. coli, Pseudomonas and Enterococci. Others have recommended ampicillin and gentamicin for the same reason [13, 14], but nephrotoxicity of the latter is a concern. Fungal urinary tract infections may occur and require specific treatment; often antifungal prophylaxis is often given during high-dose antibiotic treatment to reduce the risk of this complication. It is not uncommon for steroid doses to be increased during febrile UTIs to avoid symptoms of adrenal insufficiency.

Afebrile symptomatic UTI may be treated with oral antibiotics unless there are specific risk factors are present (renal dysfunction etc) [2, 13, 14]. Again, treatment should be specific and an oral cephalosporin may be the first choice. Whether asymptomatic UTI need to be treated remains controversial and is often an individual decision. In patients with abnormal bladder anatomy and regular catheterisation, such as those with spina bifida, colonisation is common and symptoms such as dysuria may be absent. There is no evidence or consensus on whether bacterial colonisation in these patients requires treatment, including bladder washing with antibiotics. In our centre, we currently only treat symptomatic patients with abnormal bladder anatomy and bacterial colonisation and do not use antibiotic bladder irrigation.

7 Diagnostic workup and prevention of (febrile) urinary tract infection

Non-invasive investigations include sonography in the acute infection to demonstrate or exclude dilatation of the urinary tract, tissue perfusion and bladder emptying. Diagnosis of vesicoureteral reflux into the graft may be facilitated by conventional radiological cystography (MCUG) or contrast-enhanced ultrasonography. Static dimercaptosuccinic acid scintigraphy (DMSA scan) is an elegant method of documenting renal scarring when performed after 6 months or more after graft pyelonephritis. Patients with voiding dysfunction may require further work-up including uroflowmetry or complex urodynamic studies.

Prevention and prophylaxis of febrile UTI after KTx are important. This includes antibiotic chemoprophylaxis, e.g., with trimethoprime. Most importantly, urotherapy should be offered to candidates with lower urinary tract dysfunction; in severe cases, intermittent catheterisation may be necessary. If vesicoureteral reflux into the graft is present and febrile UTI persists despite conservative measures, surgery or Deflux® injection should be discussed. Probiotics are often used in children after KTx, although there are no controlled trials on their benefits or side effects [16].

References

1 ’t Hoen LA, Bogaert G, Radmayr C, Dogan HS, Nijman RJM, Quaedackers J, Rawashdeh YF, Silay MS, Tekgul S, Bhatt NR, Stein R. Update of the EAU/ESPU guidelines on urinary tract infections in children. J Pediatr Urol. 2021 Apr;17(2):200–207. doi: 10.1016/j.jpurol.2021.01.037. Epub 2021 Feb 2. Erratum in: J Pediatr Urol. 2021 Aug;17(4):598. doi: 10.1016/j.jpurol.2021.06.022. PMID:33589366.

2 John U, Kemper MJ. Urinary tract infections in children after renal transplantation. Pediatr Nephrol. 2009 Jun;24(6):1129–36. doi: 10.1007/s00467-007-0690-0. Epub 2008 Jan 16. PMID: 18197424; PMCID: PMC2704952

3 Ranchin B, Chapuis F, Dawhara M, Canterino I, Hadj-Aissa A, Said MH, et al. (2000) Vesicoureteral reflux after kidney transplantation in children. Nephrol Dial Transplant 15:1852–8.

4 Neuhaus TJ, Schwobel M, Schlumpf R, Offner G, Leumann E, Willi U (1997) Pyelonephritis and vesicoureteral reflux after renal transplantation in young children. J Urol 157:1400–3.

5 Obata S, Nagata K, Suematsu S, Nishiyama K, Okabe Y, Kondo T, Maniwa J, Fukuta A, Kawakubo N, Yanagi Y, Miyata J, Matsuura T, Ohga S, Nakamura M, Tajiri T. The Effectiveness of Deflux® Treatment for Vesicoureteral Reflux Following Pediatric Renal Transplantation: A Single-Institution Challenging Experience. JPediatr Surg. 2024 Apr;59(4):616–620. doi: 10.1016/j.jpedsurg.2023.12.005. Epub2023 Dec 12. PMID: 38161090.

6 John U, Everding AS, Kuwertz-Broking E, Bulla M, Muller-Wiefel DE, Misselwitz J, et al. (2006) High prevalence of febrile urinary tract infections after paediatric renal transplantation. Nephrol Dial Transplant 21:3269–74

7 Goldman JD, Julian K, Practice ASTIDCo. Urinary tract infections in solid organ transplant recipients: guidelines from the American Society of Transplantation Infectious Diseases Community of Practice. Clin Transplant. 2019;33(9):e13507

8 Weigel F, Lemke A, Tönshoff B, Pape L, Fehrenbach H, Henn M, Hoppe B, Jungraithmayr T, Konrad M, Laube G, Pohl M, Seeman T, Staude H, Kemper MJ, John U. Febrile urinary tract infection after pediatric kidney transplantation: a multicenter, prospective observational study. Pediatr Nephrol. 2016 Jun;31(6):1021–8. doi: 10.1007/s00467-015-3292-2. Epub 2016 Jan 11. PMID:26754038.

9 Maraha B, Bonten H, van Hooff H, Fiolet H, Buiting AG, Stobberingh EE (2001) Infectious complications and antibiotic use in renal transplant recipients during a 1-year follow-up. Clin Microbiol Infect 7:619–25
10 Audard V, Amor M, Desvaux D, Pastural M, Baron C, Philippe R, et al. (2005) Acute graft pyelonephritis: a potential cause of acute rejection in renal transplant. Transplantation 80:1128–30.
11 Eilers E, Moter A, Bollmann R, Haffner D, Querfeld U (2007) Intrarenal abscesses due to Ureaplasma urealyticum in a transplanted kidney. J Clin Microbiol 45:1066–8.
12 Pelle G, Vimont S, Levy PP, Hertig A, Ouali N, Chassin C, et al. (2007) Acute pyelonephritis represents a risk factor impairing long-term kidney graft function. Am J Transplant 7:899–907
13 Benfield MR, McDonald RA, Bartosh S, Ho PL, Harmon W (2003) Changing trends in pediatric transplantation: 2001 Annual Report of the North American Pediatric Renal Transplant Cooperative Study. Pediatr Transplant 7:321–35.
14 Coussement J, Bansal SB, Scemla A, Svensson MHS, Barcan LA, Smibert OC, Clemente WT, Lopez-Medrano F, Hoffman T, Maggiore U, Catalano C, Hilbrands L, Manuel O, DU Toit T, Shern TKY, Chowdhury N, Viklicky O, Oberbauer R, Markowicz S, Kaminski H, Lafaurie M, Pierrotti LC, Cerqueira TL, Yahav D, Kamar N, Kotton CN. Initial empirical antibiotic therapy in kidney transplant recipients with pyelonephritis: A global survey of current practice and opinions across 19 countries on six continents. Transpl Infect Dis. 2024 Aug 26:e14362. doi: 10.1111/tid.14362. Epub ahead of print. PMID: 39185755.
15 McAteer J, Tamma PD.Diagnosing and Managing Urinary Tract Infections in Kidney Transplant Recipients. Infect Dis Clin North Am. 2024 Jun;38(2):361–380. doi: 10.1016/j.idc.2024.03.008. PMID: 38729666 Review.
16 Kizilbash SJ, Connolly H, Bartosh S, Zahr R, Al-Akash S, Chishti A, Mansuri A, Tawadrous H, Jain NG. Probiotic use in pediatric kidney transplant recipients: What are current practices, and are they evidence-based? A pediatric nephrology research consortium study. Pediatr Transplant. 2024 Aug;28(5):e14790. doi: 10.1111/petr.14790. PMID: 38837638.

CHAPTER 7.6 Vaccinations before and after organ transplantation in children

Maximilian Stich & Susanne Rieger

Heidelberg University, Medical Faculty, Department of Paediatrics I, University Children's Hospital Heidelberg, Germany

ORCIDs:
Maximilian Stich: https://orcid.org/0000-0002-6237-9058
Susanne Rieger: https://orcid.org/0009-0005-4799-713x

Recommendations for practice

The question of the benefits and risks of vaccinations in children after organ transplantation often arises. On one hand, the impaired immune system and the resulting increased susceptibility to infections represent a strong indication for many vaccinations (e.g. influenza). On the other hand, concerns persist regarding potential side effects and the risk of triggering rejection through immunostimulation. This brief guide aims to address the uncertainty that often leads to an unfounded reluctance to vaccinate organ transplant recipients.

Importance of the immunosuppressive regimen

- Immunosuppressive drugs reduce the induction and maintenance of humoral and cellular immunity.
- High-dose immunosuppression (especially MMF) is associated with a weaker vaccination response
- The level of antibody titres does not correlate reliably with immunity.

Opportunities and risks

- Sufficiently large vaccination studies for most inactivated vaccines: Side effects are rare and there is no evidence of organ rejection after vaccination with inactivated vaccines [Laws et al; Bundesgesundheitsbl. 2020; 63:588–644].

- Live vaccines are generally not recommended after organ transplantation as their safety has not been sufficiently proven. For unvaccinated patients: individual decision after thorough risk assessment.

Vaccination BEFORE organ transplantation:

As a better vaccination response is achieved before transplantation and immunity is not lost through transplantation, early vaccination before transplantation is recommended. Complete the standard vaccinations as recommended by the Standing Committee on Vaccination, Robert Koch Institute (www.rki.de):

- Measles-Mumps-Rubella-Varicella: permitted from 9 months of age (in urgent cases from 6 months of age).

Table 1 Additional recommended vaccinations

Hepatitis A	From 12 months of age (Liver transplant recipients: from 6 months of age)
Pneumococci	Age 2–17 years: sequential administration of PPSV23 (Pneumovax®) at the earliest 2 (preferably 6–12) months after PPV13 (Prevenar13®) Age ≥ 18 years: 1 dose of PCV20 (Prevenar20®) a least 6 years after PPSV23
Meningococcal ACWY	From 12 months of age: 1 dose (Nimenrix® approved from 6 weeks, but then 2nd dose + booster at 1 year)
Influenza	From 6 months of age: annual booster in autumn; for the 1st vaccination: 2nd dose after 4–6 weeks
COVID-19	From 6 months of age: annual autumn booster; Basic immunisation: ≥3 antigen contacts; of which ≥1 vaccination
Tick-borne encephalitis	If exposed to ticks in risk areas Basic immunisation: 3 doses (at intervals of 1–3 and 5–12 months)
Herpes zoster	Age ≥ 18 years and after primary VZV infection 2 doses of Shingrix® (2–6 months apart)

- Complete vaccination series with inactivated vaccines at least 2 weeks and with live vaccines at least 4 weeks (measles-mumps-rubella) or 6–8 weeks (varicella) prior to transplantation.
- Serological assessment of anti-VZV (anti-measles/mumps/rubella) and anti-HBs 4–8 weeks after completion of the vaccination series and anti-HBs annually prior to transplantation
  - Anti-HBs < 100 IU/L, re-vaccination and repeat anti-Hbs monitoring
  - Anti-HBs < 10 IU/L, determination of HBsAG and anti-HBc. If chronic HBV infection is excluded, revaccinate.

Vaccination AFTER organ transplantation

Live vaccines: are in general contraindicated after organ transplantation and require careful risk assessment in unvaccinated patients (see Laws et al.; Bundesgesundheitsbl. 2020; 63(5):588–644). But after individual risk assessment, live vaccines can also be considered for unprotected patients after organ transplantation [3].

Contraindicated vaccinations in immunosuppressed patients:

- Measles, mumps, rubella, varicella (attenuated live viruses)
- Rotavirus (attenuated live virus)
- Typhoid oral live vaccine
- Oral poliomyelitis live vaccine (OPV)
- Yellow fever (attenuated live virus)
- Tuberculosis: Bacillus Calmette-Guerin vaccine (BCG)
- Live nasal influenza vaccine

Inactivated vaccines: After organ transplantation, vaccinations can and should be given after the end of high-dose immunosuppression, usually 6 months after transplantation. An exception is the influenza vaccination, which can be given as early as 4 weeks after transplantation, depending on the season. If the basic immunisation with inactivated vaccines (standard and indication vaccines) has not been completed before transplantation, it should be completed after the end of high-dose immunosuppression, usually 6 months after transplantation.

This differs from pre-transplant vaccination:

- Tick-borne encephalitis: 4 instead of 3 vaccine doses (0,1,3,12 months) or serological control 4 weeks after the 2nd dose
- Meningococcal ACWY: 2 doses instead of 1 (interval 1–2 months)
- Hepatitis B: double the standard dose if necessary (off-label)

Table 2 Recommended booster doses of inactivated vaccines after completion of basic immunisation

Vaccine	Booster vaccination
Tetanus	every 5–10 years
Diphtheria	every 5–10 years or antibody titre < 0.1 IU/mL
Pertussis	every 5–10 years
Poliomyelitis	once at the age of 9–16 years
Hepatitis B	if anti-HBs < 100 IU/L (monitor anti-HBs titre annually and 4–8 weeks after booster vaccination)
Meningococcal B	every 5 years
Meningococcal ACWY	every 5 years
TBE	3 years after the 3rd dose, then every 5 years
Influenza	annually in autumn
COVID-19	annually in autumn
Pneumococci	Age < 18 years: every 6 years PPSV23 Age ≥ 18 years: PCV20 6 years after PPSV23

Vaccination of household contacts

Complete age-appropriate standard immunisations as recommended by the Standing Committee on Vaccination, Robert Koch Institute (www.rki.de).

Additional recommended vaccinations

- Annual influenza and SARS-CoV-2
- Tetanus, diphtheria and pertussis: booster vaccination every 10 years
- Hepatitis B
- Hepatitis A: in case of increased risk of exposure or child with LTx
- Measles, mumps, rubella, varicella in the absence of immunity (if an exanthema occurs after varicella vaccination, contact with immunosuppressed persons should be avoided until the exanthema has subsided).

Contraindicated vaccines

- Oral poliomyelitis live vaccine (OPV)
- Live nasal influenza vaccine

Travel recommendations

Before travelling

- Do not travel to countries with an increased risk of infection within the first 12 months after transplantation
- Timely health advice and vaccinations before travelling (e.g., according to the recommendations of the Standing Committee on Vaccination (STIKO) and the German Society for Tropical Medicine, Travel Medicine and Global Health e.V. (DTG) on travel vaccinations. Epid Bull 2024; 14:1–206)
- Adequate supply of medicines
- Translation of medical report/patient ID card
- Certificate of contraindication to yellow fever vaccination
- Planning for return in case of need for rapid return

During the trip

- Boiled water only
- Cooked or peeled food only
- Beware of diarrhoea:
    - Dehydration worsens kidney function

  - Altered absorption of immunosuppressive drugs: tacrolimus level↑, cyclosporine level↓
- Barrier protection against mosquito bites and sun exposure

These recommendations do not relieve the treating physician of the responsibility to make individual therapeutic decisions for each patient.

Further information: www.rki.de STIKO recommendations, Robert Koch Institute

The recommendations of the Standing Committee on Vaccination (STIKO) are also available as a free STIKO@rki app. There is also a web version of the app at www.STIKO-web-app.de, which can be used on a PC.

www.dtg.org Recommendations for travel vaccinations and malaria prophylaxis, German Society for Tropical Medicine and Global Health

References

1 Empfehlungen der Ständigen Impfkommission (STIKO) am Robert-Koch-Institut 2024: Epid Bull 2024;4:1–72. doi:10.25646/11892.3
2 Ständige Impfkommission und Deutsche Gesellschaft für Tropenmedizin, Reisemedizin und Globale Gesundheit e.V.: Empfehlungen der Ständigen Impfkommission (STIKO) und der Deutschen Gesellschaft für Tropenmedizin, Reisemedizin und Globale Gesundheit e.V. (DTG) zu Reiseimpfungen. Epid Bull 2024;14:1–206. doi:10.25646/12006.2
3 Laws HJ, Baumann U, Bogdan C, et al. Impfen bei Immundefizienz: Anwendungshinweise zu den von der Ständigen Impfkommission empfohlenen Impfungen. (III) Impfen bei hämatologischen und onkologischen Erkrankungen (antineoplastische Therapie, Stammzelltransplantation), Organtransplantation und Asplenie. Bundesgesundheitsblatt Gesundheitsforschung Gesundheitsschutz. 2020;63(5):588–644. doi:10.1007/s00103-020-03123-w

4 Niehues T, Bogdan C, Hecht J, et al. Impfen bei Immundefizienz: Anwendungshinweise zu den von der Ständigen Impfkommission empfohlenen Impfungen. (I) Grundlagenpapier. Bundesgesundheitsblatt Gesundheitsforschung Gesundheitsschutz. 2017;60(6):674–684. doi:10.1007/s00103-017-2555-4

CHAPTER 8
Haematological, osteological and metabolic complications

CHAPTER 8.1 Diagnosis and treatment of anaemia

Anja Büscher[1] & Dominik Müller[2]

[1] Department of Paediatrics II, University Hospital of Essen, Essen, Germany
[2] Department of Paediatrics, Charité University Hospital, Berlin, Germany

Background

- Definition of post-transplant anaemia (PTA): Haemoglobin concentration below the age norm after kidney transplantation (KTx).
- The prevalence of PTA is high, especially within the first year after KTx (1 month after KTx: 80–87%, 1 year: 20–48% and > 3 years: 35–57%). Females and younger children are more often affected.
- The target haemoglobin is the normal value for age and sex (Table 1).
- The aetiology of PTA is varied (see causes [below]).
- PTA is a risk factor for cardiovascular morbidity and is negatively associated with graft function, graft and patient survival and quality of life.

Causes

Reduced production of haemoglobin/erythrocytes

- Underlying disease affecting the bone marrow (e.g. cystinosis, oxalosis)
- Iron, vitamin B12 or folic acid deficiency (e.g. due to reduced dietary intake (vegans), impaired absorption or intestinal losses)
- Medications that are toxic to bone marrow: anti-infectives (e.g. valgancyclovir, cotrimoxazole), inhibitors of the renin-angiotensin-aldosterone system, immunosuppressants (antibodies such as ATG, basiliximab) and maintenance immunosuppressants (MMF, everolimus, tacrolimus, azathioprine), analgesics (metamizole).

Table 1 Age- and sex-specific reference values for haemoglobin and haematocrit in childhood

Age	Haemoglobin (g/dL)	Haematocrit (%)
1 year	10.7–13.1	33–40
2–6 years	10.8–14.3	34–41
7–12 years	11.3–14.9	37–43
13–18 years female	12.0–16.0	36–44
13–18 years male	14.0–18.0	39–47

Reference: www.laborlexikon.de/Lexikon/Tabellen/17-Blutbild_Kinder.htm

- Viral infections (parvovirus B19, human herpesvirus 6 (HHV6), cytomegalovirus (CMV), Epstein-Barr virus (EBV), hepatitis viruses, HIV)
- Acute/chronic inflammation (infection, rejection)
- Post-transplant lymphoproliferative disease (PTLD)
- Graft dysfunction (primary non-function or chronic graft failure, e.g. due to acute/chronic rejection)
- Chronic kidney disease (reduced synthesis of erythropoietin, metabolic acidosis, secondary hyperparathyroidism)

Increased loss/turnover

- Repeated blood sampling, surgery, interventions (biopsy)
- Female patients: Dysmenorrhoea, hypermenorrhoea
- Chronic intestinal bleeding (gastric or intestinal ulcers, e.g. due to glucocorticoids)
- Haemolysis (e.g. drug-induced haemolytic uraemic syndrome (cyclosporin A, tacrolimus)
- Hepatosplenomegaly (e.g. in autosomal recessive polycystic kidney disease)

Clinical symptoms

- (Mucus) skin pallor
- Tiredness, fatigue, reduced stamina
- Tachycardia, low blood pressure
- Melana
- Icterus
- Hepatosplenomegaly

Diagnostics

Medical history

- Underlying disease
- Medications (immunosuppressants, anti-infectives, analgesics, ACE inhibitors, sartans)
- Diet (e.g. vegetarianism, veganism)

Laboratory values

- Blood count with MCV, MCH, reticulocytes, Ret-Hb
- Iron, ferritin, transferrin, transferrin saturation, folate, vitamin B12
- Blood gas analysis
- Creatinine (GFR), urea, uric acid
- LDH, haptoglobin, bilirubin
- Parathyroid hormone, 25-OH vitamin D
- Virology: Parvovirus B19, HHV6, CMV, EBV (IgG, IgM, DNA), polyomavirus (BK and JC virus), hepatitis B and C serology, HIV
- Haemoccult

Diagnostic imaging

- Sonography of the abdomen (kidney transplant, liver and spleen size, ascites, intra-abdominal lymph nodes, bowel wall thickening) and neck (cervical lymph nodes, parathyroid glands)
- Oesophagogastroscopy and colonoscopy if necessary (to rule out intestinal bleeding)
- Bone marrow aspiration (if necessary)

Table 2 Drug therapy for post-transplant anaemia

Medication	Dosage[1]
Oral iron supplementation (e.g. Ferro sanol®, Ferrum Hausmann®)	2–6 mg/kg b.w. per day in 2–3 doses (at least 1 hour before or after intake of immunosuppressants)
Intravenous iron supplementation	
Sodium ferrogluconate	1–1.5 mg/kg b.w. in 50 mL 0.9% NaCl over 60 min i.v.
Iron sucrose	1–2 mg/kg b.w. in 25 mL 0.9% NaCl over 60 min i.v.
Iron carbomaltose	2–8 mg/kg b.w. in 20 mL 0.9% NaCl over 15 min i.v.
Erythropoiesis-stimulating agents	
Epoetin alpha	**Initially:** 100–300 IU/kg b.w. per week s.c. (in 1–3 doses) **Long-term:** 100 IU/kg b.w. per week s.c. (in one dose)
Darbepoietin alpha	0.45 ug/kg b.w. per week s.c. or 0.75 µg/kg b.w. every 2 weeks s.c. (in one dose)
Methoxy-polyethylenglycol-epoetin beta	1.5–3 µg/kg b.w. every 4 weeks s.c. or i.v.
Supplementation with vitamins	
Folic acid	5–10 mg/day p.o.
Vitamin B12	0.5–1 mg/week (in one dose) p.o.

Abbreviations: b.w., body weight; i.v., intravenous; p.o., per os; s.c., by subcutaneous injections

[1] Caution: higher doses may be required in case of non-response.

Treatment

Treatment depends on the underlying cause and degree of anaemia.

- Identification and, if necessary, modification of immunosuppressive or other potentially bone marrow toxic drugs
- Treatment of viral infections
- Correction of metabolic acidosis and vitamin D replacement in renal hyperparathyroidism
- Oral replacement for iron or vitamin B12/folic acid deficiency (i.v. for non-responders or severe deficiency [Table 2])
- Subcutaneous or intravenous administration of erythropoietin/analogues (dose and frequency according to response (haemoglobin). Younger patients often require higher doses per kg body weight. Dose adjustment during therapy is recommended.

References

1 Guzzo I and Atkinson MA, Pediatr Nephrol (2023) 38:3265–3273
2 Ichimaru N, et al. Transplant Proc (2016) 48:878–883
3 Krischock LA et al. Pediatr Nephrol (2016) 31:325–333
4 Galutira PJ and Del Rio D (2012) Pediatr Nephrol 27:1079–1085

CHAPTER 8.2 CKD mineral and bone disorder post-transplant

Agnieszka Prytuła[1], Claus P. Schmitt[2], Dieter Haffner[3] & Rukshana Shroff[4]

[1] Department of Paediatric Nephrology and Rheumatology, Ghent University Hospital, Ghent, Belgium
[2] Department of Paediatrics I, University Children's Hospital Heidelberg, Heidelberg, Germany
[3] Department of Paediatric Kidney, Liver, Metabolic and Neurological Diseases, Hannover Medical School, Hannover, Germany
[4] Renal Unit, University College London Great Ormond Street Hospital, London, United Kingdom

ORCIDs:
Agnieszka Prytuła: https://orcid.org/0000-0001-9551-8758
Claus P. Schmitt: https://orcid.org/0000-0003-4487-3332
Dieter Haffner: https://orcid.org/0000-0002-9601-7813
Rukshana Shroff: https://orcid.org/0000-0001-8501-1072

1 Causes and clinical spectrum of post-transplant CKD-MBD

Chronic Kidney Disease-Mineral and Bone Disorder (CKD-MBD) is highly prevalent in paediatric kidney transplant recipients, even in those with a good allograft function. The main contributing factors include pre-transplant CKD-MBD, graft function and the side effects of immunosuppressive drugs. Prior to transplantation, and starting from the early stages of CKD, every effort should be made to optimise bone health, but severe pre-transplant CKD-MBD is not a reason to delay or withhold transplantation. The clinical picture of post-transplant CKD-MBD is broad and includes bone pain, skeletal deformities, fractures, growth failure and ectopic vascular calcification.

a. First 3 months post-transplant

The earliest alteration in the pathogenesis of pre-transplant CKD-MBD is elevated levels of the phosphaturic hormone fibroblast growth factor 23 (FGF23), followed by low levels of 1,25-dihydroxyvitamin D, hypocalcaemia, hyperparathyroidism, and hyperphosphatemia [1]. During the recovery phase post-transplant, elevated levels of FGF23 and parathyroid hormone (PTH) often persist for several months, which in the presence of restored kidney function may cause *hypophosphatemia and promote impaired bone mineralisation.* In a retrospective analysis of 1,210 paediatric transplant recipients, 36% had hypophosphatemia 4 weeks post-transplant. There was no association with allograft dysfunction [2]. In addition, *hypomagnesemia* may occur as a side effect of tacrolimus due to tubular wasting.

Given that no adverse patient- or allograft outcomes have been reported to date in paediatric kidney transplant recipients with mild or moderate hypophosphatemia or hypomagnesemia, supplementation should be considered mainly in severe or symptomatic cases, bearing in mind that phosphate and magnesium supplements may cause diarrhoea and further reduce drug absorption.

b. 3 months post-transplant and beyond

After the recovery period CKD-MBD parameters often remain within reference ranges, although high PTH levels have been reported even in patients with good allograft function. At 1 year post-transplant, 56% of patients with an estimated glomerular filtration rate (eGFR) ≥ 30 mL/min/1.73 m^2 had elevated PTH levels, and the degree of hyperparathyroidism was associated with allograft dysfunction [2]. In addition, higher PTH levels have been reported in kidney transplant recipients than in pre-transplant patients with a similar eGFR [2, 3] (Table 1).

Table 1 Comparison of pre- and post-transplant PTH levels in different CKD stages

Pre-transplant	**Overall**	**Stage 2 (eGFR ≥ 60 ml/min per 1.73 m^2)**	**Stage 3a (eGFR 45–59 ml/min per 1.73 m^2)**	**Stage 3b (eGFR 30–44 ml/min per 1.73 m^2)**	**Stage 4 (eGFR 15–29 ml/min per 1.73 m^2)**
Plasma iPTH, pg/ml	51 [30, 84]	37 [26, 54]	48 [26, 70]	55 [33, 95]	74 [47, 181]
Post-transplant					
Plasma iPTH, pg/ml		55 [38, 81]	62 [40, 90]	81 [52, 122]	

Data is given as median and interquartile range; iPTH, intact PTH

In 1,237 children included in the European Society for Paediatric Nephrology (ESPN) and European Renal Association (ERA) registry, abnormal serum phosphate levels were found in 25% of patients (14% hypophosphatemia and 11 % hyperphosphatemia), and serum phosphate levels were inversely associated with eGFR. Serum phosphate levels above the recommended targets were associated with a higher risk of graft failure independent of eGFR [4].

2 Evaluation of post-transplant CKD-MBD

a. Clinical evaluation

Points to consider:

- Monitor height (length at age < 2 years), weight, skeletal deformities, and history for bone pain and fractures.
- The frequency of monitoring depends on the age, graft function, and degree of skeletal abnormalities at the time of kidney transplantation and during follow-up.

b. Laboratory evaluation

Points to consider:

- Monitor serum calcium, phosphate and alkaline phosphatase levels using age- and/or sex-specific normal ranges as well as PTH and 25-hydroxyvitamin D.
- Use trends in serum biomarkers considered together, rather than individual laboratory values, to guide therapeutic decisions.
- Tailor the frequency of monitoring to the time since kidney transplantation, the presence and severity of CKD-MBD, age, allograft function, concomitant medications, and in the early post-transplant period, also the degree of pre-transplant CKD-MBD
- Do not routinely measure 1,25-dihydroxyvitamin D levels

c. Imaging

Evidence for radiological evaluation and bone biopsy in the management of mineral bone disease in paediatric kidney transplant patients is limited.

Points to consider:
- Consider performing X-rays when the results are expected to impact on treatment decisions, i.e. in children with bone pain, suspected fractures or slipped epiphyseal dislocations, suspected avascular necrosis, to assess skeletal maturity, and in children with genetic diseases with specific bone involvement (e.g. oxalosis).
- Imaging techniques such as dual-energy X-ray absorptiometry (DXA), peripheral quantitative computed tomography (pQCT), high-resolution pQCT (HR-pQCT), magnetic resonance imaging (MRI) and ultrasound should be reserved for exceptional clinical cases and research questions.
- The risk-benefit ratio of these procedures should always be considered, particularly with regard to radiation exposure.
- Bone biopsies should be considered in paediatric transplant recipients only in rare, selected cases when clinical and biochemical findings do not explain the underlying bone disease, e.g. severe bone deformity or pain, low energy fractures, persistent hypercalcemia or hypophosphatemia, despite optimisation of treatment. Histomorphometric analysis should only be performed in centres with experience in interpreting paediatric bone biopsies.

3 Management of post-transplant CKD-MBD

a. Nutrition

Beyond 3 months from kidney transplantation maintaining serum calcium and phosphate within the normal range for age is recommended. This can be achieved by adequate dietary calcium and phosphate intake and supplementation if required. While many aspects of the diet can be liberalised after kidney transplantation, particular attention should be paid to sodium and energy intake. Transplant recipients are at high risk of hypertension, so it is important to maintain dietary sodium intake within the recommendations of the Chronic Disease Risk Reduction as a starting point, and to reduce it further in those with hypertension. In addition, renal and extra-renal sodium losses, as well as the sodium intake from medication, need to be taken into account when recommending a dietary sodium intake. In particular, sodium intake from processed and ultra-processed foods needs to be restricted.

In addition, patients tend to gain weight rapidly after kidney transplantation; so energy consumption should be carefully managed to avoid obesity and its associated complications.

b. Vitamin D - native and active

The prevalence of vitamin D deficiency persists after transplantation. The age- and CKD stage-specific recommendations for native vitamin D supplementation are considered appropriate for children after kidney transplantation [5]. Similarly, active vitamin D (alfacalcidol or calcitriol) may be used to control hyperparathyroidism or hypocalcaemia, using comparable CKD stage-specific recommendations [6].

c. Calcimimetics

Calcimimetics are not approved for use in children after kidney transplantation, but may be considered on an off-label basis in those with severe and persistent hyperparathyroidism with associated hypercalcaemia [7]. This situation may occur in those with severe pre-transplant MBD, or in those with a failing allograft.

d. Antiresorptive agents

Antiresorptive agents are not recommended in children after kidney transplantation, but may be considered in the setting of severe hypercalcaemia that persists despite withdrawal of all sources of calcium and vitamin D. Short-acting bisphosphonates such as pamidronate are preferred to long-acting bisphosphonates. In rare situations where hypercalcaemia is thought to be secondary to severe bone demineralisation, such as in patients with prolonged bed rest, denosumab may be considered.

4 Glucocorticoid-sparing immunosuppression and bone health

The benefits of glucocorticoid-sparing immunosuppression in terms of statural growth are described in Chapter 5.1. Glucocorticoid exposure is also associated with reduced bone mineral density (BMD) and increased fracture incidence, although data in paediatric patients are scarce. In a prospective longitudinal analysis of 58 recipients, Terpstra et al. reported a significant decrease in trabecular BMD after transplantation associated with greater glucocorticoid exposure, while cortical BMD increased significantly in association with greater glucocorticoid exposure and greater decreases in PTH levels [8]. Another study by Helenius et al. reported an unusually high fracture rate in 75 out of 196 paediatric solid organ transplant recipients with a 5-year follow-up. While all patients were treated with glucocorticoids, there was no association between fracture incidence and the cumulative glucocorticoid dose [9]. Overall, glucocorticoid-sparing immunosuppressive protocols should be favoured in children after kidney transplantation to improve bone health, taking into account local standards and the patient's risk profile for graft rejection including medication adherence, previous rejection and donor-specific HLA antibodies.

References

1 Drueke TB, Massy ZA. Changing bone patterns with progression of chronic kidney disease. Kidney international. 2016;89(2):289–302.
2 Prytula A, Shroff R, Krupka K, Deschepper E, Bacchetta J, Ariceta G, et al. Hyperparathyroidism Is an Independent Risk Factor for Allograft Dysfunction in Pediatric Kidney Transplantation. Kidney Int Rep. 2023;8(1):81–90.
3 Portale AA, Wolf M, Juppner H, Messinger S, Kumar J, Wesseling-Perry K, et al. Disordered FGF23 and mineral metabolism in children with CKD. Clinical journal of the American Society of Nephrology: CJASN. 2014;9(2):344–53.
4 Bonthuis M, Busutti M, van Stralen KJ, Jager KJ, Baiko S, Bakkaloglu S, et al. Mineral metabolism in European children living with a renal transplant: a European society for paediatric nephrology/european renal association-European dialysis and transplant association registry study. Clinical

journal of the American Society of Nephrology: CJASN. 2015;10(5):767–75.

5 Shroff R, Wan M, Nagler EV, Bakkaloglu S, Fischer DC, Bishop N, et al. Clinical practice recommendations for native vitamin D therapy in children with chronic kidney disease Stages 2–5 and on dialysis. Nephrol Dial Transplant. 2017;32(7):1098–113.

6 Shroff R, Wan M, Nagler EV, Bakkaloglu S, Cozzolino M, Bacchetta J, et al. Clinical practice recommendations for treatment with active vitamin D analogues in children with chronic kidney disease Stages 2–5 and on dialysis. Nephrol Dial Transplant. 2017;32(7):1114–27.

7 Bernardor J, Schmitt CP, Oh J, Sellier-Leclerc AL, Buscher A, Dello Strologo L, et al. The use of cinacalcet after pediatric renal transplantation: an international CERTAIN Registry analysis. Pediatr Nephrol. 2020;35(9):1707–18.

8 Terpstra AM, Kalkwarf HJ, Shults J, Zemel BS, Wetzsteon RJ, Foster BJ, et al. Bone density and cortical structure after pediatric renal transplantation. Journal of the American Society of Nephrology: JASN. 2012;23(4):715–26.

9 Helenius I, Remes V, Salminen S, Valta H, Makitie O, Holmberg C, et al. Incidence and predictors of fractures in children after solid organ transplantation: a 5-year prospective, population-based study. Journal of bone and mineral research: the official journal of the American Society for Bone and Mineral Research. 2006;21(3):380–7.

CHAPTER 8.3 Growth disorders

Burkhard Tönshoff[1] & Dieter Haffner[2]

[1] Heidelberg University, Medical Faculty Heidelberg, Department of Paediatrics I, University Children's Hospital, Heidelberg, Germany
[2] Department of Pediatric Kidney, Liver, Metabolic and Neurological Diseases Children's Hospital, Hannover Medical School, Germany

ORCIDs:
Burkhard Tönshoff: https://orcid.org/0000-0002-6598-6910
Dieter Haffner: https://orcid.org/0000-0002-9601-7813

1 Importance and prevalence

Growth failure is a major complication of children with chronic kidney disease (CKD). Approximately one-third of children with CKD have evidence of short stature (i.e., height < 3rd percentile for age and sex). The risk for poor growth increases with decreasing kidney function. Poor growth in children with CKD is associated with increased morbidity (e.g., increased hospitalization rate, decreased school attendance, and poorer physical function) and increased mortality. Growth failure results in adult short stature, which contributes to a lower perceived quality of life and self-esteem.

Kidney transplantation is the optimal kidney replacement therapy modality to prevent and correct growth failure, as a well-functioning allograft restores the physiological conditions required for normal growth. However, growth rates after kidney transplantation in children are highly variable and often do not fulfil the expectations of true catch-up growth, which generally is only observed in children less than five years of age [1].

2 Contributing factors

The main contributing factors to growth outcome in paediatric kidney allograft recipients are administration of growth hormone pre-transplant (positive), glucocorticoid exposure (negative), and reduced graft function (negative) [2]. The final height also depends on the age of the child at the time of transplantation, the severity of the growth failure at time of transplantation, congenital CKD, birth parameters, parental height, inadequate nutrition, metabolic acidosis, fluid and electrolyte abnormalities, anaemia, and CKD-related-mineral and bone disorders (CKD-MBD) [2, 3]. The first step to optimize growth outcome after kidney transplantation is to minimize height deficit at the time of transplantation which includes the use of growth hormone in case of persisting growth failure despite adequate nutrition and other measures contributing to growth failure in children with CKD [1]. In addition, early/preemptive kidney transplantation is a key measure as growth failure in patients on long-term dialysis treatment can be hardly overcome even with the use of recombinant human growth hormone [1]. The positive effect of living related transplantation on growth outcome reported in previous studies seems to be largely related to better graft function in these patients when compared to those with deceased donors [1].

3 Evaluation of growth

For each child with CKD, ongoing assessment of growth is based on determining height/length at every visit and to calculate annual growth velocity. These measurements can be related to age- and sex dependent growth (velocity) charts and/or converted to Z-scores of height/length measurement or growth velocity that represent the number of standard deviations from the mean values for age and sex based on data for the general population. The diagnoses of short stature and growth failure in children with CKD are based upon the following definitions:

- Short stature is defined as a length/height Z-score < -1.88 or a length/height for age < 3rd percentile.
- Growth failure is defined as height velocity Z-score < -1.88 or a height velocity for age < 3rd percentile that persists beyond three months.

4 Management - Reducing glucocorticoid exposure

Daily glucocorticoid therapy following kidney transplantation has historically been an important contributor to poor growth in children. The introduction of other immunosuppressive agents (e.g., calcineurin inhibitors [cyclosporine, tacrolimus]) and mycophenolate mofetil [MMF]), has greatly reduced the need for glucocorticoid therapy in paediatric kidney transplant recipients. Strategies to reduce the cumulative effects of glucocorticoid therapy include early or late glucocorticoid withdrawal and use of alternative immunosuppressive agents. Clinical trials and observational studies have demonstrated that steroid-sparing regimens are associated with improved growth following transplantation [4, 5]. Details regarding use of glucocorticoid-sparing immunosuppressive therapy in kidney transplant recipients are provided in chapter 5.1.

5 Management - Treatment with growth hormone

Successful kidney transplantation reverses the uremic milieu and should theoretically permit normal growth hormone (GH) secretion and function [6]. Persistent growth failure in this setting is primarily a result of reduced graft function and glucocorticoid therapy. If catch-up growth cannot be achieved by using a glucocorticoid-sparing regimen, we suggest initiating recombinant human (rh) GH therapy, particularly in children with suboptimal graft function (GFR < 50 mL/min per 1.73 m^2), in whom spontaneous catch-up growth is unlikely to occur [7, 8]. rhGH is usually prescribed only after the first year post-transplant, because spontaneous growth should be monitored for at least 12 months after kidney transplantation.

In a meta-analysis of five randomized controlled trials including 401 paediatric kidney transplant recipients, children receiving rhGH therapy had higher growth velocity compared with the control group after one year (mean standardized height difference of 0.68, 95% CI 0.25–1.11) [9]. The mean difference in growth expressed as change in height Z-score between the rhGH and control groups was 0.52 (95% CI 0.37–0.68). There was no apparent between-group difference in rates of rejection rate between the two groups (17 versus 10 percent, risk ratio 1.56, 95% CI 0.97–2.53). The study did not detect a difference in GFR between the two groups. Additional evidence supporting the benefit of rhGH in growth-delayed kidney allograft recipients was provided by a retrospective NAPRTCS study that compared the outcome of 513 paediatric kidney allograft recipients who received rhGH with 2,263 transplant patients who were not treated with rhGH [10]. The rhGH-treated group had improved growth with a mean cumulative increase in height of 3.6 cm over five years compared with controls, which resulted in higher mean final adult height Z-scores (−1.8 versus −2.6). An important limitation of the available data is that most studies were conducted in an earlier era when transplant recipients commonly received immunosuppressive regimens that included glucocorticoids. Thus, the findings in these studies may not be generalizable to the contemporary era wherein glucocorticoid-sparing regimens are generally preferred for post-transplant immunosuppression.

5.1 Goals of therapy

The goal of rhGH therapy in children with CKD is "normalization" of final height. There is some debate concerning how this goal is defined. The most commonly used definitions are either:

- Attainment of the patient's individual target height (i.e., above the lower end of the patient's mid-parental height range, or
- Attainment of a normal population-related final height (i.e., > 3rd percentile or a Z-score > −1.88). Although the former goal is certainly desirable for the individual patient, the latter approach may be economically more acceptable in view of the high cost of rhGH therapy. In our practice, the minimal therapeutic goal is a height greater than the third percentile of the general population.

5.2 Criteria for initiating rhGH

Expert panels of paediatric nephrologists and endocrinologists developed the following criteria for initiation of rhGH therapy. We generally initiate rhGH therapy if all of the following criteria are met:

- Persistent growth impairment – This is generally defined as growth delay that persists for > 3 months in infants and > 6 months in older children. As discussed below, different thresholds are used to define growth impairment for this criterion. We generally prefer early initiation of therapy (i.e., when the child's height for age is between the 3rd and 10th percentiles or height velocity is < 25th percentile for age) rather than waiting until the child meets stricter criteria for growth failure.
- Other factors that contribute to growth impairment (see above) should be addressed prior to starting rhGH.
- Kidney transplant recipients who do not have spontaneous catch-up growth by one year post-transplantation.

- Child has growth potential – Based on clinical assessment and presence of open epiphyses on radiographic bone age.
- Children with active malignancies should not receive rhGH therapy.

5.3 Timing

The optimal timing for starting rhGH therapy is uncertain. In particular, there is debate as to whether therapy should be started at an early stage when the child first shows signs of growth delay or if it should be used only once the child meets strict criteria for growth failure. In general, beginning treatment at a younger age (before six years of age) and early in the course of CKD leads to a better response to rhGH, which is more likely to result in normal or near-normal adult height.

5.4 Pre-treatment evaluation

The following baseline assessments should be performed prior to starting rhGH therapy: Laboratory tests, including blood glucose, serum creatinine, serum calcium and phosphate levels, parathyroid hormone (PTH) level, fundoscopic examination, bone age, determining pubertal status (i.e., Tanner stage).

5.5 Pre-treatment counselling

Although it might be assumed that most children with CKD who are shorter than their peers wish to be taller, the advantages and disadvantages of rhGH therapy must be discussed with the patient and their family/caregivers. In addition to reviewing the benefits and potential side effects of rhGH as outlined in this topic, counselling should include a frank discussion of the burdens of receiving daily subcutaneous injections for many years. These considerations are of particular importance for immobilized patients and those with syndromic kidney diseases [5].

5.6 Dosing

The recommended dose of rhGH for children with CKD is 0.045 to 0.05 mg/kg body weight per day given once daily (typically in the evening) via subcutaneous injection. The injection site should be changed daily to avoid lipoatrophy. The dose of rhGH used for treating children with CKD-related growth failure is greater than what is typically used for treating children with GH deficiency. This is consistent with the current understanding that CKD causes GH insensitivity. As a result, children with CKD require a higher therapeutic dose rather than simply replacement dosing as is used in children with GH deficiency.

5.7 Adverse effects

Long-term rhGH therapy is generally safe and well tolerated in children with CKD [11, 12]. Reported side effects associated with rhGH treatment in children include headaches (usually mild), idiopathic intracranial hypertension (pseudotumor cerebri), increased intraocular pressure, slipped capital femoral epiphysis, worsening of existing scoliosis, insulin resistance/glucose intolerance/type 2 diabetes. Based on the available data, treatment-associated adverse events are rare in children with CKD receiving rhGH therapy.

5.8 Monitoring for side effects

We suggest the following monitoring for patients with CKD treated long-term with rhGH [13]: We suggest monitoring for T2DM with haemoglobin A1c and/or fasting blood glucose at least annually. This is particularly important in patients with additional risk factors (e.g., concomitant glucocorticoid treatment, family history of type 2 diabetes). Most patients treated with rhGH therapy maintain normal glucose tolerance; however, there are rare reports of development of T2DM in children with CKD that appeared to be temporally related to starting rhGH therapy. In all cases, the abnormalities resolved after discontinuation of rhGH therapy.

- *Eye examination* – Children receiving rhGH therapy should have routine fundoscopic examinations to assess for signs of papilledema suggestive of idiopathic intracranial hypertension (pseudotumor cerebri). Examinations are performed every three to four months initially, and then annually if there are no concerns.

- *Monitoring for CKD-mineral bone disorder (CKD-MBD) and orthopaedic complications* – This includes: serum calcium, phosphate, and PTH levels, measured every three to four months initially; hip and knee radiographs if the patient develops symptoms concerning for slipped capital femoral epiphysis. CKD-MBD should be adequately treated before starting rhGH therapy. rhGH therapy should be withheld in patients with persistent severe secondary hyperparathyroidism (PTH > 500 pg/mL) and can be reinstituted when PTH levels return to the desired target range [14, 15]. There is not an associated deterioration of renal osteodystrophy, but rapid growth acceleration may contribute to an increased risk of slipped capital femoral epiphysis. As a result, it is advisable to obtain bone radiographs prior to initiating rhGH and to repeat the studies if symptoms occur.

5.9 Response to treatment

The response to treatment is assessed with the following: (i) measuring the growth velocity, (ii) monitoring pubertal stage, (iii) radiographic bone age, assessed annually. An adequate growth response to rhGH is defined as a growth velocity that is ≥ 2 cm/year over the baseline prior to starting therapy.

Monitoring the response to rhGH therapy in children with CKD differs from the approach used in children with GH deficiency. Specifically, insulin-like growth factor-I (IGF-I) levels are *not* routinely monitored in the CKD population whereas IGF-I levels are routinely used for guiding dose adjustments in children with primary GH deficiency. Measurement of total IGF-I levels is not informative in children with CKD because free IGF-I levels decrease with decreasing glomerular filtration rate (GFR).

5.10 Treatment failure

For patients who do not adequately respond to rhGH therapy (i.e., growth velocity < 2 cm/year over the baseline prior to rhGH therapy), the following evaluation should be performed: (i) assess patient compliance by taking a focused history since nonadherence is an important contributor to poor treatment response [16]; (ii) confirm the weight-based rhGH dose is correct, and if necessary, readjust the dose for weight gain; (iii) assess whether other nutritional or metabolic factors for poor growth are present, and if so, initiate a corrective treatment plan.

Patients with persistently poor growth despite correction of these issues may require referral to a paediatric endocrinologist for further evaluation of other possible causes of growth failure.

5.11 Duration of therapy

The optimal duration of rhGH remains uncertain. Although clinical studies have shown that the growth response is greatest in the first two years of therapy, growth velocity is persistently greater than baseline in years three through five of therapy. Dosing needs to be readjusted every three to four months to account for weight gain. In our practice, we continue rhGH therapy so long as growth velocity remains ≥ 2 cm/year above the baseline pre-treatment growth rate. Treatment is discontinued if any of the following occur [5, 13]: (i) closed epiphyses on bone radiograph, (ii) development of an active malignancy, (iii) hypersensitivity to rhGH or components of its formulation, (iv) increased intracranial pressure, (v) noncompliance that cannot be adequately addressed, (vi) severe hyperparathyroidism based on CKD stage – PTH level > 400 pg/mL for patients with CKD stage 2 through 4 and > 900 pg/mL for patients with CKD stage 5. In addition, a dose reduction (e.g., 50 percent of the usual dose) may be considered when the height goal is achieved based on mid-parental height.

References

1 Haffner D. Strategies for optimizing growth in children with chronic kidney disease. Front Pediatr. 2020;8:399

2 Jagodzinski C, Mueller S, Kluck R, Froede K, Pavičić L, Gellermann J, Mueller D, Querfeld U, Haffner D, Zivicnjak M. Growth hormone treatment in the pre-transplant period is associated with superior outcome after pediatric kidney transplantation. Pediatr Nephrol. 2022;37(4):859–869.

3 Grohs J, Rebling RM, Froede K, et al. Determinants of growth after kidney transplantation in prepubertal children. Pediatr Nephrol 2021; 36:1871.

4 Tsampalieros A, Knoll GA, Molnar AO, et al. Corticosteroid Use and Growth After Pediatric Solid Organ Transplantation: A Systematic Review and Meta-Analysis. Transplantation 2017; 101:694.
5 Drube J, Wan M, Bonthuis M, et al. Clinical practice recommendations for growth hormone treatment in children with chronic kidney disease. Nat Rev Nephrol 2019; 15:577.
6 Nissel R, Brázda I, Feneberg R, et al. Effect of renal transplantation in childhood on longitudinal growth and adult height. Kidney Int 2004; 66: 792.
7 Tönshoff B, Haffner D, Mehls O, et al. Efficacy and safety of growth hormone treatment in short children with renal allografts: three year experience. Members of the German Study Group for Growth Hormone Treatment in Children with Renal Allografts. Kidney Int 1993; 44:199.
8 Acott PD, Pernica JM. Growth hormone therapy before and after pediatric renal transplant. Pediatr Transplant 2003; 7:426.
9 Wu Y, Cheng W, Yang XD, Xiang B. Growth hormone improves growth in pediatric renal transplant recipients – a systemic review and meta-analysis of randomized controlled trials. Pediatr Nephrol 2013; 28:129.
10 Fine RN, Stablein D. Long-term use of recombinant human growth hormone in pediatric allograft recipients: a report of the NAPRTCS Transplant Registry. Pediatr Nephrol 2005; 20:404.
11 Hodson EM, Willis NS, Craig JC. Growth hormone for children with chronic kidney disease. Cochrane Database Syst Rev 2012:CD003264.
12 Fine RN, Ho M, Tejani A, Blethen S. Adverse events with rhGH treatment of patients with chronic renal insufficiency and end-stage renal disease. J Pediatr 2003; 142:539.
13 Mahan JD, Warady BA, Consensus Committee. Assessment and treatment of short stature in pediatric patients with chronic kidney disease: a consensus statement. Pediatr Nephrol 2006; 21:917.
14 Kidney Disease: Improving Global Outcomes (KDIGO) CKD-MBD Work Group. KDIGO clinical practice guideline for the diagnosis, evaluation, prevention, and treatment of Chronic Kidney Disease-Mineral and Bone Disorder (CKD-MBD). Kidney Int Suppl 2009:S1.
15 Klaus G, Watson A, Edefonti A, et al. Prevention and treatment of renal osteodystrophy in children on chronic renal failure: European guidelines. Pediatr Nephrol 2006; 21:151.
16 Akchurin OM, Schneider MF, Mulqueen L, et al. Medication adherence and growth in children with CKD. Clin J Am Soc Nephrol 2014; 9:1519.

CHAPTER 8.4 Metabolic acidosis

Agnieszka Prytuła

Department of Pediatric Nephrology and Rheumatology, Ghent University Hospital, Ghent, Belgium

ORCID:
https://orcid.org/0000-0001-9551-8758

1 Definition and types of metabolic acidosis

Metabolic acidosis is defined as plasma bicarbonate (HCO_3^-) level ≤ 22 mmol/L. It is often subdivided into low HCO_3^- levels (18.1 to 21.9 mmol/L), corresponding to mild to moderate metabolic acidosis, and very low HCO_3^- levels (≤ 18 mmol/L), corresponding to severe metabolic acidosis. The reported prevalence of mild to moderate and severe metabolic acidosis ranged from 20% to 39% and from 3% to 7%, respectively, over time in a cohort of 1911 paediatric kidney transplant recipients with up to 10 years of follow-up [1].

Post-transplant metabolic acidosis with *normal anion gap* can be classified as follows: (i) type I (distal, classic), (ii) type IVa, aldosterone resistance with low blood pressure due to hypovolaemia and hyperkalemia and (iii) type IVb, also known as pseudohypoaldosteronism type 2, with elevated blood pressure and hyperkalemia.

Experimental data suggest that calcineurin inhibitors impair mineralocorticoid transcriptional activity in the distal tubular cells and may cause aldosterone resistance, hyperkalemia, and type IV metabolic acidosis [2]. In addition, there is a strong clinical and experimental evidence that calcineurin inhibitors induce activation of salt reabsorption in the distal convoluted tubule with consequent impaired delivery of sodium to the collecting duct, thereby inducing hypervolaemia and hypertension [3, 4]. Distinguishing between different types of metabolic acidosis may be useful in tailoring and personalising treatment. In contrast to type I metabolic acidosis, type IV metabolic acidosis may respond to treatment with fludrocortisone (type IVa) or thiazide (type IVb) rather than to alkaline supplementation. In a cohort of 576 adult kidney transplant recipients with stable allograft function, 28% of patients developed type IV metabolic acidosis [5]. Paediatric data on the prevalence of different types of metabolic acidosis are not available, but persistently low HCO_3^- levels have been reported in 42% of paediatric kidney transplant recipients on alkaline therapy [1].

2 Factors associated with metabolic acidosis in paediatric kidney transplant recipients [1, 6]

- *Mild to moderate metabolic acidosis:* younger recipient age, female sex, deceased donor, tubulointerstitial kidney disease
- *Severe metabolic acidosis:* higher tacrolimus pre-dose concentration, younger recipient age, female sex, low systolic blood pressure, low estimated glomerular filtration rate (eGFR)

3 Metabolic acidosis and allograft outcome

In patients with chronic kidney disease (CKD), metabolic acidosis is associated with accelerated loss of kidney function [7, 8], and a large observational study of adult kidney transplant recipients reported an association between metabolic acidosis, graft failure and mortality [9]. These findings were not confirmed in a randomised trial analysing the effect of sodium bicarbonate supplementation on the rate of eGFR decline in 240 adult kidney transplant recipients with a mean HCO_3^- level of 21 mmol/L (placebo group) to 21.3 mmol/L (treatment group), which is mild metabolic acidosis [10]. There was no difference in eGFR decline after 2 years of follow-up, and the authors concluded that treatment with sodium bicarbonate should not be generally recommended in adult kidney transplant recipients with metabolic acidosis to preserve allograft function [10]. Given the differences in age, comorbidities, comedication, diet and distinct risk factors for metabolic acidosis such as young patient age in paediatric patients, these findings should not be directly extrapolated to a paediatric population. In a recent report including 1911 paediatric patients, there was a stepwise increase in the rate of allograft dysfunction with the severity of time-varying metabolic acidosis, as shown in Figure 1 [1].

Figure 1 Association between the degree of time-varying metabolic acidosis and time to composite endpoint defined as either graft failure or estimated glomerular filtration rate (eGFR) ≤ 30 mL/min per 1.73 m^2 or ≥ 50% decline in eGFR from eGFR at month 3 post-transplant (source: Kidney International Reports, 2024 [1]).

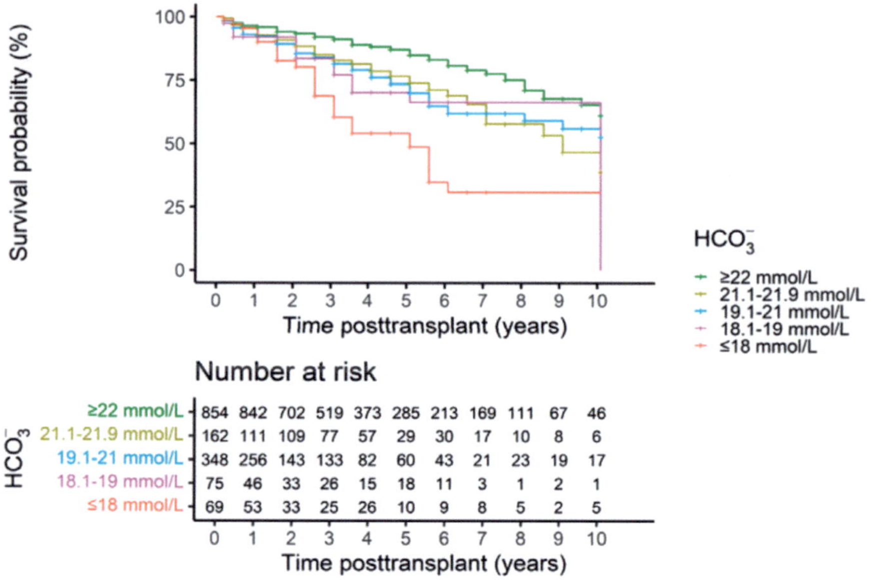

Reference: HCO_3^- ≥ 22 mmol/L
HCO_3^- 21.1–21.9 mmol/L; HR, 1.90, 95% CI, 1.27 to 2.85, $p = 0.002$
HCO_3^- 19.1–21 mmol/L; HR, 1.94, 95% CI, 1.40 to 2.67, $p < 0.0001$
HCO_3^- 18.1–19 mmol/L; HR, 2.57, 95% CI, 1.42 to 4.67, $p = 0.002$
HCO_3^- ≤ 18 mmol/L; HR, 4.09, 95% CI, 2.58 to 6.51, $p < 0.0001$

4 Metabolic acidosis and statural growth

Metabolic acidosis has been implicated as a risk factor for poor growth in paediatric CKD by causing disturbances in the growth hormone (GH)-insulin-like growth factor 1 (IGF-1) axis [11]. In animal models, metabolic acidosis inhibits GH secretion and activates catabolic pathways, leading to impaired muscle development, protein wasting and increased inflammation [12, 13]. It also inhibits osteoblast activity while stimulating osteoclasts, resulting in a defect in bone mineralisation [14]. In humans, metabolic acidosis causes a decreased IGF-1 response to circulating GH, resulting in a state of GH resistance [15]. Although treatment of metabolic acidosis has been postulated as one of the strategies to improve growth in paediatric kidney transplant recipients, there is a paucity of literature on the clinically relevant relationship between metabolic acidosis and growth failure. In a German study of 389 patients, metabolic acidosis was present in 30% of patients and showed an inverse association with body height, leg length, and sitting height [16]. More recently, in an analysis of 2,147 primary kidney transplant recipients, no statistically significant association was found between statural growth and HCO_3^- levels, and the shape of the estimated association showed a decreasing estimated growth with increasing HCO_3^-, as shown in Figure 2 [17].

Figure 2 Lack of association between plasma bicarbonate levels and statural growth expressed as Δ height relative to time between 2 consecutive visits in 2,147 primary KTx recipients analysed using Generalised Additive Mixed Models adjusted for covariates. The shape of the estimated association showed a decreasing estimated statural growth with increasing plasma bicarbonate levels.

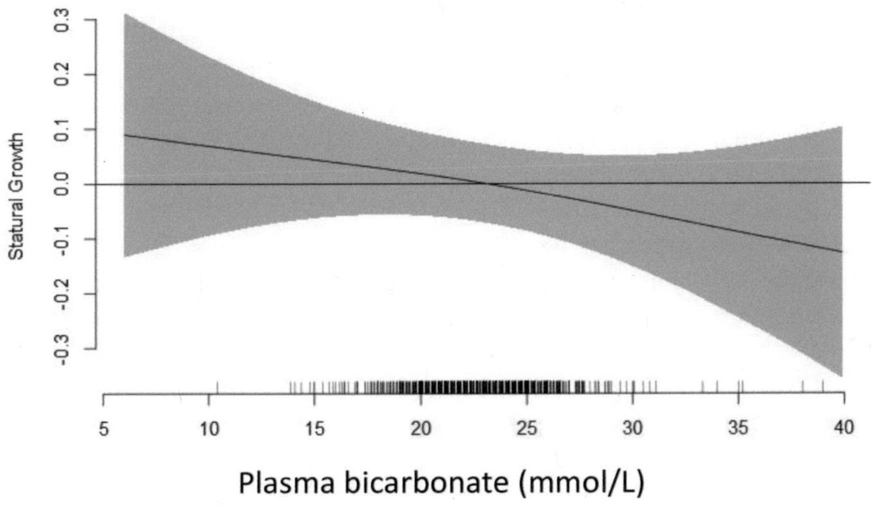

Although these findings do not support alkaline treatment in paediatric kidney transplant recipients with metabolic acidosis to attenuate growth failure, they should be confirmed in a prospective study to analyse whether mild to moderate metabolic acidosis requires treatment.

References

1 Prytula A, Shroff R, van Gremberghe I, Krupka K, Bacchetta J, Benetti E, et al. Metabolic Acidosis Is Associated With an Accelerated Decline of Allograft Function in Pediatric Kidney Transplantation. Kidney Int Rep. 2024;9(6):1684–93.
2 Deppe CE, Heering PJ, Viengchareun S, Grabensee B, Farman N, Lombes M. Cyclosporine a and FK506 inhibit transcriptional activity of the human mineralocorticoid receptor: a cell-based model to investigate partial aldosterone resistance in kidney transplantation. Endocrinology. 2002;143(5):1932–41.
3 Hoorn EJ, Walsh SB, McCormick JA, Furstenberg A, Yang CL, Roeschel T, et al. The calcineurin inhibitor tacrolimus activates the renal sodium chloride cotransporter to cause hypertension. Nature medicine. 2011;17(10):1304–9.
4 Hoorn EJ, Walsh SB, Unwin RJ, Ellison DH. Hypertension after kidney transplantation: calcineurin inhibitors increase salt-sensitivity. J Hypertens. 2012;30(4):832–3; author reply 3–4.
5 Schwarz C, Benesch T, Kodras K, Oberbauer R, Haas M. Complete renal tubular acidosis late after kidney transplantation. Nephrol Dial Transplant. 2006;21(9):2615–20.
6 Kilduff S, Hayde N, Viswanathan S, Reidy K, Abramowitz MK. Metabolic acidosis in pediatric kidney transplant recipients. Pediatr Nephrol. 2023;38(12):4165–73.
7 Dobre M, Yang W, Chen J, Drawz P, Hamm LL, Horwitz E, et al. Association of serum bicarbonate with risk of renal and cardiovascular outcomes in CKD: a report from the Chronic Renal Insufficiency Cohort (CRIC) study. American journal of kidney diseases: the official journal of the National Kidney Foundation. 2013;62(4):670–8.
8 Tangri N, Stevens LA, Griffith J, Tighiouart H, Djurdjev O, Naimark D, et al. A predictive model for progression of chronic kidney disease to kidney failure. JAMA. 2011;305(15):1553–9.
9 Park S, Kang E, Park S, Kim YC, Han SS, Ha J, et al. Metabolic Acidosis and Long-Term Clinical Outcomes in Kidney Transplant Recipients. Journal of the American Society of Nephrology: JASN. 2017;28(6):1886–97.

10 Mohebbi N, Ritter A, Wiegand A, Graf N, Dahdal S, Sidler D, et al. Sodium bicarbonate for kidney transplant recipients with metabolic acidosis in Switzerland: a multicentre, randomised, single-blind, placebo-controlled, phase 3 trial. Lancet (London, England). 2023;401(10376):557–67.
11 Brown DD, Dauber A. Growth Hormone and Insulin-Like Growth Factor Dysregulation in Pediatric Chronic Kidney Disease. Horm Res Paediatr. 2021;94(3–4):105–14.
12 Challa A, Krieg RJ, Jr., Thabet MA, Veldhuis JD, Chan JC. Metabolic acidosis inhibits growth hormone secretion in rats: mechanism of growth retardation. Am J Physiol. 1993;265(4 Pt 1):E547–53.
13 Ulrich EH, Chanchlani R. Impact of Metabolic Acidosis and Alkali Therapy on Linear Growth in Children with Chronic Kidney Disease: What Is the Current Evidence? Kidney360. 2022;3(4):590–6.
14 Jorgetti V, Drueke TB, Ott SM. Role of proton receptor OGR1 in bone response to metabolic acidosis? Kidney Int. 2016;89(3):529–31.
15 Brungger M, Hulter HN, Krapf R. Effect of chronic metabolic acidosis on the growth hormone/IGF-1 endocrine axis: new cause of growth hormone insensitivity in humans. Kidney Int. 1997;51(1):216–21.
16 Franke D, Thomas L, Steffens R, Pavicic L, Gellermann J, Froede K, et al. Patterns of growth after kidney transplantation among children with ESRD. Clinical journal of the American Society of Nephrology: CJASN. 2015;10(1):127–34.
17 Prytuła A, Reynders D, Goetghebeur E, et al. Factors associated with statural growth in pediatric kidney transplant recipients with focus on metabolic acidosis. Pediatr Nephrol 2025;40(6):2059–70

CHAPTER 8.5 Dyslipidaemia

Susanne Rieger[1], Sandra Habbig[2] & Lutz T. Weber[2]

[1] Heidelberg University, Medical Faculty, Department of Paediatrics I, University Children's Hospital Heidelberg, Germany
[2] Department of Paediatrics, University Hospital Cologne and Faculty of Medicine, University of Cologne, Kerpener Str. 62, 50937 Cologne, Germany

ORCIDs:
Susanne Rieger: https://orcid.org/0009-0005-4799-713x
Sandra Habbig: https://orcid.org/0000-0002-6511-5023
Lutz T. Weber: https://orcid.org/0000-0003-4116-598X

1 Introduction

The prevalence of dyslipidaemia in paediatric kidney transplant recipients is 10–60% [1]. In addition to immunosuppressive therapy, other comorbidities such as impaired graft function, obesity, proteinuria and diabetes mellitus contribute to its development. Dyslipidaemia causes atherosclerosis and is a classic risk factor for cardiovascular disease (CVD). Cardiovascular mortality is increased up to 1,000-fold in paediatric patients with chronic kidney disease compared to healthy controls [2]. In paediatric kidney transplant patients, CVD remains the second leading cause of mortality [3], although kidney transplantation substantially reduces several risk factors for CVD and consecutively cardiac mortality 10- to 100-fold [2]. The American Heart Association (AHA) has therefore stratified transplant recipients into the highest risk group for development of CVD [2].

2 Determination of CVD risk

(i) Identification of risk factors for CVD: family history of hyperlipidaemia, smoking status, level of physical activity, blood pressure, body mass index (BMI), fasting glucose, HbA_1C, dysregulation of the calcium/phosphate metabolism, anaemia, chronic inflammation, hyperhomocysteinaemia, albuminuria, hypothyroidism.

A positive family history of dyslipidaemia and cardiovascular disease requires a more intensive diagnostic and therapeutic approach for risk reduction.

(ii) Monitoring of blood lipids (non-fasting: triglycerides (TG), total cholesterol (TC), LDL-C (low-density-lipoprotein cholesterol), HDL-C (high-density-lipoprotein cholesterol)

- At 2–3 months post-transplant
- At 2–3 months after any change in therapy or condition that could cause dyslipidaemia
- At least 1 x per year
- Repeat lipid panel in fasting state in case of abnormal values

Table 1 Target ranges

LDL-cholesterol	≤ 130 mg/dL preferably ≤ 100 mg/dL	≤ 3.36 mmol/L ≤ 2.59 mmol/L
Total cholesterol (TC)	< 250 mg/dL	< 6.47 mmol/L
Non-HDL cholesterol	< 160 mg/dL	< 4.17 mmol/L
Triglycerides (TG)	< 400 mg/dL	< 4.56 mmol/L

(iii) Sonographic diagnosis: non-invasive measurement of carotid intima-media thickness (cIMT) as a surrogate for cardiovascular damage (reference values [6]).

3 Prophylactic options:

Therapeutic lifestyle changes (TLC) [7]:

- Dietary advice (e.g., rapeseed or olive oils, trans-fat-free margarines)
- Physical activity advice: Children: ≥ 60 minutes of active play daily; Adolescents: 3 to 4 times a week moderate physical activity (e.g., 20–30 minutes of walking, swimming, supervised activity within ability) and resistance exercise training (i.e., exercises that cause muscle contraction against an external resistance)
- Limit screen time (computer + video games and TV) to ≤ 2 hours per day as recommended by the WHO
- Weight loss

- Stop smoking
- Optimal treatment of hypothyroidism and diabetes, if present

4 Therapeutic options

Step 1:
(i) Therapeutic lifestyle changes (TLC) [7]
- Physical activity guidance: see above
- Diet with < 30% of calories from fat, < 7% of calories from saturated fat, 10% from polyunsaturated fat, cholesterol < 200 mg/d, avoidance of trans-fatty acids according to prescription of registered paediatric dietitian, used judiciously in case of failure to thrive
- Diet with whole grains, high fibre foods, legumes, fruits and vegetables
- Reduce obesity (refer to obesity clinic)

(ii) Adjustment of immunosuppressive therapy (balance with risk of rejection) [8]:
- Steroid withdrawal/minimisation
- Cyclosporin A withdrawal/minimisation/change to tacrolimus
- mTOR inhibitor withdrawal/minimisation

Step 2:
Start statin therapy in children aged > 8–10 years (> 6 years for rosuvastatin) if LDL-C target is not achieved within 6 months with therapeutic lifestyle changes.

General recommendations
- Start with the lowest recommended dose and increase in small increments, no more than every 4 weeks.
- In general, be aware of the frequent drug interactions of statins – *check if combined with any drug.*
- Monitor serum CK (especially if muscle pain occurs) and liver enzymes; caution: rhabdomyolysis; interrupt treatment if severely ill, avoid intensive sun exposure.
- Effectiveness: Statin therapy reduces LDL-C by about 30% (+ 15% additional reduction with ezetimibe)

Preferred statins depend on concomitant immunosuppressive regimen:

- No interaction between statins and mycophenolate mofetil and methylprednisolone
- Cyclosporin A: In general, strongest interactions between statins and cyclosporin A (see chapter 4.3); simvastatin and rosuvastatin are contraindicated, strong interaction with pravastatin, and atorvastatin.
- Tacrolimus: Potentially clinically relevant, moderate interaction between tacrolimus and pravastatin/simvastatin.
- Everolimus: No interaction with pravastatin or atorvastatin.

Table 2 HMG-CoA reductase inhibitor (statin) dosing in paediatrics

Medication name	Lowest available tablet strength	Approved at the earliest from	Noteworthy
Fluvastatin	20 mg	9 years	• No relevant interaction with tacrolimus • Potentially clinically relevant moderate interaction with cyclosporin A
Pravastatin	10 mg	8 years	• No relevant interaction with everolimus • Potentially clinically relevant moderate interaction with tacrolimus • Clinically serious interaction with cyclosporin A – avoid combination
Rosuvastatin	5 mg	6 years	• Contraindicated in comedication with cyclosporin A or if CCR <30 ml/min/1.73 m^2 BSA
Atorvastatin	10 mg	10 years	• No relevant interaction with tacrolimus • No relevant interaction with everolimus • Clinically serious interaction with cyclosporin A – avoid combination
Simvastatin	5 mg	♂ > Tanner II ♀ 1 year post menarche	• Potentially clinically relevant moderate interaction with tacrolimus • Contraindicated in comedication with cyclosporin A

Information adapted from manufactures' prescribing information; prescribing is at your own responsibility.

Fluvastatin might therefore be a good choice for combination therapy with calcineurin inhibitors. Fluvastatin is approved in Germany for the treatment of heterozygous familial hypercholesterolaemia from the age of 9 years.

Alternative treatment options:

- Ezetimibe (blocks intestinal absorption of cholesterol; combination with statins possible): 10 mg/day in patients >10 years: safe, well tolerated and effective. Most common adverse events: diarrhoea, myopathy. Cautiousness in cases of elevated transaminases/hepatic disease; caution: eGFR < 30 mL/min/1.73 m^2 increases exposure to ezetimibe. Caution against the combination with cyclosporin A (interaction).
- Omega-3 fatty acids (fish oil capsules + vitamin E; if triglycerides > 400 mg/dL (> 4.56 mmol/L); initial dose 1 g/day, which can be increased after a few weeks, if necessary; well tolerated.
- Bile acid sequestrants (e.g., cholestyramine): May be used in combination with statins. Caution: May reduce absorption of fat-soluble vitamins and mycophenolate mofetil.
- Use of sevelamer (lowers LDL-C) as a prophylactic or therapeutic option in hyperphosphatemia [9] (caution: reduces exposure to mycophenolic acid).

Newer agents: Evolocumab: human monoclonal antibody that inhibits PSCK9 and thus LDL receptor degradation → enhances removal of circulating LDL cholesterol; approved for children ≥10 years of age with homozygous familial hypercholesterolaemia (HFH). No effect on CYP450, P-glycoprotein or OATP pathways, so limited potential for drug-drug interactions. Monthly injection. Limited but encouraging experience to date: safe and effective in one randomised trial, 104 children aged 10–17 years with HFH received evolocumab, follow-up 24 weeks [10]; 1 study in 13 adult kidney transplant recipients, follow-up 6 months: effective, stable kidney function, proteinuria and immunosuppression, no other safety concerns reported [11]. Most common adverse events: nasopharyngitis (7.4%), upper respiratory tract infection (4.6%), back pain (4.4%), arthralgia (3.9%).

Figure 1 Screening and management of paediatric kidney transplant recipients aged ≥ 8 years, adapted from [7]

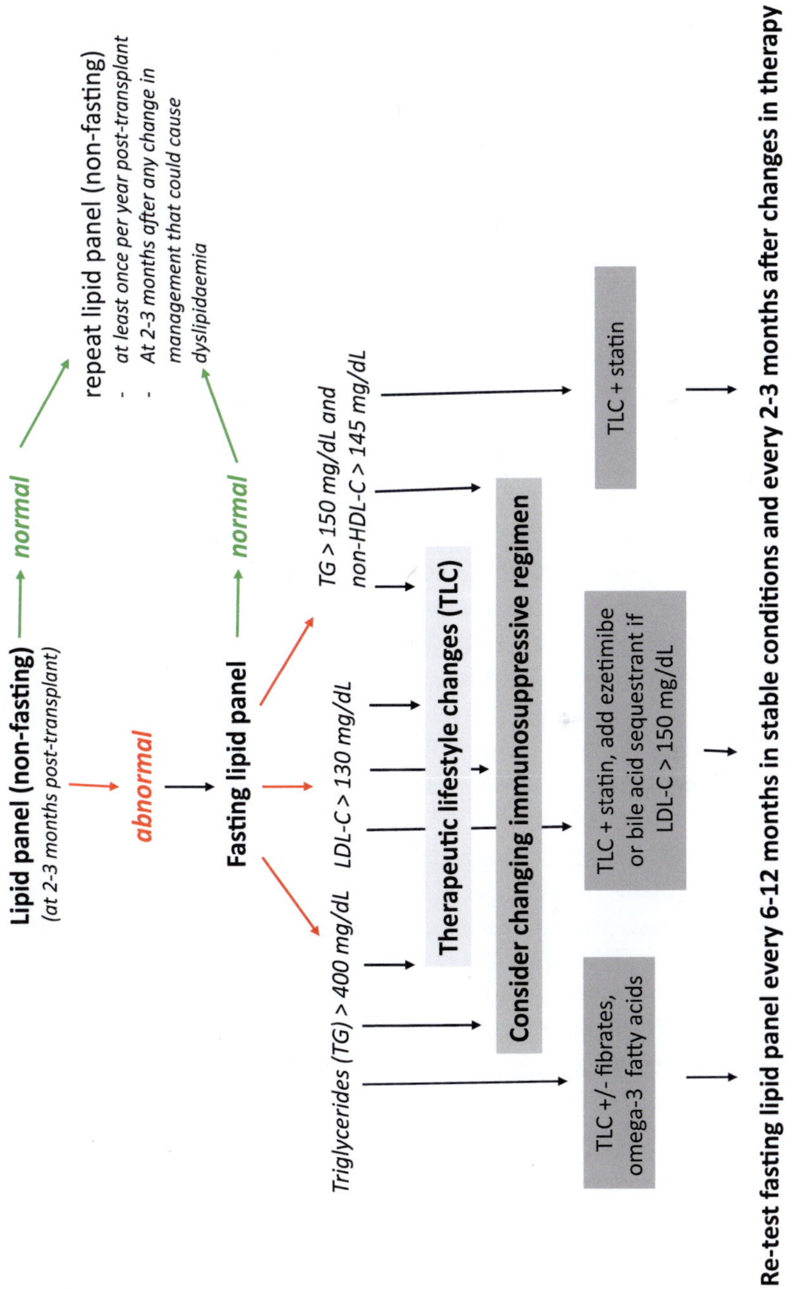

References

1 Kasap B (2011) Sirolimus in paediatric renal transplantation. Pediatr Transplantation, 15:673–685
2 de Feranti SD et al (2019) Cardiovascular Risk Reduction in High-Risk Patients; A scientific Statement From The American Heart Association. Circulation 139; e603–e634
3 North American Pedatric Renal Trials and Collaborative Studies (2014) Annual Report. https://web.emmes.com/stdy/ped/annlrept/annualrept2014.pdf
4 KDIGO Clinical Practice Guideline for lipid Management in Chronic Kidney disease (2013) Kidney International Supplements, 3 (3):249–305
5 Kavey R-E.W. et al. (2006) Reducing cardiovascular risk in high-risk paediatric patients. Circulation, 114:2710–2738
6 Jourdan C, Wühl E, Litwin M, Fahr K, Trelewicz J, Jobs K, Schenk JP, Grenda R, Mehls O, Tröger J, Schaefer F (2005) Normative values for intima-media thickness and distensibility of large arteries in healthy adolescents. J Hypertens. 2005 Sep;23(9):1707–159
7 Bock M et al (2021) Management of dyslipidemia in pediatric renal transplant recipients. Pediatric Nephrology (2021) 36:51–63
8 Habbig S, Volland R, Krupka K, Querfeld U, Dello Strologo L, Noyan A, Yalcinkaya F, Topaloglu R, Webb NJ, Kemper MJ, Pape L, Bald M, Kranz B, Taylan C, Höcker B, Tönshoff B, Weber LT. (2017) Dyslipidemia after pediatric renal transplantation – The impact of immunosuppressive regimens. Pediatr Transplant, https://doi.org/10.1111/pedtr.12914
9 Pieper AK, Haffner D, Hoppe B, Dittrich K, Offner G, Bonzel KE, John U, Fründ S, Klaus G, Stübinger A, Düker G, Querfeld U (2006) A randomized crossover trial comparing sevelamer with calcium acetate in children with CKD. Am J Kidney Dis. 2006 Apr;47(4):625–35
10 Santos RD et al 2020 Evolocumab in Pediatric Heterozygous Familial Hypercholesterolemia. N Engl J Med. 2020 Oct 1;383(14):1317–1327. doi: 10.1056/NEJMoa2019910. Epub 2020 Aug 29
11 Amaro JM et al (2024) Management of Dyslipidemia with Evolocumab in Kidney Transplant Recipients. Transplantation 108(5):e74–e76, May 2024. DOI: 10.1097/TP.0000000000004942

CHAPTER 8.6 Post-transplant diabetes mellitus

Daniela Choukair

Heidelberg University, Medical Faculty, Department of Paediatrics I, University Children's Hospital, Heidelberg, Germany

ORCID:
https://orcid.org/0000-0002-1631-3883

Introduction

Post-transplant diabetes mellitus (PTDM) is associated with an increased risk of cardiovascular morbidity, increased mortality and decreased graft survival [1]. The incidence varies from 10% to 74% in adults [2] and from 3% to 20% in children [3].

Definition

Hyperglycaemia in the first days and weeks after transplant surgery should be differentiated from PTDM, which should be diagnosed at the earliest six weeks to six months after transplantation and in the setting of stable immunosuppressive therapy [1, 2]. According to the diagnostic criteria of the American Diabetes Association (ADA), PTDM is present when one of the following criteria is met [1, 2, 4]:

- Randomly elevated plasma glucose ≥ 200 mg/dL with symptoms of diabetes mellitus (DM) such as polyuria, polydipsia or unexplained weight loss.
- Fasting plasma glucose ≥ 126 mg/dL after a fasting period of at least eight hours.
- Two-hour plasma glucose ≥ 200 mg/dL during a standardised oral glucose tolerance test (OGTT).
- HbA1c ≥ 6.5%.

Causes and risk factors

Risk factors that predispose to type 2 DM in the non-transplant population have also been identified as risk factors for post-transplant patients [2]:

- Overweight (> 90th BMI percentile) and obesity (> 97th BMI percentile)
- African American or Latino heritage
- Impaired glucose tolerance or pre-diabetes prior to transplantation
- Positive family history of DM
- Genetic predisposition, such as variants in the *HNF-1B* gene [5]

Specific risk factors for kidney transplant patients [1]:
- HLA mismatch especially on HLA-DR
- Male gender
- Deceased donor organ
- Hepatitis C infection
- Risk constellation for cytomegalovirus (donor CMV seropositive/recipient CMV seronegative)
- Polycystic kidney disease as primary kidney disease
- Perioperative hyperglycaemia
- Immunosuppressive therapy

Immunosuppressants:
Glucocorticoids [3]:
- Diabetogenic effect is dose-dependent and can cause weight gain
- Reduced binding of insulin to its receptor and increased gluconeogenesis in the liver.
- The effect of steroid-free immunosuppression on the reduction of PTDM is unclear. Steroid-free immunosuppression appears to have little effect on the development of PTDM compared to low-dose steroid medication [6]. In a group of paediatric kidney transplant patients, the use of steroid-based immunosuppression at discharge was not a risk factor for the subsequent development of PTDM [7]

Calcineurin inhibitors [1]:
- Tacrolimus (Tac): direct toxic effect on ß-cells, resulting in reduced secretion of insulin

- Ciclosporin A (CsA): Dysfunction of ß-cells with reduced insulin secretion (animal study)
- The diabetogenic effect of Tac is more pronounced than that of CsA [1]

mTOR inhibitors:
diabetogenic effect, as ß-cell proliferation is reduced [1], but no increased incidence of PTDM is described in other studies [8]

Antiproliferative agents:
Mycophenolate mofetil (MMF) or azathioprine (AZA) tend to have a protective effect with regard to the development of PTDM. It is unclear whether this is a direct effect or whether glucocorticoids and calcineurin inhibitors can be spared through the use of antiproliferative agents [3].

Diagnostics

Glucose metabolism should be carefully assessed before transplantation. After transplantation, the management of PTDM includes close monitoring of glucose metabolism and, in individual cases, modification of immunosuppressive therapy, treatment of DM and reduction of other cardiovascular risk factors in patients with impaired glucose metabolism. The KDIGO guidelines recommend weekly monitoring of glucose metabolism for the first four weeks after transplantation, then quarterly and annually after the first year following transplantation [9].

HbA1c and fasting glucose are commonly used to assess glucose metabolism. The high false-negative rate of fasting glucose and HbA1c must be taken into account [1]. In addition, after glucocorticoid administration in the morning, spontaneous glucose levels are elevated, especially in the afternoon and evening [10]. Therefore, the gold standard for the diagnosis of PTDM is the OGTT [11]. It can also be used to identify patients with impaired glucose tolerance and initiate appropriate screening. Continuous glucose monitoring (CGM) systems are increasingly being used to monitor treatment [12]. PTDM requires multidisciplinary care by an experienced diabetes team [2] and screening for diabetes complications should be included in transplant aftercare.

Therapy

Postoperative hyperglycaemia after transplantation occurs in about 60% of adults [13] and requires insulin therapy, mostly intravenously initially [2]. If PTDM is diagnosed during outpatient follow-up, modification of immunosuppression should always be weighed against the risk of potential rejection. Glucocorticoid therapy should be reduced as soon as possible, although steroid-free immunosuppression is not mandatory [1]. However, a switch from tacrolimus to ciclosporin may be considered in cases of difficult-to-control diabetes [1]. According to the current KDOQI recommendations, drug therapy for diabetes should be initiated immediately and should be accompanied by lifestyle changes such as increased physical activity, dietary changes, weight loss and treatment of other cardiovascular risk factors [14].

When selecting antidiabetic drugs, it is important to consider the potential for interaction with immunosuppressants, and some drugs are contraindicated in cases of impaired GFR [2]. Data on the safety and efficacy of these drugs in PTDM are sparse in adults [2] and not available in children. The group of drugs used in adults with PTDM, such as dipeptidyl peptidase 4 (DPP4) inhibitors, thiazolidinediones, sulfonylureas, meglitinides and alpha-glucosidase, are not approved for use in children in Germany [1].

New classes of drugs, such as sodium-glucose co-transporter 2 (SGLT2) inhibitors and glucagon-like peptide-1 (GLP-1) receptor agonists, are now an integral part of the guidelines for the treatment of type 2 diabetes in adults with chronic kidney disease [14, 15]. Both classes of drugs have been shown to reduce cardiovascular risk and the progression of kidney disease [15]. In Germany, there are still official limitations on the eGFR up to which SGLT2 inhibitors can be used. Based on small studies in transplant patients, the use of SGLT2 inhibitors appears to be safe [16]. However, it should be noted that there may be a transient increase in creatinine and urogenital infections; euglycaemic ketoacidosis may occur, and discontinuation of SGLT2 inhibitors is required in the event of prolonged fasting periods or acute illness [17].

In Germany, SGLT2 inhibitors are approved for children aged 10 years and older; their use in children with an eGFR < 60 ml/min/1.73 m^2 has not been tested. Publications on the use of SGLT2 inhibitors in paediatric kidney transplant patients are not yet available. As PTDM often involves a combination of insulin resistance and insulin deficiency, insulin deficiency should always be ruled out before using this group of drugs to minimise the risk of life-threatening ketoacidosis.

In one case series, kidney transplant patients were treated with GLP-1 receptor agonists and liraglutide appeared to be safe and effective in these adults [18]. The benefits of these agents include facilitation of weight loss in obesity, absence of hypoglycaemia, improvement in insulin sensitivity, and substantial independence from eGFR (particularly with liraglutide). Due to the initial main side effects of inappetence, nausea and very rarely vomiting, the dose must be increased slowly with close monitoring of immunosuppressive drug levels. GLP-1 receptor agonists are approved for use in children from 12 years of age and may be considered as combination therapy in obese children with type 2 DM, although long-term data on cardiovascular risk reduction are lacking [19]. No data are available on their use in paediatric kidney transplant patients.

Paediatric societies continue to recommend metformin as the first-line treatment for type 2 DM in children [19]. If GFR is impaired, the benefit of metformin must be carefully weighed against the risk of lactic acidosis. Insulin therapy should be initiated if fasting blood glucose is > 200 mg/dL, metabolic decompensation is present, oral antidiabetic medications are ineffective, or HbA1c is persistently > 10% [19]. Comprehensive patient education should be provided and therapy should be monitored by an experienced multidisciplinary diabetes team. Continuous blood glucose monitoring is helpful as steroids are taken by transplant patients in the morning and a significant rise in blood glucose levels is observed in the late afternoon or early evening.

Although current recommendations for the treatment of type 1 diabetes mellitus no longer include medium-acting sustained-release insulin (usually NPH insulin (neutral protamine Hagedorn)), it can be given in the morning in PTDM in order to control the steroid-induced rise in blood glucose levels in the late afternoon or early evening [20]. Alternatively, detemir can be used, which has a similar efficacy profile. In the evening, a long-acting insulin analogue such as glargine, Glargine U300® or degludec is recommended to control the morning blood glucose rise and minimise the risk of nocturnal hypoglycaemia [20]. Rapid-acting insulin analogues such as insulin aspart or insulin lispro are recommended for prandial substitution. Insulin pumps are a useful therapeutic option, but are rarely used. Only human insulin or insulin analogues should be used in children [20].

Despite the ongoing development of new antidiabetic agents, and in the absence of recommendations from professional societies for the treatment of PTDM in children, it can be concluded from the reviewed studies that insulin therapy is recommended for the treatment of PTDM after intensive patient and parent education and care by an experienced paediatric diabetes team.

Depending on the severity of the hyperglycaemia, insulin therapy should be individualised. SGLT2 inhibitors and GLP-1 receptor agonists may be considered on a case-by-case basis after weighing the benefits and risks.

Complications

Children and adolescents with PTDM after organ transplantation have a threefold increased risk of death compared with healthy peers [21]. Cardiovascular mortality increases significantly when other risk factors such as arterial hypertension or hyperlipidaemia are also present. Patients with PTDM also have an increased risk of developing serious infections or sepsis, particularly urinary tract infections, pneumonia and cytomegalovirus infections [2]. Diabetic sequelae such as ophthalmological and neurological complications should not be neglected [19].

Summary

PTDM is defined as (i) fasting glucose ≥ 126 mg/dL, or (ii) symptoms of hyperglycaemia with random blood glucose of ≥ 200 mg/dL, or (iii) 2-hour glucose during an oral glucose tolerance test ≥ 200 mg/dL, or (iv) HbA1c ≥ 6.5%. The incidence of PTDM in children varies from 3% to 20%. Glucocorticoids, calcineurin inhibitors and mTOR inhibitors have a diabetogenic effect, with tacrolimus showing an increased risk of PTDM compared with ciclosporin. In patients with PTDM, modification of immunosuppression should always be weighed against the risk of potential rejection. In addition to the recommendations for lifestyle changes, diabetes should be treated promptly with medication.

The current consensus guideline for adults with PTDM recommends an individualised therapy with metformin, SGLT2 inhibitors, GLP-1 receptor agonists, DPP4 inhibitors and insulin, taking into account the risk-benefit ratio. In Germany, DPP4 inhibitors are not approved for use in children with diabetes mellitus. Metformin is still approved by the paediatric diabetes associations for the treatment of type 2 diabetes mellitus, but must not be used in cases of severely impaired renal function because of the risk of lactic acidosis. SGLT2 inhibitors are approved in Germany for children from 10 years of age and have a favourable risk profile for cardiovascular complications. Side effects such as life-threatening euglycaemic ketoacidosis must be taken into account when prescribing them.

GLP-1 receptor agonists are approved in Germany for use in children 12 years and older to facilitate weight loss in obesity. Gastrointestinal side effects, which may interfere with the absorption of immunosuppressive drugs, must be considered. There are no expert recommendations for the treatment of PTDM in children. Early insulin therapy in children with PTDM is reasonable, especially as insulin therapy is approved for use in children and does not interact with immunosuppressants. This therapy requires intensive patient education and should be supervised by an experienced paediatric diabetes team. In individual cases, the use of SGLT2 inhibitors and GLP-1 receptor agonists may be considered on a risk-benefit basis. Screening for long-term complications of PTDM should be included in transplant aftercare.

References

1 Sharif A, Chakkera H, de Vries APJ, Eller K, Guthoff M, Haller MC, et al. International consensus on post-transplant diabetes mellitus. Nephrol Dial Transplant. 2024;39(3):531–49.
2 Shivaswamy V, Boerner B, Larsen J. Post-Transplant Diabetes Mellitus: Causes, Treatment, and Impact on Outcomes. Endocr Rev. 2016;37(1): 37–61.
3 Grundman JB, Wolfsdorf JI, Marks BE. Post-Transplant Diabetes Mellitus in Pediatric Patients. Horm Res Paediatr. 2020;93(9–10):510–8.
4 2. Classification and Diagnosis of Diabetes: Standards of Medical Care in Diabetes-2021. Diabetes Care. 2021;44(Suppl 1):S15–s33.
5 Bellanné-Chantelot C, Chauveau D, Gautier JF, Dubois-Laforgue D, Clauin S, Beaufils S, et al. Clinical spectrum associated with hepatocyte nuclear factor-1beta mutations. Ann Intern Med. 2004;140(7):510–7.
6 Kasiske BL, Snyder JJ, Gilbertson D, Matas AJ. Diabetes mellitus after kidney transplantation in the United States. Am J Transplant. 2003;3(2):178–85.
7 Woodle ES, First MR, Pirsch J, Shihab F, Gaber AO, Van Veldhuisen P. A prospective, randomized, double-blind, placebo-controlled multicenter trial comparing early (7 day) corticosteroid cessation versus long-term, low-dose corticosteroid therapy. Ann Surg. 2008;248(4):564–77.

8 Montero N, Quero M, Melilli E, Pérez-Sáez MJ, Redondo-Pachón D, Bestard O, et al. Mammalian Target of Rapamycin Inhibitors Combined With Calcineurin Inhibitors as Initial Immunosuppression in Renal Transplantation: A Meta-analysis. Transplantation. 2019;103(10):2031–56.
9 KDIGO clinical practice guideline for the care of kidney transplant recipients. Am J Transplant. 2009;9 Suppl 3:S1–155.
10 Hecking M, Werzowa J, Haidinger M, Hörl WH, Pascual J, Budde K, et al. Novel views on new-onset diabetes after transplantation: development, prevention and treatment. Nephrol Dial Transplant. 2013;28(3):550–66.
11 Kurnikowski A, Nordheim E, Schwaiger E, Krenn S, Harreiter J, Kautzky-Willer A, et al. Criteria for prediabetes and posttransplant diabetes mellitus after kidney transplantation: A 2-year diagnostic accuracy study of participants from a randomized controlled trial. Am J Transplant. 2022; 22(12):2880–91.
12 Tauschmann M, Forlenza G, Hood K, Cardona-Hernandez R, Giani E, Hendrieckx C, et al. ISPAD Clinical Practice Consensus Guidelines 2022: Diabetes technologies: Glucose monitoring. Pediatr Diabetes. 2022;23(8): 1390–405.
13 Cohen E, Korah M, Callender G, Belfort de Aguiar R, Haakinson D. Metabolic Disorders with Kidney Transplant. Clin J Am Soc Nephrol. 2020; 15(5):732–42.
14 Mottl AK, Nicholas SB. KDOQI Commentary on the KDIGO 2022 Update to the Clinical Practice Guideline for Diabetes Management in CKD. Am J Kidney Dis. 2024;83(3):277–87.
15 Sarafidis P, Ferro CJ, Morales E, Ortiz A, Malyszko J, Hojs R, et al. SGLT-2 inhibitors and GLP-1 receptor agonists for nephroprotection and cardioprotection in patients with diabetes mellitus and chronic kidney disease. A consensus statement by the EURECA-m and the DIABESITY working groups of the ERA-EDTA. Nephrol Dial Transplant. 2019;34(2):208–30.
16 Lim JH, Kwon S, Jeon Y, Kim YH, Kwon H, Kim YS, et al. The Efficacy and Safety of SGLT2 Inhibitor in Diabetic Kidney Transplant Recipients. Transplantation. 2022;106(9):e404–e12.
17 Zinman B, Lachin JM, Inzucchi SE. Empagliflozin, Cardiovascular Outcomes, and Mortality in Type 2 Diabetes. N Engl J Med. 2016;374(11): 1094.
18 Liou JH, Liu YM, Chen CH. Management of Diabetes Mellitus With Glucagonlike Peptide-1 Agonist Liraglutide in Renal Transplant Recipients: A Retrospective Study. Transplant Proc. 2018;50(8):2502–5.

19 Shah AS, Zeitler PS, Wong J, Pena AS, Wicklow B, Arslanian S, et al. ISPAD Clinical Practice Consensus Guidelines 2022: Type 2 diabetes in children and adolescents. Pediatr Diabetes. 2022;23(7):872–902.
20 Cengiz E, Danne T, Ahmad T, Ayyavoo A, Beran D, Ehtisham S, et al. ISPAD Clinical Practice Consensus Guidelines 2022: Insulin treatment in children and adolescents with diabetes. Pediatr Diabetes. 2022;23(8):1277–96.
21 Chanchlani R, Kim SJ, Dixon SN, Jassal V, Banh T, Borges K, et al. Incidence of new-onset diabetes mellitus and association with mortality in childhood solid organ transplant recipients: a population-based study. Nephrol Dial Transplant. 2019;34(3):524–31.

CHAPTER 8.7 Arterial hypertension

Anette Melk[1], Elke Wühl[2] & Tomas Seeman[3, 4]

[1] Department of Paediatric Nephrology, Hepatology, Metabolic and Neurology Diseases, Hannover Medical School, Hannover, Germany
[2] Heidelberg University, Medical Faculty Heidelberg, Department of Paediatrics I, University Children's Hospital Heidelberg, Germany
[3] Department of Paediatrics, 2nd Faculty of Medicine, Charles University Prague, Prague 5, Czech Republic
[4] Department of Paediatrics, University Hospital Ostrava and Faculty of Medicine of University of Ostrava, Ostrava, Czech Republic.

ORCIDs:
Anette Melk: https://orcid.org/0000-0002-8164-6318
Elke Wühl: https://orcid.org/0000-0002-1205-2620
Tomas Seeman: https://orcid.org/0000-0003-1371-3096

Introduction

Arterial hypertension is a common complication in children after kidney transplantation (prevalence 60–90%) and is an important risk factor for graft failure and increased cardiovascular morbidity and mortality in children. Therapeutic control of hypertension is often inadequate; 50–80% of treated transplanted children have persistent hypertensionand isolated nocturnal hypertension is a common finding.

Diagnosis

Ambulatory 24-hour blood pressure monitoring (ABPM) is the method of choice to diagnose hypertension and blood pressure rhythm disturbances in transplanted children. It should be performed once a year in all transplanted children and 3–6 months after any change in antihypertensive therapy. Regular clinical follow-up should always include standardised office blood pressure measurement (ESH Guidelines 2016) at each outpatient visit. In addition, home blood pressure measurements are recommended and should be encouraged. Regular checks for hypertension-mediated organ damage (HMOD) should be carried out including echocardiography (once a year), albuminuria/proteinuria (once a month) and fundoscopy (especially in high-risk patients, to be included in the annual check by an ophthalmologist).

Antihypertensive medication

No controlled trials have been conducted on the treatment of hypertension in transplanted children. In transplanted adults, the antihypertensive effects of different classes of antihypertensive drugs are comparable, with ACE inhibitors/angiotensin receptor blockers also having antiproteinuric effects.

All five basic classes of antihypertensive drugs can be prescribed (calcium channel blockers, diuretics, beta-blockers, ACE inhibitors, angiotensin receptor blockers). Some antihypertensive drugs approved for the use in children are listed in table 1. The choice of drugs is empirical, but in certain conditions and comorbidities the use of specific antihypertensive drugs may be beneficial (e.g. ACE inhibitors/angiotensin receptor blockers for concomitant proteinuria or left ventricular hypertrophy, or diuretics for volume or salt overload). Combination antihypertensive therapy is often required to achieve adequate blood pressure control. In severe, refractory hypertension, use of additional antihypertensive drug classes (e.g., mineralocorticoid receptor antagonists (MRA), $alpha_1$-blockers, centrally acting agents or vasodilators) may be required.

Contraindications: Same as for antihypertensive therapy in non-transplanted children (e.g., ACE inhibitors/angiotensin receptor blockers in renal graft artery stenosis). It should be kept in mind that graft function in transplanted children may be more sensitive to dehydration events than in children with native kidney CKD. In girls with child-bearing potential RAAS blockers can be prescribed, but contraceptive measures are mandatory.

Goal of therapy: The target blood pressure for transplanted children and adults is not known and the recommended limits are based on expert consensus (EBM level C). The office blood pressure target should be at least < 95th percentile for both systolic and diastolic blood pressure. For ABPM, the target blood pressure should be < 95th percentile for both day and night. There is currently no data on whether a target blood pressure of < 90th percentile or even lower (as recommended for children with native kidney CKD) is more beneficial for transplanted children.

Table 1 Antihypertensive medications with clinical experience in children

Antihypertensive drug class	Generic name	Recommended daily dose	Divided in
ACE-inhibitors	Captopril*	Up to 6 mg/kg/day	3 doses
	Enalapril	up to 0.6 mg/kg/day	2 doses
	Ramipril*	1.5 to 6 mg/m^2/day	1 dose
	Lisinopril*	0.08–0.6 mg/kg/day (max.40mg/day)	1 dose
Angiotensin-receptor blockers	Losartan	0.7 to 1.4 mg/kg/day	1 dose
	Irbesartan	6–12 years: 75 to 150 mg/day	1 dose
		≥ 13 years: 150 to 300 mg/day	1 dose
	Candesartan	0.15–0.5 mg/kg	
Beta-Blockers	Propranolol	0.5 to 6 mg/kg/day	2–3 doses
	Atenolol	1 to 2 mg/kg/day	1–2 doses
	Metoprolol	0.5 to 2 mg/kg/day	1–2 doses
Calcium channel blockers	Nifedipine SR, GITS*	0.5 to 3 mg/kg/day	3–4 doses
	Amlodipine*	0.6 to 0.15 mg/kg/day	1 dose
	Felodipine	0.5 to 1 mg/kg/day	1 dose
	Isradipine	0.5 to 1 mg/kg/day	1 dose
Diuretics	Hydrochlorothiazide	0.5 to 3 mg/kg/day	2 doses
	Furosemide	1 to 3 mg/kg/day	2–3 doses

Although every effort has been made to confirm the recommended doses by consulting appropriate references, manufacturers' prescribing information is frequently updated and should be consulted.

*Antihypertensive drugs for which clinical experience in kidney transplanted children exists based on published studies

References

1 Arbeiter K, Pichler A, Stemberger R, Mueller T, Ruffingshofer D, Vargha R, Balzar E, Aufricht C (2004) ACE inhibition in the treatment of children after renal transplantation. Pediatr Nephrol 19:222–226
2 Lurbe E, Agabiti-Rosei E, Cruickshank JK, Dominiczak A, Erdine S, Hirth A, Invitti C, Litwin M, Mancia G, Pall D, Rascher W, Redon J, Schaefer F, Seeman T, Sinha M, Stabouli S, Webb NJ, Wühl E, Zanchetti A. 2016 European Society of Hypertension guidelines for the management of high blood pressure in children and adolescents. J Hypertens. 2016 Oct;34(10): 1887–920.
3 Opelz G, Wujciak T, Ritz E for the Collaborative Transplant Study (1998) Association of chronic kidney graft failure with recipient blood pressure. Kidney Int 53:217–222
4 Opelz G, Dohler B, Collaborative Transplant Study (2005) Improved long-term outcomes after renal transplantation associated with blood pressure control. Am J Transplant 5:2725–2731
5 Seeman T, Vondrák K, Dušek Effects of the strict control of blood pressure in pediatric renal transplant recipients – ESCORT trial. J. Pediatr Transplant. 2019 Feb;23(1):e13329.
6 Seeman T, Feber J. Should ACE inhibitors or calcium channel blockers be used for post-transplant hypertension? Pediatr Nephrol. 2021 Mar;36(3): 539–549.
7 Seeman T, Myette RL, Feber J (2023): Hypertension in pediatric kidney transplantation. Pediatr Transplant. 2023 Aug;27(5):e14522.
8 Sugianto RI, Grabitz C, Bayazit A, Duzova A, Thurn-Valsassina D, Memaran N, Doyon A, Canpolat N, Kaplan Bulut I, Azukaitis K, Obrycki Ł, Anarat A, Büscher R, Caliskan S, Harambat J, Lugani F, Ozcakar ZB, Paripović D, Ranchin B, Querfeld U, Schaefer F, Schmidt BMW, Melk A. Stricter Blood Pressure Control Is Associated With Lower Left Ventricular Mass in Children After Kidney Transplantation: A Longitudinal Analysis of the 4C-T Study. Hypertension. 2023 Sep;80(9):1900–1908.
9 Sugianto RI, Schmidt BMW, Memaran N, Duzova A, Topaloglu R, Seeman T, König S, Dello Strologo L, Murer L, Özçakar ZB, Bald M, Shenoy M, Buescher A, Hoyer PF, Pohl M, Billing H, Oh J, Staude H, Pohl M, Genc G, Klaus G, Alparslan C, Grenda R, Rubik J, Krupka K, Tönshoff B, Wühl E, Melk A. Sex and age as determinants for high blood pressure in pe-

diatric renal transplant recipients: a longitudinal analysis of the CERTAIN Registry. Pediatr Nephrol. 2020 Mar;35(3):415–426.
10 Tian Z, Bergmann K, Kaufeld J, Schmidt-Ott K, Melk A, Schmidt BMW. Left Ventricular Hypertrophy After Renal Transplantation: Systematic Review and Meta-analysis. Transplant Direct. 2024 May 17;10(6):e1647.

CHAPTER 8.8 Recurrence of primary kidney disease

Nele Kanzelmeyer[1] & Sebastian Loos[2]

[1] Medical University Hannover, Department of Pediatric Kidney, Liver, Metabolic and Neurological Diseases, Hannover Medical School, Hannover, Germany
[2] University Medical Centre Hamburg, Department of Paediatrics, Hamburg, Germany

ORCIDs:
Nele Kanzelmeyer: https://orcid.org/0000-0002-4865-4906
Sebastian Loos: https://orcid.org/0000-0002-8620-042X

1 Focal segmental glomerulosclerosis (FSGS)

Pathophysiology: Podocyte damage leads to mesangial matrix proliferation, allowing protein leakage and resulting in sclerosis and scarring of the glomerulus [1].

Frequency: FSGS is one of the most common diseases to recur with rates ranging from 30% to 60%, increasing to 86% after re-transplantation. In genetic forms of FSGS, recurrence occurs very rarely [2].

Clinical appearance: FSGS presents with nephrotic-range proteinuria shortly after transplantation. Gross haematuria is rare, although microscopic haematuria may occur [3].

Monitoring: Frequent monitoring of urine protein-to-creatinine ratio.

Therapy: Plasmapheresis is postulated to reduce the circulating permeability factor. It may be used with or without rituximab [4]. Supportive measures: Sodium and protein restriction, blood pressure control, use of RAAS inhibitors, and management of dyslipidaemia. SGLT2 inhibitors may offer kidney protection, but evidence is limited. Diuretics for oedema and adequate nutrition [5].

2 C3 glomerulopathy (C3G)

Frequency: The recurrence rate of C3 glomerulopathy after kidney transplantation varies, but studies suggest that it may occur in up to 50% of patients [6].

Pathophysiology: The high risk of recurrence after kidney transplantation is due to the continued activation of the complement system, which is damaging even in the new kidney. Some patients may have genetic predispositions that affect complement regulation, increasing the likelihood of recurrence in the transplanted kidney.

Monitoring: Close monitoring is essential for early detection and management of recurrence in transplant recipients with a history of C3 glomerulopathy:

1. Clinical monitoring: Assessment of kidney function, proteinuria, and haematuria.
2. Kidney biopsy: If there are signs of recurrence, a kidney biopsy is the most definitive way to diagnose C3-glomerulopathy.
3. Complement studies: Testing for complement levels (C3, sC5b-9, C3d, autoantibodies (C3/C4/C5Nef, anti-CFH), etc.) can provide insight into the ongoing complement activation that is a hallmark of C3-glomerulopathy [7].

Therapy: Treatment of recurrent C3 glomerulopathy after kidney transplantation typically involves several approaches:

1. Immunosuppressive therapy: Adjustment of immunosuppressive medication can help control the immune response. This may include increasing the dose of existing medications or adding new agents.
2. Plasmapheresis: This procedure can be used to remove pathogenic factors, including complement components and antibodies, from the blood. It may be effective in reducing recurrence and controlling symptoms.
3. Complement blocker therapy: Monoclonal antibodies blocking the terminal complement cascade such as eculizumab or ravulizumab have limited efficacy [7]. New more specific complement inhibitors such as iptacopan or pegcetacoplan might have better efficacy and will soon achieve regulatory approval [8].
4. Supportive care: Control of blood pressure and proteinuria and close monitoring of kidney function are essential to prevent further damage.

3 IgA nephropathy (IgAN)

Pathophysiology: IgAN is the most common primary glomerulonephritis worldwide and is characterised by impaired IgA1 glycosylation (due to galactose-deficient IgA1, immune complex deposition, genetic predisposition [e.g. *C1GALT1* or *IGAN1*] or familial predisposition) [9].

Frequency: Recurrence is highly variable time-dependent. The cumulative incidence in a large retrospective study was 19% at 10 years und 23% at 15 years [10, 11].

Clinical appearance: Patients with recurrent IgAN usually present with persistent microscopic haematuria. New or worsening proteinuria or, occasionally, an increase in the serum creatinine may also be seen [12].

Monitoring: In IgAN, increased urinary protein excretion indicates a higher risk of disease progression [13].

Therapy:
1. Glucocorticoid withdrawal may increase the risk of recurrence in IgAN [14].
2. ACE inhibitors/AT1 antagonists to reduce proteinuria and blood pressure [15]. Treatment of cardiovascular risk factors [16].
3. Standard immunosuppressive regimens (e.g., tacrolimus, mycophenolate, corticosteroids) have limited effect on the risk of recurrence.
4. High-dose glucocorticoids may be considered for treatment of aggressive glomerulonephritis. Experimental options include rituximab [17] and SGLT2 inhibitors as nephroprotective agents [18].

4 Atypical/complement-mediated haemolytic uremic syndrome

Pathophysiology: Many patients with atypical haemolytic uraemic syndrome (aHUS) have underlying genetic mutations affecting complement regulation (e.g., in the genes encoding for CFH, CFI etc.). In addition, aHUS can be triggered by anti-FH antibodies. Persistent dysregulation of the complement system before and/or after transplantation is associated with a high risk of recurrence in the transplanted kidney.

Frequency: Depending on the underlying cause, recurrence of aHUS after kidney transplantation occurs in approximately 30% to 50% of cases [19]. Close monitoring and proactive management, including the peri-transplant use of complement inhibitors such as eculizumab or ravulizumab can help to reduce the risk of recurrence and improve outcomes for transplant recipients [20].

Prevention: Preventing the recurrence of atypical haemolytic uremic syndrome (aHUS) after kidney transplantation involves a multifaceted approach:

1. Genetic screening: Identifying patients with genetic mutations associated with aHUS can help tailor prevention strategies. Understanding a patient's specific genetic risk can guide management.
2. Complement inhibitors, plasmapheresis: Drugs such as eculizumab or ravulizumab may be used to prevent or treat recurrence. If these are not available, plasmapheresis might be considered.
3. Adequate immunosuppression: It is important to ensure optimal immunosuppressive therapy post-transplant. This may help to prevent an immune response that could trigger aHUS or a recurrence of anti-FH antibody-induced aHUS.
4. Monitor for early signs: Regular monitoring of urine (proteinuria, haematuria), kidney function, and blood tests for haemolysis (such as LDH and haptoglobin) and thrombocytopenia, can help detect early signs of recurrence.
5. Kidney biopsy: If there are no laboratory signs of recurrence, a kidney biopsy can provide definitive evidence of thrombotic microangiopathy (TMA).

Therapy: Treatment of recurrent aHUS after kidney transplantation typically involves several strategies: A complement inhibitor is now the considered to be the first-line treatment. It can help to prevent further complement-mediated damage and control haemolysis. Plasmapheresis may be used, if complement inhibitor therapy is not available or to remove circulating factors contributing to aHUS, such as complement components or antibodies.

Patient education: Educating patients about recognising early signs of recurrence, including urine testing, and the importance of adherence to follow-up care can facilitate prompt intervention.

5 Lupus nephritis (LN)

Pathophysiology: LN is a manifestation of systemic lupus erythematosus (SLE) and results from an immune dysregulation with autoantibody and immune complex formation.

Frequency: LN recurs in approximately 2–11 % of cases after kidney transplantation [21, 22]. It manifests at a median of 4.3 years [23].

Clinical features: Proteinuria, microhaematuria, deterioration of graft function [21]. Systemic manifestations of SLE recurrence such as arthralgias, skin lesions, fatigue and serological activity (e.g. increased anti-dsDNA antibodies) may also occur.

Monitoring: Monitor proteinuria and (micro-)haematuria. Complement levels (C3 and C4), anti-dsDNA antibodies and ANA indicate serological activity. Kidney biopsy is required if a relapse is suspected [24].

Therapy: Treatment of recurrent LN follows the same guidelines as for the primary disease: High-dose steroids to control acute inflammation. Mycophenolate mofetil (MMF) as preferred maintenance therapy. Calcineurin inhibitors (tacrolimus, cyclosporine) may be used in combination with MMF. Cyclophosphamide for aggressive relapses or lupus nephritis (class III/IV). Rituximab is used in refractory cases and reduces the production of autoantibodies. Eculizumab in severe cases with complement activation. Supportive therapy with ACE inhibitors/AT 1 antagonists to reduce proteinuria; control blood pressure, cholesterol levels and cardiovascular risk factors. In the presence of antiphospholipid syndrome, consider anticoagulation to prevent thrombotic events.

6 Primary hyperoxaluria (PH1)

Pathophysiology: Primary hyperoxaluria is a genetic disorder affecting oxalate metabolism in the liver. If isolated kidney transplantation is performed, the underlying metabolic defect persists, resulting in continued overproduction of oxalate leading to (rapid) recurrence in the transplant. Therefore, sequential or combined liver and kidney transplantation (SLKT/CLKT) are current transplantation strategies [25]. Alternative approaches using isolated kidney transplantation under pyridoxine and/or siRNA therapy in responsive patients may be considered [25]. If a patient has a significant pretransplant oxalate burden, oxalate may be deposited in the transplanted kidney even after SLKT/CLKT. Oxalate levels may remain elevated even years after transplantation.

Monitoring/therapy: Therefore, certain measures should be taken after transplantation:

1. Short-term management: Lowering oxalate levels is critical to prevent recurrence after transplantation. Therefore, haemodialysis/-filtration may be necessary after transplantation, especially if graft function is delayed.
2. Long-term management: Hydration and urine alkalisation should be optimised even years after transplantation. In patients with isolated kidney transplantation on pyridoxine and/or siRNA therapy it is imperative to continue these therapies. Plasma and urinary oxalate levels should be monitored after transplantation. Ultrasound should be used to assess for kidney stones or calcifications. If there are significant signs of recurrence, a biopsy may be performed to check for oxalate deposits in the renal tissue.

References

1 Eddy AA, Symons JM (2003) Nephrotic syndrome in childhood. Lancet 362 (9384):629–639. https://doi.org/10.1016/S0140-6736(03)14184-0

2 Cormican S, Kennedy C, O'Kelly P, Doyle B, Dorman A, Awan A, Conlon P (2018) Renal transplant outcomes in primary FSGS compared with other recipients and risk factors for recurrence: A national review of the Irish Transplant Registry. Clin Transplant 32 (1). https://doi.org/10.1111/ctr.13152

3 Tejani A, Stablein DH (1992) Recurrence of focal segmental glomerulosclerosis posttransplantation: a special report of the North American Pediatric Renal Transplant Cooperative Study. J Am Soc Nephrol 2 (12 Suppl): S258–263. https://doi.org/10.1681/ASN.V212s258

4 Fuentes GM, Meseguer CG, Carrion AP, Hijosa MM, Garcia-Pose A, Melgar AA, Torres MN (2010) Long-term outcome of focal segmental glomerulosclerosis after pediatric renal transplantation. Pediatr Nephrol 25 (3):529–534. https://doi.org/10.1007/s00467-009-1361-0

5 Floege J, Barbour SJ, Cattran DC, Hogan JJ, Nachman PH, Tang SCW, Wetzels JFM, Cheung M, Wheeler DC, Winkelmayer WC, Rovin BH, Conference P (2019) Management and treatment of glomerular diseases (part 1): conclusions from a Kidney Disease: Improving Global Outcomes (KDIGO) Controversies Conference. Kidney Int 95 (2):268–280. https://doi.org/10.1016/j.kint.2018.10.018
6 Patry C, Webb NJA, Feisst M, Krupka K, Becker J, Bald M, Antoniello B, Bilge I, Gulhan B, Hogan J, Kanzelmeyer N, Ozkaya O, Buscher A, Sellier-Leclerc AL, Shenoy M, Weber LT, Fichtner A, Hocker B, Meier M, Tonshoff B (2024) Kidney transplantation in children and adolescents with C3 glomerulopathy or immune complex membranoproliferative glomerulonephritis: a real-world study within the CERTAIN research network. Pediatr Nephrol 39 (12):3569–3580. https://doi.org/10.1007/s00467-024-06476-5
7 Vivarelli M, Barratt J, Beck LH, Jr., Fakhouri F, Gale DP, Goicoechea de Jorge E, Mosca M, Noris M, Pickering MC, Susztak K, Thurman JM, Cheung M, King JM, Jadoul M, Winkelmayer WC, Smith RJH, for Conference P (2024) The role of complement in kidney disease: conclusions from a Kidney Disease: Improving Global Outcomes (KDIGO) Controversies Conference. Kidney Int 106 (3):369–391. https://doi.org/10.1016/j.kint.2024.05.015
8 Heidenreich K, Goel D, Priyamvada PS, Kulkarni S, Chakurkar V, Khullar D, Singh R, Bale C, Zipfel PF (2024) C3 glomerulopathy: a kidney disease mediated by alternative pathway deregulation. Front Nephrol 4:1460146. https://doi.org/10.3389/fneph.2024.1460146
9 Wyatt RJ, Julian BA (2013) IgA nephropathy. N Engl J Med 368 (25): 2402–2414. https://doi.org/10.1056/NEJMra1206793
10 Choy BY, Chan TM, Lo SK, Lo WK, Lai KN (2003) Renal transplantation in patients with primary immunoglobulin A nephropathy. Nephrol Dial Transplant 18 (11):2399–2404. https://doi.org/10.1093/ndt/gfg373
11 Moroni G, Longhi S, Quaglini S, Gallelli B, Banfi G, Montagnino G, Messa P (2013) The long-term outcome of renal transplantation of IgA nephropathy and the impact of recurrence on graft survival. Nephrol Dial Transplant 28 (5):1305–1314. https://doi.org/10.1093/ndt/gfs472
12 Kessler M, Hiesse C, Hestin D, Mayeux D, Boubenider K, Charpentier B (1996) Recurrence of immunoglobulin A nephropathy after renal transplantation in the cyclosporine era. Am J Kidney Dis 28 (1):99–104. https://doi.org/10.1016/s0272-6386(96)90137-7

13 Park S, Baek CH, Cho H, Yu MY, Kim YC, Go H, Kim YH, Lee JP, Min SI, Ha J, Moon KC, Kim YS, Ahn C, Park SK, Lee H (2019) Glomerular crescents are associated with worse graft outcome in allograft IgA nephropathy. Am J Transplant 19 (1):145–155. https://doi.org/10.1111/ajt.14908
14 Leeaphorn N, Garg N, Khankin EV, Cardarelli F, Pavlakis M (2018) Recurrence of IgA nephropathy after kidney transplantation in steroid continuation versus early steroid-withdrawal regimens: a retrospective analysis of the UNOS/OPTN database. Transpl Int 31 (2):175–186. https://doi.org/10.1111/tri.13075
15 Oka K, Imai E, Moriyama T, Akagi Y, Ando A, Hori M, Okuyama A, Toki K, Kyo M, Kokado Y, Takahara S (2000) A clinicopathological study of IgA nephropathy in renal transplant recipients: beneficial effect of angiotensin-converting enzyme inhibitor. Nephrol Dial Transplant 15 (5):689–695. https://doi.org/10.1093/ndt/15.5.689
16 Courtney AE, McNamee PT, Nelson WE, Maxwell AP (2006) Does angiotensin blockade influence graft outcome in renal transplant recipients with IgA nephropathy? Nephrol Dial Transplant 21 (12):3550–3554. https://doi.org/10.1093/ndt/gfl506
17 Lafayette RA, Canetta PA, Rovin BH, Appel GB, Novak J, Nath KA, Sethi S, Tumlin JA, Mehta K, Hogan M, Erickson S, Julian BA, Leung N, Enders FT, Brown R, Knoppova B, Hall S, Fervenza FC (2017) A Randomized, Controlled Trial of Rituximab in IgA Nephropathy with Proteinuria and Renal Dysfunction. J Am Soc Nephrol 28 (4):1306–1313. https://doi.org/10.1681/ASN.2016060640
18 El Karoui K, Fervenza FC, De Vriese AS (2024) Treatment of IgA Nephropathy: A Rapidly Evolving Field. J Am Soc Nephrol 35 (1):103–116. https://doi.org/10.1681/ASN.0000000000000242
19 Le Quintrec M, Zuber J, Moulin B, Kamar N, Jablonski M, Lionet A, Chatelet V, Mousson C, Mourad G, Bridoux F, Cassuto E, Loirat C, Rondeau E, Delahousse M, Fremeaux-Bacchi V (2013) Complement genes strongly predict recurrence and graft outcome in adult renal transplant recipients with atypical hemolytic and uremic syndrome. Am J Transplant 13 (3):663–675. https://doi.org/10.1111/ajt.12077
20 Siedlecki AM, Isbel N, Vande Walle J, James Eggleston J, Cohen DJ, Global a HUSR (2019) Eculizumab Use for Kidney Transplantation in Patients With a Diagnosis of Atypical Hemolytic Uremic Syndrome. Kidney Int Rep 4 (3):434–446. https://doi.org/10.1016/j.ekir.2018.11.010

21 Wong T, Goral S (2019) Lupus Nephritis and Kidney Transplantation: Where Are We Today? Adv Chronic Kidney Dis 26 (5):313–322. https://doi.org/10.1053/j.ackd.2019.08.007

22 Mojcik CF, Klippel JH (1996) End-stage renal disease and systemic lupus erythematosus. Am J Med 101 (1):100–107. https://doi.org/10.1016/s0002-9343(96)00074-5

23 Contreras G, Mattiazzi A, Guerra G, Ortega LM, Tozman EC, Li H, Tamariz L, Carvalho C, Kupin W, Ladino M, LeClercq B, Jaraba I, Carvalho D, Carles E, Roth D (2010) Recurrence of lupus nephritis after kidney transplantation. J Am Soc Nephrol 21 (7):1200–1207. https://doi.org/10.1681/ASN.2009101093

24 Stone JH, Millward CL, Olson JL, Amend WJ, Criswell LA (1998) Frequency of recurrent lupus nephritis among ninety-seven renal transplant patients during the cyclosporine era. Arthritis Rheum 41 (4):678–686. https://doi.org/10.1002/1529-0131(199804)41:4<678::AID-ART15>3.0.CO;2-7

25 Michael M, Harvey E, Milliner DS, Frishberg Y, Sas DJ, Calle J, Copelovitch L, Penniston KL, Saland J, Somers MJG, Baum MA (2024) Diagnosis and management of primary hyperoxalurias: best practices. Pediatr Nephrol 39 (11):3143–3155. https://doi.org/10.1007/s00467-024-06328-2

CHAPTER 9
Aftercare and Outcome

Burkhard Tönshoff[1] & Lars Pape[2]

[1] Heidelberg University, Medical Faculty Heidelberg, Department of Paediatrics I, University Children's Hospital, Heidelberg, Germany
[2] Department of Paediatrics II, University Hospital of Essen, Essen, Germany

ORCIDs:
Burkhard Tönshoff: https://orcid.org/0000-0002-6598-6910
Lars Pape: https://orcid.org/0000-0002-3635-6418

1 Aftercare

Intensive follow-up care at specialist paediatric transplant facilities, in collaboration with a paediatrician or family doctor, is crucial for the success of a kidney transplant. Certain examinations should be carried out routinely at regular intervals to detect complications early (Table 1). It is also important to check medication adherence, particularly among adolescent patients.

2 Outcome

According to data from the North American Pediatric Renal Trials and Collaborative Studies (NAPRTCS), the one-year survival rate for patients receiving a kidney from a living or deceased donor is currently 98% and 97%, respectively, while the five-year survival rate is 96% and 93%, respectively [1]. The most common causes of death are infection (40%), cardiopulmonary disease (13%), and malignancy (10%). Overall, however, the prognosis for patients undergoing kidney transplantation in childhood is significantly better than for those receiving long-term dialysis therapy. Transplant survival rates have improved considerably in recent years, particularly for deceased kidney transplants. According to recent data from the CTS registry, paediatric patients in Europe, North America and Australia can currently expect a 5-year transplant survival rate of 90% after living donation and 86% after deceased donation (Figure 1). The recently published data from the Cooperative European Paediatric Renal Transplant Initiative (CERTAIN) registry in conjunction with Eurotransplant data also show a

Table 1 Aftercare examinations following kidney transplantation in children

1. At every visit
   - Clinical examination: weight, length, blood pressure, physical examen (painful graft)
   - Laboratory tests:
     - Blood count with differential blood count and thrombocytes
     - Serum: creatinine, urea, cystatin C, electrolytes including magnesium and phosphate, glucose, blood gases in venous blood, trough levels of the immunosuppressants tacrolimus, cyclosporin A, mycophenolic acid, everolimus
     - Urine: dipstick, protein/creatinine ratio, albumin/creatinine ratio, cytology, culture if necessary. If correct urine collection is possible: 24-hour urine for protein excretion and protein/creatinine and albumin/creatinine ratio, creatinine and urea clearance
2. Every 3 months (in addition to 1.):
   - Laboratory tests: Reticulocytes, PTH, protein, uric acid, enzymes (AP, GPT, GOT, CHE, γGT, LDH), bilirubin, cholesterol, triglycerides, quantitative PCR for CMV, EBV, BKPyV (in the first 2 years post-transplant, depending on individual risk profile)
3. Annually (in addition to 1. and 2.):
   - Laboratory tests:
     - Glucose (fasting), HbA_{1C}, iron, ferritin, transferrin, cholesterol (HDL, LDL), triglycerides, creatin kinase, immunoglobulins, testosterone, oestradiol,
     - anti-HBS antibodies, anti-HC-AK, HC-DNA using quantitative PCR, antibody titres (IgG) for vaccine-preventable pathogens (mumps, measles, rubella, varicella, hepatitis A, hepatitis B), donor-specific HLA antibodies (more frequently than annually if there is a high immunological risk),
   - X-ray: left hand: if symptoms X-ray of other parts of the skeleton
   - Sonography of the kidney transplant and of the kidneys, Doppler sonography of the kidney transplant artery
   - ECG, echocardiography, ambulatory blood pressure measurement over 24 hours
   - Ophthalmological examination: cataract, glaucoma, fundus?
   - Dermatological status
   - Dental status
   - Stage of puberty

Figure 1

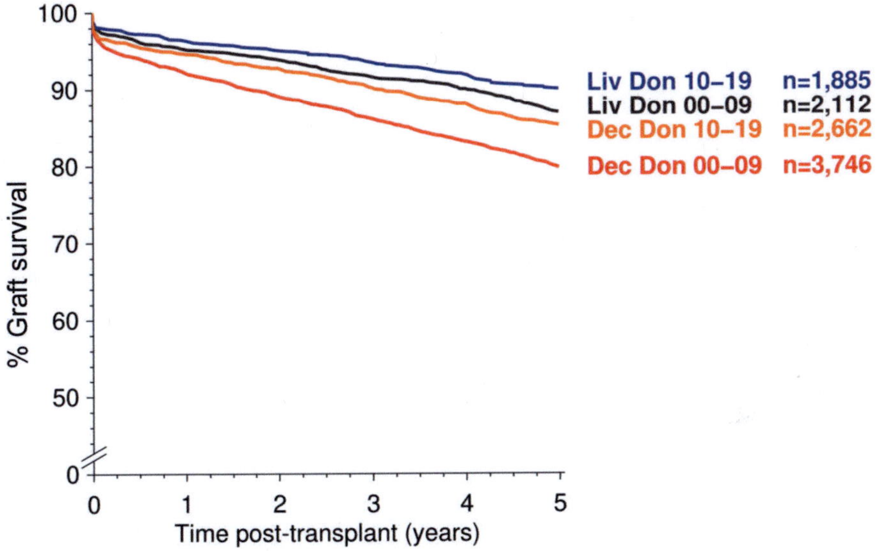

Figure 2

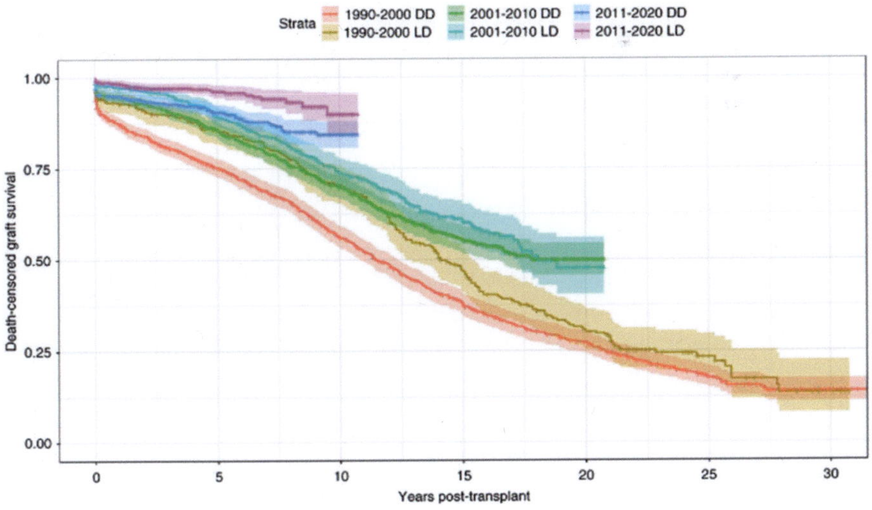

lower risk of premature graft loss after living kidney donation compared to deceased donation (Figure 2). In addition, analogous to the CTS data, this analysis showed a further improvement in treatment outcomes after both living and deceased donation in the cohort that received their transplant in the period 2011–2020 compared to the cohort in the period 2001–2010 [2].

2.1 Factors influencing kidney transplant survival

The following factors influence the survival of kidney transplants in children and adolescents:

- transplant source (deceased or living donation);
- pre-emptive transplantation or previous dialysis therapy;
- the age of the donor and recipient;
- the extent of HLA compatibility;
- sensitisation with the development of preformed HLA antibodies;
- a long cold ischaemia time;
- delayed kidney transplant function;
- acute and chronic rejection;
- intercurrent infections, particularly opportunistic ones;
- non-adherence;
- the recipient's underlying kidney disease and its possible recurrence in the transplant.

Non-immunological factors are also important, particularly arterial hypertension, pronounced secondary hyperparathyroidism, and inadequately treated metabolic acidosis.

The success of kidney transplants in children and adolescents depends on the recipient's age. While the results for children under five years of age were unsatisfactory around 20 years ago, the survival rate for kidney transplants in this age group is now comparatively good, thanks to improvements in surgical techniques and postoperative management (see Figure 3). Adolescents and young adults have the poorest five-year survival rates following a kidney transplant. According to an analysis of the NAPRTCS registry, the five-year survival rate for kidney transplants after living donation was 85% for children under five, 85% for those aged six to 12, and 79% for those aged over 12. Similar results can be seen in the Collaborative Transplant Study (CTS) registry (Figure 3). The poorer re-

Figure 3

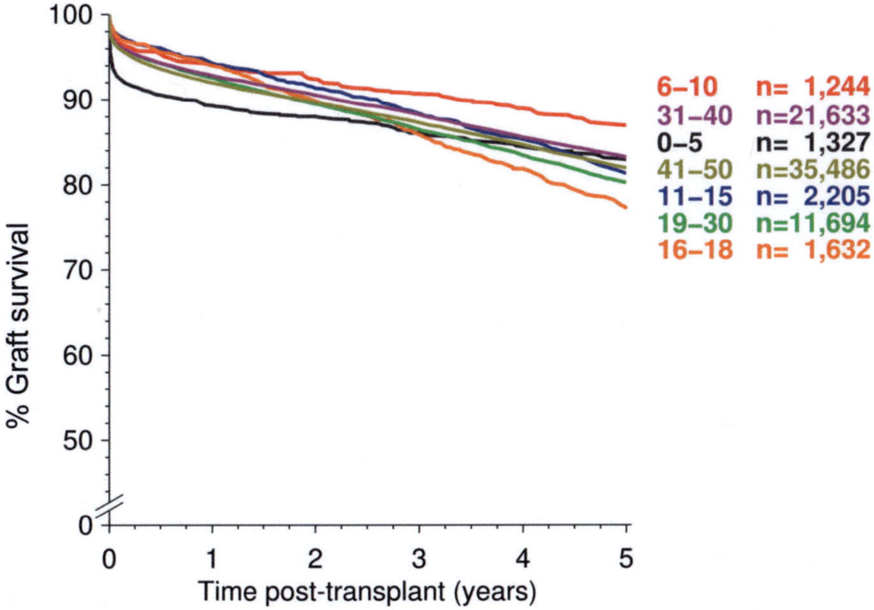

sults observed in adolescents and young adults are largely due to non-adherence to regular use of immunosuppressive medication and to the transition to adult medical care during this vulnerable life phase.

As with adults, good HLA compatibility between the recipient and donor is associated with a higher survival rate for kidney transplants, whether the donor is living or deceased. The best results are achieved with an identical HLA profile. However, children and adolescents rarely have HLA-identical adult siblings who can be considered as donors. Therefore, the vast majority of living donations come from a parent, resulting in a haploidentical HLA match between parent and child. An optimal HLA match is also important to avoid sensitisation in young recipients who will require multiple transplants throughout their lifes [3]. In the Eurotransplant region, most paediatric kidney transplant centres therefore define one match on the HLA-DR locus and one match on the HLA-A or HLA-B locus as the minimum requirement for acceptance of a deceased kidney transplant offer.

References

1 Tönshoff B, Becker JU, Pape L. Nierentransplantation, pp. 243–74. In: Nierenerkrankungen im Kindes- und Jugendalter, Dötsch J, Weber LT (Hrsg.), Springer Berlin, 2025

2 Coens F, Knops N, Tieken I, Vogelaar S, Bender A, Kim JJ, Krupka K, Pape L, Raes A, Tönshoff B, Prytula A; CERTAIN Registry. Time-Varying Determinants of Graft Failure in Pediatric Kidney Transplantation in Europe. Clin J Am Soc Nephrol. 2024;19(3):345–354

3 Coens F, Reynders D, Goetghebeur E, Tieken I, Vogelaar S, Krupka K, Raes A, Claas F, Tönshoff B, Prytula A. Incidence and determinants of graft failure and death with functioning graft after re-transplantation. Pediatr Nephrol 2025;40(12):3761–3774

CHAPTER 10
Rehabilitation

Eberhard Kuwertz-Bröking & Miriam Zimmering

Rehabilitation Centre Ederhof, Iselsberg-Stronach, Austria

ORCID:
Eberhard Kuwertz-Bröking: https://orcid.org/0000-0001-6399-0126

Introduction

Kidney transplantation in childhood and adolescence is the only renal replacement therapy that can enable a largely normal life. To achieve this, these patients require specialised long-term aftercare. Structured rehabilitation programmes play a key role in this. While good outpatient aftercare focuses on managing physical problems, it often falls short in addressing the full range of follow-up needs. In addition to the side effects of immunosuppressive therapy, patients may face complications such as arterial hypertension, hyperlipoproteinemia, cardiovascular disease, obesity, diabetes mellitus, bacterial and viral infections and neoplasia, all of which can affect long-term graft survival and limit participation in social life. There is also a risk of gradual loss of organ function, which may eventually require dialysis again.

The mental stability of the transplanted child can be negatively affected by difficulties in accepting the new organ, inadequate coping with the illness and the demands of ongoing medical treatment, and fears and worries about the future. These factors can also affect the function of the transplant. This also applies to the child's social integration into the natural living environment, acceptance by peer groups, self-confidence and overall quality of life [1]. Non-adherence to medication plays an important role in the survival of the transplanted organ, especially in adolescents. Up to 1/3 of the adolescents do not take their immunosuppressive medication regularly in this phase of life. The risk of organ loss is particularly high during the transition period between the ages of 17 and 24 years [2].

Children with complex congenital syndromes, who previously had no treatment options, now have a better chance of survival. An increasing number of these children are treated with peritoneal dialysis from infancy and receive a transplant (often a live donation from a parent) by the age of 2–3 years. In many cases, these children have additional extrarenal symptoms such as physical and mental disabilities associated with significant developmental delays in motor, cognitive, language, social and emotional areas. This places increasing demands on parents in terms of care and expertise.

A child's chronic illness causes a variety of emotional stresses, not only for the child's parents but also for the child's siblings. Because one or both parents are very involved with the sick child, siblings and the other parent may feel neglected. This can lead to family dysfunction. This highlights the importance of early rehabilitation: parent coaching should go hand in hand with efforts to stabilise the child's physical and emotional well-being.

Approximately 30% of children and adolescents in Germany receive a living kidney donation. The donor must learn to protect the remaining single kidney (e.g. through annual follow-up examinations) [3]. Donors may not always regain their previous physical, mental and work capacity. They may also feel a strong sense of responsibility for the transplanted child, especially at a time when young people are seeking independence from their parents. This can lead to additional stress, making rehabilitation important for donors as well [4].

Aims of rehabilitation

The main aim of rehabilitation is to improve participation in family, school, social life and eventually work life and to improve life quality. This includes:

- Strengthening the patient's ability to manage their illness, improving coping mechanisms and organ acceptance
- Improving and stabilising medication adherence
- Preventing or reducing the impact of secondary complications
- Improving physical and mental performance
- Improving psychosocial well-being
- Addressing the special relationship between the donor and the recipient in the case of living donation
- Promote age-appropriate autonomy
- Stabilise and optimise nutritional status
- Provide education for patients and parents, tailored to the type of rehabilitation, transition

Ideally, rehabilitation should lead to a comprehensive and significant stabilisation of the patient's health status, with a focus on preventing rapid deterioration of the transplant function or even organ loss.

Implementing rehabilitation

In paediatrics, it is important to consider the wider context of the child. In the case of inpatient rehabilitation, the primary caregiver is admitted to the hospital as a "co-therapist". However, the aim should be to involve all family members in the rehabilitation programme.

During the course of congenital kidney disease and subsequent transplantation several stages of rehabilitation are beneficial: during infancy, school age and adolescence. Final rehabilitation should take place between the ages of 15 and 18 years, depending on the individual's developmental stage, and should include a transition programme that fully prepares the young person for adulthood and a long life with the transplanted organ.

Older adolescents and young adults with developmental delays or who are still in school or in vocational training can continue to receive paediatric rehabilitation until the age of 27 years.

Rehabilitation for children from 1 to 14 years of age (or longer in special cases, e.g. developmental delay, physical and mental disability) should be carried out as "Family Oriented Rehabilitation (FOR)", involving as many family members as possible. With the increasing number of young children undergoing transplantation (e.g. early nursery school age), the additional offer of family-oriented infant rehabilitation is very useful. All FORs should aim for groups of families to be admitted to the rehabilitation clinic at the same time and then generally attend rehabilitation together for 4 weeks. Longer periods of rehabilitation are also possible (e.g. 6 weeks).

Adolescents aged 15–18 years and young adults should receive rehabilitation unaccompanied in larger groups specifically designed for this age group, depending on their developmental age and comorbidity. If parents have their own rehabilitation needs, such as in the case of living donors, they should be admitted to the same clinic at the same time if a rehabilitation measure is approved by the funder.

Based on preliminary findings, the rehabilitation clinic develops a personalised treatment plan that includes medical, psychological, educational, physiotherapeutic, occupational and sports therapy services as required. In addition, the children and young people and their siblings receive a qualified education in core subjects in consultation with their home school. Rehabilitation is therefore not dependent on school holidays.

Motivation for rehabilitation

The motivation of children and adolescents to participate in rehabilitation depends not only on their age, but also on the motivation of their caregivers, who are actively involved in the child's care as co-therapists. The willingness to accept all therapy offers (which are always mandatory) is essential for the overall success of rehabilitation. Providing patients and families with sufficient information about the goals of rehabilitation, the course of rehabilitation and the conditions and possibilities of the rehabilitation clinic is an important motivational aid.

The rehabilitation team

The interdisciplinary rehabilitation team includes professionals from the fields of nursing, psychology, physiotherapy, occupational therapy, speech therapy, dietetics, education and social work as well as medical specialists. Sports instructors and specialist teachers should also be part of the team.

The medical management of a rehabilitation facility requires many years of competent and constantly updated specialist knowledge, oriented towards the specifics of congenital and acquired nephrological diseases, dialysis treatment and kidney transplantation. Close cooperation between the rehabilitation clinic and the referring physician or centre is necessary.

Diagnostic and therapeutic services

Medical care:

- Continuous medical care by nurses and doctors throughout rehabilitation is essential. Where appropriate, staff should be experienced in dialysis therapy (particularly peritoneal dialysis and, where possible, haemodialysis), which should also be available during rehabilitation.
- Short-term blood tests for serum sodium and potassium, blood gas analysis, prompt determination of essential serum parameters and level checks

(immunosuppressive drugs), urinalysis, 24-hour blood pressure measurement, sonography, ECG.
- Lectures and training on nephrological diseases, organ functions, immune system, immunosuppressive drugs, concomitant medication after transplantation, post-transplant infections, transition training

Educational services:
- Individual patient care based on clinical picture and co-morbidities
- Individual and group care for parents and siblings
- Learning support for school-age children
- Active leisure activities
- Occupational therapy to improve functioning in daily activities
- Encouraging and supporting interaction between all patients and families, both with and independently of the rehabilitation team

Psychological services:
- Psychosocial assessment, including standardised and validated tests
- Behavioural assessment, family interaction
- Assessment of adherence, disease acceptance, self-confidence, self-responsibility
- Individual and group psychological interventions, crisis management.

Physiotherapy and sports therapy:
- Psychomotor skills, activation of muscle activity during sport and play, also as part of leisure activities
- Improving physical performance, coordination and balance
- Stabilisation of body awareness
- Relaxation programmes

Nutrition therapy and advice including tube feeding
- Ensuring an individualized and healthy diet
- Practical training in a teaching kitchen

Legal regulations

In Germany, the rehabilitation for children and young people is a social service covered by the statutory health insurance or the German Pension Insurance. The necessary legal basis for this is formulated in the German Social Code (SGB IX: Rehabilitation and Participation of People with Disabilities) and in the respective social codes of the individual rehabilitation providers.

These regulations are intended to take account of the special needs of children with disabilities, including emotional disabilities.

The Flexible Pensions Act, which came into force in December 2016, established legal regulations for the rehabilitation of children and adolescents. Children's rehabilitation is defined as a compulsory benefit if the child's chronic illness affects his or her participation in school and vocational training and thus also has affects his or her ability to earn a living in the future. Children are entitled to be accompanied if this is necessary for the implementation or success of the child's rehabilitation. This also applies to the admission of family members if their involvement in the rehabilitation process is necessary. Inpatient services are generally provided for four weeks. The four-year period between two rehabilitation measures, which applies to adults, does not apply to children.

References

1 Reichwald Klugger E: Psychosoziale Betreuung bei chronischer Niereninsuffizienz. In: Schärer K, Mehls O, Hrsg., Pädiatrische Nephrologie. Springer Verlag Berlin, Heidelberg 2002

2 Watson, AR (2000). Non-compliance and transfer from pediatric to adult transplant unit. Pediatric Nephrology, 14, 469–472.

3 Lentine KL, Kasiske BL, Levey AS, Adams PL, Alberú J, Bakr MA, Gallon L, Garvey CA, Guleria S, Li PK, Segev DL, Taler SJ, Tanabe K, Wright L, Zeier MG, Cheung M, Garg AX (2017) KDIGO clinical practice guideline on the evaluation and care of living kidney donors. Transplantation 101(8S Suppl 1):S1–S109

4 Gerbig D, Koehler M, Krautzig S, Degenhardt S (2017) Informationen und Stellungnahme der Kommission Rehabilitation, Transition und Altersmedizin der DGfN (Deutsche Gesellschaft für Nephrologie) zur stationären Rehabilitation bei chronisch Nierenkranken, Nierentransplantierten und Nierenlebendspendern. Nephrologe 12:438–442

5 Kidney Disease (2017) Improving global outcomes (KDIGO) living kidney donor work group. KDIGO clinical practice guideline on the evaluation and care of living kidney donors. Transplantation 101:S1–S109
6 Weber LT (2011) Pediatric renal diseases after transfer/transition to adult care. Nephrologe 6:9–21

CHAPTER 11
Child development in the context of renal replacement therapy

Jenny Prüfe

Department of Paediatrics II, University Hospital of Essen, Essen, Germany

ORCID:
https://orcid.org/0000-0001-7565-295X

Development describes a change in human experience and behaviour that builds up over time. It should be noted that the permanent decline in abilities, such as occurs in neurodegenerative diseases, is also considered as development. In the context of chronic kidney disease and renal replacement therapy, a number of factors can exert an influence on the course of development. These can be divided into three categories. In general, the earlier and more extensively the disease affects the developing organism, the greater the difficulties and abnormalities that can be observed.

1. General effects of impaired kidney function, such as

- systemic inflammation,
- consequences of acidaemia and uraemia,
- sympathetic overactivity,
- hypertension and vascular changes.

While some of these factors can be alleviated by transplantation, others persist post-transplantation and continue to exert an influence. Immunosuppressive therapy, which almost always includes a potentially neurotoxic calcineurin inhibitor and corticosteroids, may introduce additional influencing factors.

2. Extra-renal manifestations of kidney disease, such as

- syndromic diseases without structural brain changes (e.g. Alport syndrome, HUS),
- syndromic diseases with structural brain changes (e.g. Joubert syndrome),
- metabolic diseases (e.g. cystinosis, oxalosis),
- systemic diseases with kidney involvement (e.g. vasculitis, SLE)

It is important to note that individuals with congenital nephrotic syndrome may have severe developmental problems even in the absence of kidney dysfunction. The significant loss of protein can result in a deficiency of essential nutrients required for normal physiological development.

3. Environmental factors such as
- Reduced play and learning opportunities due to hospitalisation
- Traumatic experiences
- Changed parental behaviour
- Physical stigmatisation
- Difficult social contacts

Possible impacts on different areas of development are listed in Table 1.

The above risks and impairments have been shown to increase the likelihood that people with childhood-onset ESRD will

- have lower grades and educational attainment
- lack school-leaving qualifications
- become unemployed
- live on benefits
- have a delayed transition to independent living
- live in a partnership [2, 3, 4].

In the light of these findings, it is imperative to prioritise the early identification of developmental disorders and delays at an early stage and to address them through targeted interventions. This can be achieved by:

1. Regular paediatric developmental screening to detect abnormalities
2. In-depth developmental psychology and/or neuropaediatric assessment to differentiate abnormalities, initiate differential diagnosis and develop support plans
3. Connection to multi-professional diagnostics and treatment in a socio-paediatric centre (SPC)

The support measures can be summarised as follows:

Table 1 Possible developmental abnormalities associated with renal replacement therapy

Area of development	Possible abnormalities
Sensors	• Hearing impairment (e.g. Alport) • Visual impairment (e.g. cystinosis) • Dizziness • Pain • Tactile-kinaesthetic abnormalities • Proprioceptive-vestibular abnormalities (positional sensitivity)
Motor skills	• Orofacial weakness with sucking and swallowing difficulties and articulation problems • Muscular hypotonia with trunk instability • Disproportionately short stature with impaired development of movement sequences • Organic brain movement disorders (e.g. Joubert syndrome)
Language	• Delayed speech development with a reduced understanding of cause and effect • Interaction problems • Phonetic disorders
Cognition	• Global intellectual disability • Memory problems • Concentration disorders • Reduced processing speed • Executive dysfunction
Social-emotional development	• Attachment disorders (e.g. in the case of prolonged intensive care after birth) • Repeated trauma and trauma-related disorders • Isolation, hospitalisation, (anxiety including fear of the future • Depression • Behavioural problems (e.g. obsessive-compulsive or oppositional behaviour)

Special educational early intervention

- Applicable in the first 3 years of life or before the start of KiTa (note: differences between districts)
- Early start important
- Direct developmental support and training of parents
- Integration of appropriate facilities in case of visual or hearing impairment
- Funded in Germany through "Eingliederungshilfe"/integration assistance (social benefit according to SGB IX § 46),
- Requires a certification of need by treating paediatrician

Therapeutic measures

- Physiotherapy (e.g. strengthening, tone regulation, training of physiological movement patterns)
- Occupational therapy (e.g. sensory integration, body awareness, stimulus regulation)
- Speech therapy (e.g. tube weaning, swallowing training, articulation support)
- Psychotherapy (e.g. for trauma, depression, interactional disorders)

All of these therapies require a doctor's prescription and regular reviews of their usefulness and success.

Psychological and educational interventions

- Inconsistent research on cognitive outcome after transplantation.
- Cognitive decline after transplantation has also been described [5].
- Heterogeneous developmental profiles with circumscribed cognitive problems despite normal intelligence (e.g. concentration, attention or processing speed) are common.
- Early neuropsychological diagnostics and analysis of performance profiles are needed to initiate targeted support and compensate for disadvantages.
- Use of hospital schooling and home schooling for extended periods of absence (e.g. following transplantation)
- Involvement of specialist staff from relevant special educational needs schools to determine compensation for disadvantages at school (also applies to children without certified special educational needs).

References

1 Gesell A, Amatruda C (1941) Developmental Diagnosis. Normal and abnormal child development. Harper & Row, New York

2 Groothoff JW, Grootenhuis MA, Offringa M, Stronks, K, Hutten GJ, Heymans, HS (2005). Social consequences in adult life of end-stage renal disease in childhood. The Journal of paediatrics, 146(4), 512–517. https://doi.org/10.1016/j.jpeds.2004.10.060

3 Kärrfelt HM, Berg UB (2008). Long-term psychosocial outcome after renal transplantation during childhood. *Pediatric transplantation, 12*(5), 557–562. https://doi.org/10.1111/j.1399-3046.2007.00859.x

4 Harshman LA, Ward RC, Matheson MB, Dawson A, Kogon AJ, Lande MB, Molitor SJ, Johnson RZ, Wilson C, Warady BA, Furth SL, Hooper SR (2023). The Impact of Pediatric CKD on Educational and Employment Outcomes. *Kidney360, 4*(10), 1389–1396. https://doi.org/10.34067/KID.0000000000000206

5 Lullmann O, van der Plas E, Harshman LA. Understanding the impact of paediatric kidney transplantation on cognition: A review of the literature. Pediatr Transplant. 2023 Dec;27(8):e14597.i: 10.1111/petr.14597. Epub 2023 Sep 4. PMID: 37664967; PMCID: PMC11034761.

CHAPTER 12
Social-legal aspects in paediatric kidney transplantation

Jenny Prüfe

Department of Paediatrics II, University Hospital of Essen, Essen, Germany.

ORCID:
https://orcid.org/0000-0001-7565-295X

From the moment of diagnosis, chronic terminal kidney disease becomes a lifelong companion for the child and their family. Although the therapy changes with the transplant, the child remains chronically ill and requires ongoing medical support. In Germany, chronically ill people are entitled to a range of material, financial and non-material forms of compensation for the disadvantages they face. In the case of minors, applications must be submitted by their legal representatives. Advice on social entitlements and assistance in claiming them is provided by the social services staff at the treatment centres. Families often benefit, if the attending physician also has information about possible sources of assistance and can make specific referrals. An overview of this is provided in this chapter.

The entitlements of those affected are derived from the books of social legislation, which also regulate the procedures for applying for and granting these entitlements. The most important of these are:

SGB V → Statutory health insurance benefits and their relationship to service providers ("gesetzliche Krankenversicherung")
SGB VI → Statutory pension insurance benefits, e.g. relevant for rehabilitation benefits ("gesetzliche Rentenversicherung")
SGB VIII → Child and Youth Welfare, e.g. relevant for services for integration assistance for children with (impending) mental disabilities and child day care services ("Kinder- und Jugendhilfegesetz")
SGB IX → Rehabilitation & Participation (Rehabilitation and Severely Disabled Persons Act and Integration Assistance/"Bundesteilhabegesetz")
SGB XI → long-term care insurance, e.g. relevant for claims and benefits in the event of a need for long-term care (e.g. aids) ("gesetzliche Pflegeversicherung")

In detail, this results in the following benefits to which patients may be entitled after a kidney transplant. We have not included specific reimbursement rates, as these are regularly adjusted. In addition, we have not listed all services that are theoretically possible, but only those that play a role in everyday clinical practice and require a doctor's prescription or certificate.

Benefits from statutory health insurance

Patient transport is regulated in conjunction with the patient transport guidelines. This implies that there must be a medical necessity to justify the prescription and that the mode of transport is selected accordingly. While this can generally be assumed in the case of dialysis treatment, the medical necessity after transplantation is determined by the patient's immune status and any other pre-existing impairments. In the event of an uncomplicated course of treatment, travel costs associated with "post-inpatient treatment" are covered for a period of three months following the transplantation. Other relevant health conditions, e.g. for patients with complex illnesses, must be examined separately.

In principle, trips for outpatient treatment require prior authorisation, i.e. a doctor's prescription must be submitted to and approved by the payer before the trip begins. Exceptions are made for patients who are certified on their Disability Pass as having exceptional walking disabilities, blindness or helplessness on their severely disabled person's pass, as well as for patients with care level 4 or 5, and care level 3 in combination with a permanent mobility impairment. Trips made in the family's own car are only partially reimbursed according to the German SGB V. However, trips to the hospital and outpatient clinic should be documented and confirmed by the centre so that they can be taken into account for tax purposes.

In the case of hospitalisation, it should be noted that visits are generally not reimbursable. The situation is different if the presence of the parents – regardless of the child's age – is medically or psychologically necessary. This applies for example, to educational discussions or medical crises and should be certified by a doctor.

If medically necessary, *a parent or legal guardian* may also be *admitted* during an inpatient stay [1]. Co-admission is considered medically necessary if separation from the parent/primary carer would otherwise jeopardise the success of treatment. The health insurance companies decide up to what age the need for co-admission of a parent is considered to be age-related (usually around the age of 9 years). If the parent cannot be accommodated in the patient's room due to lack of space, the costs of a nearby guesthouse or hotel may be covered if the medical necessity is certified and proof of the costs incurred is submitted to the health insurance company.

If a child's illness prevents their parent from working, they can claim wage replacement benefit (also known as child sickness benefit) for a limited number of days per child per year. To qualify for wage replacement benefit, a doctor's certificate confirming the child's illness must be submitted.In cases where the child's prognosis is limited to a few weeks or months – as outlined in § 45 Para. 4 SGB V – the entitlement to wage-replacement benefit is unlimited.

If there is another child under the age of 12 years living in the household or a disabled child who is dependent on assistance, the provision of *household assistance* may be granted for a maximum of 8 hours per day to help the family with its domestic tasks, provided that one of the parents also takes care of the child.

Preventive care and rehabilitation measures are also covered. A distinction is made between father/mother/child rehabilitation, child rehabilitation and family-orientated rehabilitation (FOR). After transplantation, family-oriented rehabilitation (FOR) is given the highest priority, as it is not only aimed at the sick child but also offers support to the parents and healthy siblings. In contrast, paediatric rehabilitation focuses on the chronically ill child. Parents may be allowed to accompany their child on the programme, but siblings are not included. It is important to note that all the benefits described here apply within the framework of statutory health insurance. Different rules may apply to privately insured persons and recipients of benefits.

Benefits from the statutory pension insurance scheme

The pension insurance fund is responsible for measures for rehabilitation and participation in working life. Like the health insurance fund, it is responsible for covering the costs of rehabilitation measures. While the health insurance fund and the pension insurance fund may share the costs of rehabilitation before the patient enters working life, the pension insurance fund becomes the main provider of benefits as soon as the patient is in vocational training, military or civilian service and the aim of the rehabilitation is to maintain or restore the patient's ability to work.

In contrast to the health insurance system, the pension insurance system's right to request and choose a measure is primarily limited to contracted centres. If the pension insurance fund does not name a suitable contract centre from the patient's point of view, a medical report is required for the selection of a place of rehabilitation outside the contract centres. The statutory pension insurance funds also provide benefits for participation in working life according to §§ 49–54 SGB IX as well as in the introductory procedure and vocational training area of the workshops for disabled people according to § 57 SGB IX (see below).

Child and youth welfare services

Child and youth welfare services are by no means limited to educational assistance and the protection of children's welfare. Child and Youth Welfare also acts as a rehabilitation organisation for children and young people who are threatened or affected by so-called "mental disabilities". In accordance with the provisions of SGB IX, the Youth Welfare Office is empowered to provide integration assistance in the event of an (imminent) mental disability, e.g. for educational and therapeutic services outside the remit of other organisations. This is the case, for example, when children and young people develop mental or behavioural problems as a result of specific learning difficulties. In the case of manifest concentration disorders, dyscalculia or dyslexia, learning therapy can be applied for as an educational-therapeutic measure, the costs of which are covered by the Youth Welfare Office.

The Youth Welfare Office also provides services to support children in day care centres and with childminders. This includes creating the conditions for a child with a kidney transplant to attend a day care centre, such as a crèche, day care centre or kindergarten. In addition, if necessary, the Youth Welfare Office provides support with inclusion, for example by providing integration assistants.

Rehabilitation and participation services

The primary objective of the Ninth Chapter of the Social Code (SGB IX) is to regulate entitlements and measures for people with severe disabilities in order to enable them to participate in society. According to Section 2 of SGB IX, a person is considered to be severely disabled if he or she has a degree of disability of at least 50% and his or her place of residence, habitual abode or employment falls within the scope of this Code. This status applies to all persons who have undergone a kidney transplant, as the degree of disability is at least 50% after a recovery period of two years post-transplant.

Official recognition of this status and the issue of a severely disabled person's card is based on an application to be submitted by the person's legal guardian. The resulting benefits depend on the degree of disability determined and any additional characteristics recognised. These include tax allowances of varying amounts, reduced/free use of public transport, assistance under the Housing Assistance Act and housing benefit, reduction or exemption from telephone and radio licence fees, and special provisions in employment law, e.g. protection against dismissal, holiday entitlement and retirement age.

It is of the utmost importance that the application is supported by careful medical documentation, even if it is made by legal representatives and with the support of social services. This is essential for the accurate recognition of the applicant's health problems. If the above-mentioned documents are not available at the time of submission, they will be requested by the administrative staff of the pension offices. They check whether the criteria in the appendix to § 2 of the Versorgungsmedizin-Verordnung/"Versorgungsmedizinische Grundsätze" are met. The more detailed the patient's health impairment is described in the doctor's letter, the more accurately the application can be processed. In addition to the transplant and kidney function, additional effects of the underlying disease (e.g. visual impairment in cystinosis, liver dysfunction in ARPKD, hearing impairment in Alport, bronchopulmonary dysplasia in LUTO, cardiac hypertrophy, brain malformations, movement disorders, cognitive impairment, short stature, nutritional and failure to thrive disorders, etc.) should also be explicitly listed. In addition, diseases independent of the kidney disease should be included. A look at the guidelines will help to understand the terminology and concepts familiar to case workers.

The main benefit groups resulting from SGB IX are benefits for medical rehabilitation, including early intervention and support for self-help; participation in working life, including sheltered workshops; maintenance or supplementary benefits; benefits for participation in education and social participation, including assistance benefits, mobility benefits and special aids.

Care insurance benefits

For the purposes of this book, “vulnerable people” are those who have health-related impairments to their independence or capabilities and who therefore require assistance from others. Such persons must be unable to compensate for or cope with physical, cognitive or mental impairments or health-related burdens or demands independently. The need for care must be permanent, be expected to last for at least six months and meet the criteria of § 15 (§ 14.1 SGB XI).

A kidney transplant alone does not usually lead to a need for long-term care. Instead, the Medical Service of the Health Insurance Funds (MDK) uses an assessment procedure to determine the extent to which a person is able to act independently in defined areas. The modules that are tested include (i) mobility, (ii) cognitive and communicative abilities, (iii) behavioural and psychological problems, (iv) self-care, (v) coping with the demands and stresses of the illness or therapy, and (vi) organisation of everyday life and social contacts.

There are two exceptions to the approach used for adults when determining the level of care for children. Firstly, for children up to the age of 11, a comparison is always made with healthy peers, as children are still developing certain skills. In the case of children with disabilities, the level of care is determined on the basis of the child’s specific needs. The question is therefore whether the child’s ability to care for himself or herself is below the norm for his or her age. Secondly, since healthy infants and toddlers are also dependent on comprehensive care, there is a “natural” need for care regardless of whether there is a complex illness. To take this into account, children under 18 months who need care are classified one level of care higher than adults.

The primary factors that determine the need for care after kidney transplantation in childhood and adolescence are therefore additional impairments associated with syndromic kidney disease. These may include global developmental disorders, associated epilepsy, motor/movement disorders or sensory impairments. In addition, the general challenges associated with kidney disease may also contribute to the level of care. These may include incontinence, the need for tube feeding, complex therapeutic regimens involving frequent medication administration, out-of-home therapeutic services and frequent visits to the doctor, or regular monitoring of bodily functions.

The level of care, which can range from 0 to 5, determines the range of benefits available, including care allowance, care benefits in kind (such as basic care services provided by professional carers), combined benefits (which combine cash benefits and benefits in kind, including care aids and consumables), and benefits to protect the carer (such as pension and accident insurance for carers).

There are also entitlements to short-term and/or respite care to reduce the burden on family carers. It should be noted that successful kidney transplantation in the absence of a syndromic disorder with developmental delay can significantly reduce and often even eliminate the need for care.

Summary

Even after a kidney transplant, a person remains chronically ill and severely disabled. The social services provide advice on social rights and help to enforce them. Many services require a medical prescription. Even if the social services provide support in this respect, the taxi licence/transport prescription, rehabilitation application and prescription of medical aids remain activities for which doctors are responsible and which may be relevant to the budget and recourse. Payers often rely on medical reports and expert opinions. The more complete and accurate these are, the more accurate the implementation and the lower the risk of appeals.

References

1 Roters in: Kasseler Kommentar, Sozialversicherungsrecht, SGB V, status: August 2019, Section 11 marginal number 22.

CHAPTER 13
Transition to adult care

Jenny Prüfe

Department of Paediatrics II, University Hospital of Essen, Essen, Germany.

ORCID:
https://orcid.ord/0000-0001-7565-295X

Nowadays, most children with chronic kidney disease (CKD) stage 5 and kidney transplantation survive into adulthood. As a result, healthcare transition from paediatric into adult (nephrological) care becomes necessary. Transition is a deliberate process designed to support the development of young patients and help them become self-reliant adults who understand and actively manage their condition. During this process patients gradually take responsibility for their own health care in line with acquired skills and competencies, while their main caregivers step back and become supervisors rather than actors. "Transfer", on the other hand, refers a specific point in time when care is handed over from one health care provider (paediatrician) to another (nephrologist).

The 5 Ws of transition can be summarised as follows:

- **Who:** paediatric (renal) patients and their carers
- **What:** a focused process to help patients and their families acquire the knowledge and skills needed to manage the chronic condition, including the medical, psychosocial, educational and vocational aspects of living with progressive chronic kidney disease
- **When:** as soon as possible, but no later than 12 years of age, until the patient is transferred out (usually around 18 years of age)
- **Where:** in out-patient clinics and, in later stages, in collaboration with the continuing adult nephrologist
- **Why:** to improve long-term outcomes by helping patients to take responsibility for their own health needs.

With regard to age, it is important to recognise that the age of transition is often determined by the prevailing legal and regulatory framework. This is a highly unfavourable situation, as readiness for transition cannot be determined by a calendar age. Rather, it depends on a number of factors, including the child's development, social network, health stability and the success of several years of preparation. To illustrate, a child may not begin the transition process at the age of 12 years because the centre does not have the resources to facilitate early transition, or because the child and parents are not ready. Similarly, a patient may be transferred out at the age of 18 years, despite the presence of suboptimal conditions, because of compelling regulatory reasons. This highlights the importance of more flexible processes and regulations to allow for paediatric patients to be transferred when they are ready, regardless of age.

The aims of transition are (i) educating the patient about the disease and treatment, (ii) facilitating the patient's decision making, and (iii) supporting future caregivers to ensure optimal health care. According to the German S3 guideline on transition [1], the following aspects should be considered:

1. An individualised transition plan should be drawn up, with planned actions individually defined and timed;
2. Readiness for transition should be assessed in a detailed clinical interview;
3. The timing of transition should not be strictly linked to the patient reaching legal adulthood (18th birthday), but should take into account patient and condition specific needs (e.g. complex condition requiring more than one health care transition);
4. The transition process should include education of the patient and, where appropriate, their parents/carers on relevant aspects of the disease and the transfer itself;
5. An interdisciplinary approach to transition should be taken, including allied health professions and non-medical specialists specific to the patient and health condition;
6. At the time of transfer, a structured medical letter should be provided to the patient and future caregivers, including details of the history and course of the illness, psychosocial needs, and any findings relevant to previous and/or future treatment;
7. A designated transition key worker should accompany and oversee the transition process and act as a point of contact for all others involved;
8. To improve adherence, low-threshold services should be used as reminders and sources of information through appropriate internet services, apps, SMS, email and/or telephone where available;
9. In younger adolescents, parents/caregivers should generally be involved in the transition process. Where appropriate and agreed with the patient,

parents/carers should be involved beyond the transition. For patients with cognitive impairment, parent/carer involvement is mandatory;
10. The offer of a joint consultation or case discussion involving both the paediatrician and the continuing adult physician should be considered;
11. To support the transition process, several of the elements described in the guidelines should be effectively combined rather than applied in isolation;
12. Conversations about transition should begin as early as possible and be developmentally appropriate;
13. Issues relevant to adolescents, such as sexuality, family planning, sleep-wake patterns, use of alcohol, nicotine and illegal substances, and their interaction with the disease and its treatment, should be addressed during the transition process;
14. Screening for mental health and psychological distress should be an integral part of the treatment routine;
15. Sufficient time should be allocated for detailed transition discussions in paediatrics, but also with the future health care provider;
16. Responsibility for disease management should be gradually transferred from parents to the young person;
17. Counselling should be offered to young people on professional and social issues related to the chronic condition;
18. Young patients should be referred to self-help groups and patient organisations that are relevant to them. Self-help groups and patient organisations can be involved in shaping the transition process.

Transition is a complex process that involves patients, parents, healthcare providers and various members of the multidisciplinary care team all working towards the same goal. However, there can be various barriers to successful transition. Such barriers may arise at different levels. Being aware of these barriers can help to alleviate them. A selection of possible barriers is shown in Table 1.

Table 1 Barriers to successful transition to adult care

Individual barriers (patient level)	**Social barriers (parents, peers, school and work)**	**Structural barriers (health care system)**	**Professional level (health care professionals**
Striving for normality	Overprotective parenting	Lack of resources (finance, staff, transition clinics)	Specific paediatric conditions not part of adult nephrologist training (syndromes and congenital conditions)
Increased risk-taking behaviour as part of adolescent's development	Negligent parenting	Lack of transition staff and structures	Complex conditions requiring more than one speciality in adult care
Limited executive function/impulse control/action planning	Parents not transferring responsibility	Lack of professional interaction	Challenges in learning about rare conditions
Cognitive impairment	Peers challenging behaviour	Lack of psychosocial support in adult care	Workload: more patients – less time per patient
Lack of autonomy and self-care skills	Lack of social support and acceptance	School/working hours interfere with medical needs and physician office hours	Little education about adolescent medicine and treatment of a still developing body
Lack of disease and treatment specific knowledge		Rigid timing of transition (age not readiness)	

Optimal transitional care is provided in a clearly structured way. However, there are no comprehensive transitional programmes in Germany. Although the KfH (Kuratorium für Dialyse und Nierentransplantation e.V.) offers patients the opportunity to participate in "Endlich Erwachsen" (Finally Adult), this programme is a valuable addition, but it is disconnected from the patient's routine care. In the UK, 'Ready – Steady – Go' is an established generic tool to facilitate transition, regardless of the underlying medical condition. It provides a structured training programme alongside regular clinic visits and promotes an individualised approach to empowering patients [https://www.readysteadygo.net/rsg.html].

To avoid overwhelming the patient, the time of transfer should be planned carefully and too many changes should be avoided at once. Ideally, the transition itself should be gradual, with joint or alternating appointments and a gradual transfer of responsibility from the paediatrician to the nephrologist. In this way, both doctors and patients can get to know each other and refer back to each other until they feel comfortable handing over care. The timing should not be based on age but on ability: a patient may be ready for transfer at any time when:

- Allograft function is stable
- Health literacy and medication adherence are well established
- Patient is emotionally stable (no acute adverse life events)
- Social functioning is established (school completed, supportive environment)
- Health services are established (nephrologist appointed for ongoing care, health insurance coverage is secured).

Successful transition is a time-consuming and costly process. But it will result in a competent patient, a confident adult nephrologist and a favourable medical outcome with stable allograft function. To achieve this, the combined efforts of patients and professionals are essential.

References

1 Gesellschaft für Transitionsmedizin. S3-Leitlinie: Transition von der Pädiatrie in die Erwachsenenmedizin. Version 1.1 vom 22.04.2021. Verfügbar: https://www.awmf.org/leitlinien/detail/ll/186-001.html (01.06.2024)

Printing and Binding
Libri Plureos GmbH
Friedensallee 273, 22763 Hamburg, Germany